HEALTH IS

ENCYCLOPEDIA
A TO Z
OF
OVER THE COUNTER
NATURAL
REMEDIES
AND
GOOD FOOD

RONNIE PLANT

Published by St John Publishing.
Wellington Bridge, Co. Wexford, Ireland.

Printed in Republic of Ireland by Staybro Printing Limited.
19 Annesley Place, Fairview, Dublin 3
email: staybro@indigo.ie

ISBN 0-9551051-0-2

CONTENTS

ACKNOWLEDGEMENTS AND THANKS

Over forty years ago I had several ailments, leading to weakness and ill health of mind and body. This was due entirely to my lifestyle. Since then the seeds, the words, experiences, leading to accumulation of knowledge, have been recorded in yearly diaries. These and many files are filled with information gleaned and collected.

Much of this came when building up a Naturopathy practice, when many visited my home, telephoned and sought information or advice regarding health problems. During this time I made friends, received much thanks, letters and 'thank-you' cards.

Many have been helped, advised, often cajoled, coaxed, even with bitter or hard hitting words on occasions, in order to get the message across. Those who smoked and gave up, lost weight, changed their diets or lifestyle, learned about the need for necessary sleep, natural remedies and thousands of other health giving things have been an inspiration to keep records and diaries.

It was never my intention to write about my experiences or the knowledge gained from the many to whom I refer. I have been prevailed upon. Frequently the instruction or the remarks have been to 'put it on paper'. Very often I have been told: "You should share the knowledge" or words to that effect. "You should write a book" is a favourite, almost a cliché. I now pass on the advice given, feedback, results and much more.
Some remedies worked for some, others for others, some did not work at all, being like placebos. Over the times referred to, many reliable, trust worthy natural treatments, supplements and health aids were prescribed and used, as is now done. Others are long forgotten about because they did not bring results.

My late brother-in-law, friend, mentor and fishing companion, Dr. Con O'Riordan, is remembered with gratitude. All those years ago when I was ill, this good man took me aside and set me on the path to better health. At the time I had this mannish attitude towards health and life in general. When I look back, the realisation is, that I knew little about either. Dr. O'Riordan was very knowledgeable about Diet, which is unusual for most GPs. He told me that they received no training about the subject. He was also informative about the natural way of living, homeopathy and the need for sleep and exercise, especially as one becomes older. He was regarded highly as a good and caring physician. He died as a result of what was a minor car accident. Indirectly, through myself, he has helped and continues to help thousands who have turned to the natural way of thought and living.

I owe much to my daughter Geraldine who ran a health food business. Thanks is due to Tomás Hayes for his valuable experience and advice when setting out to put this Encyclopedia into words also to Margaret Lowndes for sorting the grain from the chaff, so to speak, as she toiled at the word processor for hours on end. To Marie Cleary, Fiona Kearney, Marette O'Rourke-O'Brien and the many friends, I am grateful for the help and encouragement. To Charlie Keegan, whose journalism experience was wonderful, I am indebted. To Ken Broughall, Sarah Broughall, Keith Dollin and the team at Staybro, what is there left to say. To those whom I cannot name, whose information is within these pages, my acknowledgements and thanks are passed on. I dedicate the writings, musings and collection on natural health information in the Encyclopedia, to my wife Freda, whose help and patience made it possible. Over many years, having been both a prompter and tutor, this kind person has listened to the problems of a host of different personalities, including myself. Many have said, as I do here, "Thank you Freda". My especial thanks are extended to my first cousin David Neilson, better known as Roy Cropper of Coronation Street fame. David has given an amount of his valuable time to assisting, especially in the launch of the Encyclopedia. Thank you David – or do I say Roy?

I hope that you, the reader, will find much of interest, including aids to well being, in the search for Better Health.

Ronnie Plant

THE EUROPEAN UNION AND NATURAL VITAMINS, MINERALS AND FOOD SUPPLEMENTS.

For some years the bureaucrats and mini-dictators who are the European Commission, commonly known as the E.U., have being drawing up and formulating plans to control NATURAL food supplements, vitamins, and minerals.

Thanks to the organisation 'The Alliance for Natural Health' standing up for the rights of the many who use these wholly-pure products by taking the matter to the Courts, there will be little change. All users will be able to obtain most of them in the foreseeable future. It has certainly been a major victory for opponents of another E.U. Directive; those who wish to use entirely safe products, as supplied down the years by the Health Food Stores

Almost 1.5 million users signed petitions presented to the governments in both the U.K. and Ireland, decrying the unnecessary interference of the E.U. There are many millions too who would have signed if asked or requested to do so. The producers of health-giving and natural goodness do not have the resources of the allies of the domineering drug companies to promote or fight their cause.

It is widely acknowledged that the all-powerful multinational drug industry, also the various medical and pharmaceutical organisations and associations, are within the circle behind this premeditated interference. They wield enormous power within the country's Government. They have easy - one can add all too excessive - access to our politicians and those who presumably govern. Their influence over them is and will be unknown. The employment given, turnover of money, taxes paid, also indirect service and work, leads to their having well-organised lobbies, also health and industry quangos. All have tremendous influence - very much more than people realise. In recent years there has been a huge swing away from synthetic, conventional drugs. The reality is that all too much of it does not work, very often causing or leading to further illness or ill effects.

The pharmacies and their providers, the mighty and world dominant drug companies, see their customers turn to the natural alternative remedies. Because of this they now wish to control what is normally sold by the Health Food Stores.

Only a little over 10 years ago, when I asked for a branded natural remedy, a pharmacist held me up to ridicule in front of other of her customers, when she almost sarcastically told me: "We don't stock that stuff, it's only a passing phase". Her words I have never forgotten. Now they stock an amount of these excellent food supplements and curative remedies - herbal, homeopathic and others. They realise that billions are being spent on them. An often annoying and little-known fact is that very few pharmacy assistants know anything about these invaluable natural things, often plugging or promoting drug manufacturers' medication instead. They should have trained personnel who understand natural remedies, more especially the supplements being offered for sale.

The safe, natural products about which I write, have not caused any of the problems witnessed, written and heard about - many of them never reported - through the use of modern medicines or pills. Some have led to fatalities. Frequently much distress is caused by their use, misuse and over-use, often through wrong or over-prescribing decisions, but much more by their make-up or chemical ingredients.

THE VAST MAJORITY OF THOSE WHO USE NATURAL SUPPLEMENTS, VITAMINS AND MINERALS, REALISE THAT NATURAL IS BEST.

These writings are not intended as a substitute for professional advice. Anyone who has a medical condition or is concerned about their health is advised to consult with a qualified practitioner, homeopathic doctor, herbalist, complimentary therapist or health food store personnel.

Parents should carefully check the instructions or seek advice from qualified person, such as health food store personnel, before administering to or allowing children to use complementary medicine or natural remedies. There are many children's natural remedies available.

THE FOOD, DRINKS, PHARMACEUTICAL DRUGS AND HEALTH SERVICE MERRY - GO - ROUND

Those who rule our country are frequently criticised about the various problems we face or which arise. Much is ill founded, not the fault of our legislators. In many instances the complainer would do well to put into practice the motto: "Don't find fault, find a remedy", instead of blaming others.

Where our health services are concerned, the Government rightly stands accused, but for the wrong reasons. We hear the calls of: "Gimme, Gimme, Gimme", as those connected with the funding of the health organisations seek and obtain more and more money from the Treasury, the financial purse-holders.

This year, the UK and Ireland will hand out well over €110 billion to those who are responsible for organising the Health Departments of the two countries. Even this figure is increasing regularly as the call for more money continues. Astronomical figures are predicted as being necessary for the requirements some five years hence. It is as if being poured into a black hole. Those in authority know that we have a health crisis. They wring their hands and talk. Obesity is a problem we hear of. We have other major problems, which are largely ignored. They must be fools if they can't see that it is because of the lifestyle, the eating, drinking and sedentary habits of the majority, that we are a sick nation.

There is too the excessive use of pharmaceutical drugs, most of them of little if any asset to better health. Many people are taking up to twenty medicinal preparations daily. Certain of these are probably nullifying others. Who does anything about the blatant overuse or prescribing? The MERRY-GO-ROUND continues, out of control, while those who are paid to administer give lip service, taking no apparent action.

Many of those who are ill, those who eat and drink sugary, fat and additive-filled 'foods' and 'drinks', mixing them with medicinal preparations, must take much of the blame, because: **'Your Health Is Your Responsibility, You Are What You Eat And Drink'**.

Our legislators do nothing to advise people about the need to read the ingredients labels or lists. They certainly will not tell us to reject what is offered as additive-filled 'food' and 'drink'. There is little warning or advice of the dangers of alcohol and medicines being taken together. Drinking when taking the contraceptive pill is an example of this. We hear little about the need for exercise, proper sleep pattern or Diet.

Against the wills of the majority, those in Council Chambers put Chlorine and Fluoride - both chemicals, both toxic - into our water. We are advised to drink plenty of the foul-tasting liquid, without any idea of the consequences.

It can be repeated that little common sense prevails amongst many who are responsible, including those in Government. They are on the Merry Go Round, like dogs chasing their tails. They know we are a sick nation, doing, as already stated, little to ease the problem. The boat will not be rocked. The blind eye is turned where cartels are visible, where quangos are numerous and extremely powerful.

We are told of extra millions being allocated to the health administrators, only to be gobbled up by the provision of more offices and the appointment of more managerial, supervisory and office staff. The regulatory and executive side is already over-staffed, one could safely SAY out-of-control. Visit any of these places to see the air of business, as reams of paper are produced and distributed, all-too- much of which is unnecessary. Note the exorbitant expenses paid out to bureaucrats.

The taxpayer, who has been and is paying for all of this, accepts it without a word of dissension. Our legislators are certainly not tackling the problem. We read of money foolishly spent, of doctors being paid millions for ghost patients - yes some long-departed from this life - of the enormous expenses paid for questionable reasons, of bad planning. The powerful Medical Board, the doctors Trade Union, refuses to pay, or rather repay, the falsely obtained monies, as those in authority stand idly by. If a layperson did this they would in all probability be charged with what could be construed as a criminal offence. Here is another example of our weak-kneed mandarins remaining silent.

We learn of analysis and studies carried out, sometimes costing many millions, and then being left unused, shelved. **It appears that nobody is responsible to anybody. A concentrated, combined, united effort is needed to tackle the problems of what people eat and drink, and also of what they are being offered as medicine. The foods and drinks industry must be investigated, and taken to task. The processors, the additive-producers, the supermarkets, should explain as to why all these artificial fillers are needed. It certainly cheapens the 'food'. Who wants cheap 'food' if it is not nutritious, edible, good? The purchaser should read the ingredients labels and refuse to buy the bulked-up, unnatural, and often inferior 'foods' and 'drinks' we are offered. Everyone should realise that it is cheaper to prevent illness than to cure it. They must learn that pure, natural, additive, preservative and colour-free food is as medicine. Only the best is good enough for the intricate human body.**

The Pharmaceutical drug conglomerates must be taken to task too. They must be asked many questions, not least why they refuse to have little or nothing to do with the natural things suitable as medicine and cure. Why have they neglected the many things where patents have run out? Aspirin is a prime example in this regard. This, and Penicillin are probably the two greatest of the small number of extremely successful treatments produced. Here is an example of the natural and chemical working together. Why not more? The usual kind of defence will be that they need to make what are exorbitant profits in order to research further. We have far too much of their pain-stoppers on the market, very

few of them cures. Their charges and resultant profits are obscene.

An eminent Professor tells us "The influence of the Pharmaceutical Industry has led to inappropriate prescribing by doctors. This influence has led to demonstrable harms, including less effective, wasteful and sometimes harmful prescribing practices". The Professor spoke of her concerns at what she termed "A growing conflict of interest". She added "The marketing budgets of drug companies exceed twice that spent on research and development, constituting about one third of revenue expenditure". The president of the Pharmaceutical Association, which represents the drug industry, refuted these claims. HE WOULD, WOULDN'T HE? All are cogs in the 'FOOD', 'DRINKS', PHARMACEUTICAL DRUGS AND HEALTH SERVICE MERRY-GO-ROUND.

Those who are in authority must be held responsible for not acting to sort out the many accountable for the dire situation within the Health Service. They sit back hoping the problem will go away, as daily it becomes even worse. The Gimme, Gimme, Gimme cry is answered by giving more money.

The problem will not go away. It must be tackled properly, in a cohesive and business-like manner. We hear about democracy. Simply because of the fear to rock the boat those democratically elected will not do so. Votes would be lost, many would lose their cushy jobs, trade unions would be antagonised, and the carousel would come off the rails. I am not against legitimate business. It is extremely satisfying to see manufacturers progress and grow. Ethics seemingly no longer exist in much of the food, drinks, chemical drug, and pharmaceutical industries. Profits have ousted them.

Health mandarins or bureaucrats, with little if any business perception or experience, are endeavouring to run the muddle, which is the Health Service. As set out elsewhere in this Guide, what is needed to restore stability, confidence and eventually a healthy Health Service is a level headed, no nonsense businessman, a company doctor and I don't mean a medical one. He should be enabled to bring in his chosen personnel to help run the industry and turn it around. It is a sickness industry in every parlance. Medical qualifications are unnecessary to get the system back on track.

We are entitled to ask those who supposedly govern, and to receive from them, answers to some very pertinent questions. Just simple, honest answers will do, with no evasive or political jargon.

- Do we continue to throw money away as we do now, with no satisfactory end in sight?
- Are we to become an even sicker nation?
- Are we expected to accept and purchase the all-too-much, non-sustaining stuff offered as 'food' and 'drinks' also synthetic chemical medicines and drugs?

- Are we to continue down the road of ill health, without any attempt to educate all about the need to avoid the unnatural things we are expected to put into our bodies?
- Are we to allow the mighty drug and pharmacy industry, the 'food' and 'drinks' producers also the medical profession, to dictate to us as they do now?
- Are they to be allowed to manufacture, promote and prescribe, without curb on an industry, which offers pills and medicines as if they were sweets or soft drinks?
- Do we continue to give in to those interested only in profits, big business, or is the health of our people to be given high priority?
- Are we to sit on the fence, so to speak, and watch the Merry-Go-Round continue unchecked?
- Are we to watch the spineless, namby-pamby politicians who aimlessly run the health service continuing to do so?
- Are we to continue allowing the bureaucrats and the many others who benefit, to manipulate the billions of Euros and Pounds involved, much of it ILL spent, in every sense of the word?

ARE WE TO BECOME SICKER THAN EVER, ALLOWING THE QUEUES TO GET LONGER, WITH MONEY SEEMINGLY EXPECTED TO COME FROM THE BOTTOMLESS PURSE, OR WILL SOME GOOD PERSON SHOUT HALT, DOING SOMETHING LOGICAL TO PUT A BRAKE ON THE MERRY-GO-ROUND?

Reading this Encyclopedia might lead one to remark something to the effect that: 'THERE DOES NOT APPEAR TO BE FOOD OR DRINK WITHOUT ADDITIVE, ANYTHING NATURAL"
How wrong one can be to think this way? There is an almost endless list of all that is pure, natural, good and nutritious. It just needs a little thought. Read this Guide to learn much about what is natural and pure, all of which helps to keep one in better health, especially the main caption, DIET.

THE STORY OF A FAMILY WHO ATE THEIR WAY TO ILL HEALTH

Some time ago a husband and wife, both in their fifties and both in ill health, visited us. They were typical of many who visit their doctor regularly. One was on twelve tablets daily, the other on eleven. Psoriasis, depression, cholesterol, blood pressure, prostate trouble, arthritis, stress and kidney problems were all mentioned. Out of over 1,000 ailments, many of them niggling, referred to in this Encyclopedia, those mentioned are just a sample. The natural remedies for these, with no harmful or side effects, are given under the relevant captions listed A - Z.

On being questioned about their Diet, it was amazing, appalling, - one can add frightening - to discover that these two nice, intelligent people, as well as many of the hundreds of thousands who are ill and on medication, are a huge drain on our health services. Why? I am convinced that it is because of what they eat and drink, what they allow to enter their bodily system, their lifestyle.

On being questioned further they spoke freely about their Diet, also their sedentary habits, being inactive, taking little exercise. A walk of a few hundred metres with the dog was the norm. They told of how they did not drink milk because it contained fat, not being aware of the necessity for calcium and other nutrients found in milk, whether fat-free or otherwise.

Yoghurt was a favourite. Like most yoghurts on display it was not natural. The particular brand they used contained: Strawberry Puree (6%), Sugar, Glucose Syrup, Modified Starch, Flavouring, Fruit Concentrate, Guar Gum, Acidity Regulator, Citric Acid, Sodium Citrate. They did not like the natural yoghurts. "They were not tasty," they said. *Turn to Yoghurt caption.*

The sugar bowl had been put away, as they had given up taking sugar in tea or coffee. Unwittingly, however, they had sugar intake in many other ways.

They used what was termed 'Low-fat margarine'- a sales gimmick, which contained, among other additives: Water, Hydrogenated Vegetable Oils, Salt, Emulsifier, Mono and diGlyceride of Fatty Acids, Flavourings and Synthetic Vitamins. Being brainwashed by the advertising of the food conglomerates into the low-fat way of thinking, there is little awareness of additives in this kind of spread, or of the goodness of butter when used sparingly. Butter is pure and natural, nothing taken away except the buttermilk, with nothing added, when unsalted. *Turn to Butter also Margarine captions.*

My friends gave no thought to the kind of cooking oil used in the deep-fat fryer. It could have been Diesel oil for all they knew. The majority of oils offered for cooking are refined, processed, pressed and repressed, over-heated, distilled, bleached, deodorised and much more. Pure, fresh, cold-pressed, unrefined cooking oils are natural. *See both captions Cooking Oils, also Cooking Oils, How They Are Produced.* Olive oil is the elixir of pure oil. It must not be used in deep fat frying. This is sufficient warning of the advisability to leave the deep-fat fryer in wraps. Cheap cooking oils can be expensive health wise. Much of what my above-mentioned friends ate was fast food and micro waved, which is a deplorable practice.

Coffee was taken regularly, at and between meals. This caffeinated drink is no asset to well being. *Turn to Coffee also Caffeine captions.*

They had been advised to drink plenty of tap water from the town supply. *This contained the toxic chemicals Chlorine and Fluoride. Turn to both these captions..*

When they purchased items taken from the shelves of the supermarket, it never occurred to them to read the ingredient's labels. Surveys show that less than nine out of 10 people, even though aware of the lists, do not look at them. "They would not understand them," they said.

For breakfast the family had a well advertised energy giving mixture, which is highly-processed, additive-filled, sugarised and made attractive to the taste buds. Amongst their make-up were: Sugar, Glucose Syrup, Fructose, Hydrogenated Vegetable Oil, Humectants, Maltodextrin, Calcium Carbonate, Sodium Alginate, Cellulose, Xanthan Gum, Locust Bean Gum, Modified starch, Flavourings, Salt, Potassium Hydrogen Carbonate, Acetic acid, Esters of Mono, and diGlycerides of Fatty acids, also Glyceryl Monostearate Distearate, Anthocyanins, Citric acid, Calcium phosphate, Malic acid and Vitamins, which like many of the additives are factory-produced. If the 'food' was not foodless these would not be required in the make up of the transformed and treated so-called breakfast sustenance.

The breakfast also consisted of what is eaten by many, fried or grilled. The bacon and sausages, as well as containing some Meat, included Water, Rusk, Pork, Fat, Salt, Diphosphates and Triphosphates, Sodium Sulphite, Flavour Enhancer Monosodium Glutamate, Dextrose, Sodium Ascorbate, Lactose, Sodium Nitrite, and Smoke flavourings, the addition of which has been curtailed by order of the EU, because of their overuse, which constitutes a health hazard.

White breads, used as loss leaders at point of sale in the supermarkets, which can sometimes taste like cotton wool, were used daily. These contained: Salt, Water, Acetic Acid, Esters Of Mono and diGlycerides of Fatty Acids, Flour Treatment Agents, Sodium Stearoyl, Lactylate, Calcium Propionate, Dextrose and other Antioxidants.

The low, or so called low-salt being used, contained Lysine Hydrochloride, Anti-caking agents and Flavour enhancers Monosodium Glutamate and Disodium Guanylate mixed with Disodium Inosinate which are given as E621 and E635. This makes it more complicated for the user, who does not realise what the E numbers stand for. In my kitchen the sea salt used is just salt – additive-free, from the health food store. *Turn to Salt caption.*

They described how lunch often consisted of packet soup - where the label shows: Lactose, Potato Starch, Hydrogenated Vegetable Oil, Onion Powder, Salt, Malto Dextrin, Rice Flour, Flavour Enhancers - Monosodium Glutamate, Disodium Isominate, Disodium Guamylate, Colours, Flavouring and sugar. Included were factory-produced vitamins. Also on the menu for lunch were smoked kippers. The fish is dipped in, or covered with, a coloured smoke-flavour agent, again factory-produced. The natural flavour of actual smoke is seldom used, as the labour-saving cheap method has taken precedence. Our friends did at least have fresh vegetables and potatoes frequently.

Dessert often came in small plastic containers, again purchased in the supermarket. The contents made doleful reading, with a big question mark over their nutritional value. Included were: Water, Fruit Cocktail 12% - including Cherries with the Colour Erythrosine, Sugar, Sponge, Polyglycerol, Esters of Fatty Acids, Mono-and diGlycerides of Fatty Acids, Tetrapotassium Diphosphate, Calcium Orthophosphates, Sodium Hydrogen Carbonate, Xanthan Gum, Dextrose, Modified Starch, Skimmed Milk Powder, Acidity Regulators, Citric Acid, Tri Sodium Citrate, Carotene, Flavourings, Stabilisers, Sodium Alginate, Guar Gum, Carob Gum, Preservative Potassium Sorbate - altogether some 40 ingredients to produce an after-meal sweet.

Sometimes they bought sandwiches from their supermarket or sandwich bar. The ingredient description is usually printed on the packaging. Seldom is this small print, which shows the makeup on the label, looked at. Here again much is additive-laden. What appears to be and should be, a nice, fresh sandwich is very often not simply pure or natural. When I pointed this out to the purchasers - my friends - they were amazed, not realising what they had been eating. Perhaps another reason why, like themselves, so many feel lethargic, run down, with little energy and more serious ailments. *Turn to Sandwich caption if you wish to learn more about the makeup of what we often think is a nice, fresh sandwich.*

A popular item, which they purchased regularly, was Pork, Onion and Tomato Sliced Roll. This contained: Pork 66%, Water, Potato Starch, Salt, Soya Protein Concentrate, Seasoning Which Contained Monosodium Glutamate, Hydrolysed Vegetable Protein, Allura Red Colour, Onion 2.3%, Tomato 2%, Dextrose, Sodium Triphosphate, Sodium Polyphosphate, Sodium Diphosphate, Sodium Nitrite, Sodium Nitrate, Yeast Extract And Sodium Ascorbate.

Doctors and other 'experts', whom we read of from time to time, advising that there is no need for vitamins, minerals or food supplements, must be stupid. How can a balanced diet be maintained or proper sustenance be provided, when eating the kind of mixtures referred to here.

At night when watching television, which they do regularly, Lucozade, Coke and crisps were taken. The drinks contained: Carbonated Water, Sugar, Colour E150,

Phosphoric Acid, Citric Acid, Lactic Acid, Flavourings, including Caffeine, Sodium Benzoate, Sodium Bisulphite, Ascorbic Acid, with the colour Sunset Yellow E110 in the Lucozade. The crisps had additives of Vegetable Oil, Cheese Flavour, Monosodium, Disodium 5 Ri:bonucleotides, Colours, Salt and Soya Oil.

My two friends gave much information about the lifestyle and that of their family when I visited their house. Two daughters live with them, one of them - a single parent - has a small baby. They too attended the doctor regularly, also being on medication, which consisted of eleven different drugs or medicines. The baby's mother, being grossly overweight, was on a diet similar to her parents. She was told by the pharmacy assistant to use the products advised for the low carb Atkins Diet. In my opinion, one must eat a well-balanced mix of purely natural foods, free from additives, preservatives, colours and chemicals to enjoy better health, also to help lose weight. This is explained fully, and perhaps annoyingly repeated, in this Guide. Low-protein and high carbohydrates are a recipe for ill health. The Diet must be nutritionally balanced.

The Atkins concoction purchased and being taken, consisted of: Water, Milk Protein Concentrate, Genetically Modified Soya Bean Oil, Alkalised Cocoa, Cellulose Gel, Magnesium Chloride Hexahydrate, Tricalcium Phosphate, Dipotassium Hydrogen Phosphate, Magnesium Hydrogen Phosphate Trihydrate, Dipotassium Phosphate, Potassium Chloride, Potassium Citrate, Maltodextrin, Sodium Citrate, Sodium Ascorbate, Ferric PyroPhosphate, Vitamin E, Zinc Sulphate Monohydrate, Nicotinamide, Biotin, Vitamin A, Sodium Selenite, Calcium D-Pantothenate, Pyridoxine Hydrochloride, Potassium Iodide, Thiamine Mononitrate, Folic Acid, Copper Sulphate Pentahydrate, Vitamin D, Riboflavin, Manganese Sulphate Monohydrate, Vitamins B12, and K, Chromium Chloride Hexahydrate, Sodium Molybdate Dihydrate, Flavouring, Lecithin, Sucralose , Carrageenan stabiliser.

The result of taking all this when also taking any medicinal preparation, is best left to the imagination. The long-term consequences cannot be foretold or known. OVER 95% OF DIETERS WHO FOLLOW THESE WHIMSICAL DIETING IDEAS REVERT TO THEIR ORIGINAL WEIGHT.

We see headlined in the media: 'Atkins Mania' has died away. Another dieting craze, one of dozens we have heard of over the years, has been left aside, as we await the next fallacy. It was hailed as a wonder, with many column inches devoted to it. All have been moneymakers for those who set out their theories, those who sold their books and the various products. Again many are wiser, having derived little if any benefits, failing to notice that the health of the devotee was again well down the agenda. It was all about money.

The child was being fed with a well-known brand of liquid infant food, which on the carton had a sell-by-date of 12 months hence. The ingredients would put any intelligent or health-caring person off on reading them, if one had the patience to do so fully. They are: Demineralised Water, Skimmed Milk, Lactose, Vegetable Oils,

Citric Acid, Calcium Hydroxide, Vitamin C, Potassium Hydroxide, Tri Calcium Phosphate, Tri Sodium Citrate, Sodium Chloride, Choline Chloride, Tourine, Iron, Lactate, Vitamins E & A, Zinc, Sulphate, Vitamin D, Niacin, Vitamin B12, Copper Gluconate, Pantothenic Acid, Vitamin K, Manganese Sulphate, Potassium Iodide, Sodium Selenite. Very much of this was factory made 'food'. When this list was read out, they remarked how it had never occurred to them that the 'baby food' contained anything like this. *Turn to Baby Foods caption.*

On the table were cheeses, orange squash and jam. The cheeses included the additives Annatto colouring or dye, Sodium Polyphosphate. Disodium Diphosphate, Sodium Phosphate, Phosphoric Acid with Stabilisers E410 and E417.

The jam was branded "Weight Watchers" with the fruit content shown as 26%. In the make up were: Sugar, Acidity Regulators, Citric Acid, Sodium Citrates, Stabiliser, Flavouring, Preservative, Potassium Sorbate, Calcium Chloride, Ascesulfame Potassium, Aspartame and Anticyanins. It also contains or is a source of Phenylalanine, which is one of the essential amino acids to be taken in combination with the other 20 plus found in the complete blend. This can be harmful when taken singly. Here is another example of the blatant overuse of additives, many of them chemicals. It certainly makes for a cheaper product. There is no comparison between this preserve and spread with 100% fruit with no added-sugar, being purely natural and easily available.

The orange squash, being extremely cheap, was being used as if it were pure orange. How were these people to know that it is additive-filled, certainly not natural, if - like the vast majority of people - they do not read the ingredients label? Here is what it contained: Water, Reconstituted Orange Fruit from concentrate 10%, Citric Acid, Sodium Citrate, Flavourings, Sweeteners: Aspartame, Sodium Saccharin, Preservatives: Potassium Sorbate, Sodium Metabisulphite, Stabiliser; Carboxymethylcellulose, Ascorbic Acid, Colour. It also had a source of Phenylaline also Sulphites. The sell-by-date was 12 months forward from the date of purchase. Imagine drinking a water based-plastic bottle stored drink, a year after purchasing, even if kept in cool conditions!

Their refrigerator was filled with 'foods' and 'drinks', which were additive-laden. I noticed nothing natural, as I pointed out the various items included in the tins, cartons, fizzy 'drinks', margarine, jams, peanut butter, pâté, shrink-wrapped meats, sausages and other processed items. To list the added ingredients would more than fill the page. One shelf was filled with tins and bottles of alcoholic drinks. Only on examining some of the labels did I realise that there was no list of the make-up of the liquids.

It is farcical that all 'foods' and 'drinks'' must legally display the ingredients, while alcoholic beverages - some of them harmful to the body - especially if taken in excess, can escape the law. This can only lead one to the conclusion that the mighty drinks lobby have dictated to

those who profess to police our food and drinks safety. The excuse that they might be giving away trade secrets or formulas should not be accepted. Let them display the chemical, factory-made, non-edible make up, with all being warned of what is being taken. I repeat: "It is absurd that what are called soft drinks must display the ingredients, when the alcohol-filled liquids are outside this rule".

Frequently we hear or read of the danger of certain additives, preservatives, colour etc., with directives being issued as to their uses. Often they are withdrawn, even after years of use and of our being told that they were safe.

How many know that children should not eat foods containing certain additives or use toothpaste containing fluoride?

Fluoride, as already mentioned, is a toxic chemical. Now our health bureaucrats advertise, telling us that children under the age of two must not use toothpaste - no use of the words Fluoride or Fluoridated toothpaste. This is despicable, because all children from the earliest age possible should be taught to clean their teeth properly, especially with Fluoride-free toothpaste. Natural toothpastes are available from health food stores or other outlets. Typical of the dental health mentors they have found a way around the fact that Fluoride is being used against the wills of many - those who realise its dangers to health. They do not tell us not to use Fluoride as in toothpaste. This would, of course, be contrary to the Governments determination to promote and force upon us the toxic waste material, which is Fluoride. The easy way is to say: "Children under the age of two must not use toothpaste". Only a politically minded guru would come up with the contemptible idea that small children should not clean their teeth. Why not be truthful about the harm of the Fluoride additive? We are being indirectly told of its harm. Why not the full story?

An example of the many doubts which arise over the use of unnatural ingredients is that of the toxic Aspartame, made up from two amino acids, being over 200 times sweeter than sugar. There have been many complaints about the product, as those for and against its use denigrate or defend its harm or otherwise, according to their interests, whether it be better health or the pursuit of monetary gain. *Turn to Aspartame caption.*

The relevant Food Safety Authorities tell us that all of these additives are safe. They told us this before and some were not safe. How can they have the audacity to tell us this when it is unknown how a mixture of food and drink additives, chemical, or unnatural, mostly factory made, enters the human system? Combined with all-too-many pills and synthetic drugs prescribed, there is no way of knowing of their consequences, long or short-term.

The husband, wife, daughters and child - the family I write about - were on thirty- four different kinds of medication. They had a mini-medicine chest. All

these chemicals were being taken into their bodies with no realisation of what the after-effects might be, of what harm they might do, taken long-term. Imagine the ingredients of all these synthetic chemical medicines taken with the factory-made food ingredients I have listed as being eaten. Imagine the system trying to absorb these.   Who questions this?   Who regulates this? The answer is apparently: NOBODY.

Three different doctors whom they attended were involved. Not one of these medics mentioned the words Food or Diet to these people who were sick, both physically and mentally. There were no questions asked about their lifestyle. What a deplorable Health Service we have!

It could be said that the many who live their lives as the people mentioned here have been doing, have only themselves to blame. This is so to a limited degree. They should at the very least be questioned, spoken with and advised by their doctor about their lifestyle, including what they eat and drink. It is blatantly obvious that PREVENTION is not the responsibility of, or within the vocabulary of, those who direct our Health Service, including the majority of General Practitioners.

Today as these words were being set down, I had a visit from an elderly couple, both unwell. They sought advice because they are highly disillusioned with the medication being prescribed by their doctor. The lady was on nineteen forms of medication, which included a nebulizer.   The man was on nine tablets or capsules. Many whom I speak with are being prescribed far too much, which could safely be said is indiscriminate. This seldom happened some years ago. Why should it be allowed to happen now? There is apparently no control over this kind of prescribing, whatever about diagnosing!

Frequently we are being informed of the harmful medicines being dispensed, of licenses being withdrawn because of their dangers. We are told of the doubts about other pharmaceutical drugs, including painkillers, weight loss and skin treatment prescriptions, also anti-depressants. Some doubtful products are big sellers. Dr David Graham of the US Food & Drug Administration, the body responsible for ensuring drug safety there, is on record as saying: "We have case reports of people dying clutching their inhalers".

If only the purveyors of these products would turn their attention to the many things natural which are in abundance in our world, including unadulterated, additive free   foods and drinks written about and advised in this Guide, all would have immense relief from sickness and ill health.

Despite questions being asked and drugs being withdrawn, we have denials from executives and spokespersons of the giants in the drug industry, who seek to distance their companies from the relevant watchdogs. The safety 'experts' opinions are regarded as damaging to their business. WHY? Yes, WHY were these products allowed on the market in the first instance? They cannot have been properly tested or appraised. Another instance, like all too many, where those who seek medical help are used for exploratory tests.

Sometimes it is difficult for the drug companies to obtain a licence for their product in order to market it. The questions regarding suitability or otherwise are often unanswered until the public are used as part of the testing procedure. This is totally wrong and should not be allowed. There is much evidence to sustain this view.

It is also obvious that removal of products, which should not be there, is very difficult, certainly not without resistance or fight back by the maker. Their aim is to sell, to make money. Sad to relate it seems to be at any cost in too many instances. Some 30 years ago over 75% of what the farmer produced was sold in shops. Now we are told that it is in the region of 9%, excluding milk, meat and dairy products. Much of what we eat is factory-made, chemicalised, and additive-filled, over-processed.

The latest word from the food industry is Functional. Yes, Functional foods, and this includes Probiotics. *Turn to Functional Foods caption.* The trade has been informed that this will be big business in the future. It has been highlighted in the trade magazine in front of me. I don't think there is a need to ask or answer the question "Big Business for whom?" **They have let it be known that:: It can be health enhancing. They do not use the words 'will be'.** Functional means practical or working. If much of the foods we are offered now are not functional why should their sales be allowed?

Going back 25, 35, 45 years ago - before the fast and factory-made chemical, 'food' and 'drinks' additive-filled fare became readily available and before the enormous influx of pharmaceutical drugs and medicines - there were no hospital waiting lists. There were no queues in the doctors' waiting areas, no waiting lists for beds, no trolleys with patients waiting in corridors. There was little delay in obtaining treatment. There was no need to offer advice to take a well-balanced Diet. The big question in this regard today is: "If what we eat is additive-filled, how do we find the right balance?" It is easy to find additive-free, natural foods. It requires just a little effort on the part of those who wish to have better health, a feel-good factor. It also means reading the ingredients labels. Additive-free foods are in the health food store and supermarkets. One just has to look for them.

'LOOKING FOR NON- CONVENIENCE FOODS IS SOMETIMES A LITTLE INCONVENIENT'!

Much of the ill health with which we are plagued -some serious, a huge amount of it niggling, energy-sapping - can be put down to the partaking of chemicals and additives in the 'foods' and 'drinks' we are offered, and also the over-prescribed, all-too- easily obtained, medicinal preparations. Much of what is natural and health-giving is far from the line of thought of the money-orientated, profit-seeking manufacturers.

Those who run our health services, including the medical profession, have

conveniently forgotten the maxim of the Father of medicine. Hippocrates said: "Let food be your medicine and medicine be your food" It should be remembered that everything was natural then. To this advice could be added the need for exercise, sufficient and proper sleep pattern. Combined they work wonders for one's health.

No so long ago pride was taken in the ability to cook delicious appetising food. A recent survey shows that only 32% people can prepare and cook a meal. A total of 19% could not make a snack like beans on toast while. 6% could not even boil an egg. We are told that these figures have been tolerant or sparing to those interviewed. Simple meals of natural food are easy to prepare. Many cannot do so. *The family gathering at the table to eat - sitting and talking together - is almost unknown. Fast food on the run, or snacks in front of the television are mostly the meals of the day. Many dine out, not knowing what they are eating. We are offered foreign dishes such as Thai, Chinese, French and others. The national dishes of health- giving Lancashire Hot Pot, Irish Stew, Saddle of Lamb, Bacon & Cabbage, the simple meal of Cottage Pie or the many traditional-cooked foods are fast becoming unknown, seldom on the menu. Tourists remark on the change, commenting:: "We are losing our national identity", many complaining about the food as they come away disappointed. Stir-fries, Pasta, Quiches, Pizzas and Burgers appear to be the meal of today. As already written, they would certainly be more appetising if naturally produced, additive-free, and unprocessed.*

The Health Industry is just that, as is the Food Industry - a multi billion, all-powerful industry, where the health of our people is far down their agenda. A doctor said recently - and I quote his words: "It is very provable that having people ill and keeping them that way, is the primary motivating factor behind modern medicine."

Within these industries the power within and outside Government, with all-powerful lobbies and quangos, is inexplicable. Food, medicine, drinks and alcohol producers cannot be trusted. Public confidence in the Pharmaceutical industry is at an all-time low. Few realise the vastness, the enormous increase in the size of the food ingredients, medicinal, also pharmaceutical and additive-manufacturing concerns. Regularly we read or learn of their growth into multi-national conglomerates.

What I have told you, the reader, in this chapter, about the serious health and financial implications of the Food, Drinks, Pharmaceutical Drugs, and Health Service has been at the prompting of the family who were most unwell, now with vastly improved health. Here were some extremely nice people, caught up in the carousel, the Merry-Go-Round, to whom they owe no thanks for their very much-improved state of well being.

Having been advised to change their Diet and lifestyle, now reading the ingredients labels, eating healthy foods, they are changed people. They use greens, fruit, natural food and drinks and take regular exercise. With good and proper sleep pattern, they are a changed family. The two daughters are now in employment. Neither, they or the little girl require medication from the doctor. The parents have almost eliminated their intake of pills. All this some two years after change of diet, lifestyle, and becoming food and health conscious. They have made reference to me on several occasions about the DIET caption in this Guide, saying how they have found the recommendations helpful. It is also available in booklet form, which they use for reference.

THE CHILD'S MOTHER LOST 20 LBS. (9KG) OVER 10 MONTHS AND HOPES TO LOSE AS MUCH MORE. DOING SO SLOWLY HAS AIDED THE RETURN TO VERY MUCH BETTER HEALTH. HERE IS ONE FAMILY WHO UNHESITATINGLY STATE: "IT NEVER OCCURRED TO US TO READ THE INGREDIENTS LABELS. WE DID NOT KNOW THAT FOOD CONTAINED OTHER THAN NATURAL INGREDIENTS. WE DID NOT REALISE THAT WE COULD DO WITHOUT THE DOCTOR TO GET BACK TO BEING HEALTHY". THESE ARE THEIR WORDS

Many chemists have now decided that they should be stockists of natural remedies. They have condescended to turn to the natural. It is almost unbelievable. They just had to; as they could no longer resist the call for alternative, non-habit forming, no side effect remedies. Most annoying to the discerning, is the matter of display by the pharmacist, of natural remedies, including herbal, homoeopathic, or food supplements. Being eager to promote and sell their high-profit synthetic products, as made by the giant drug companies, certain of these and other chemical medicines or tablets are cunningly placed in with the natural product. All-too-often they speak with those who seek an aid to better health, at the same time recommending their chemical medication. Be discretionary. Support your health food shop to be sure you are being sold natural remedies or products.

OUR BODIES CANNOT COPE WITH THE 'FOOD'

Over the past 30 years there has been a huge increase in the addition of the thousands of manufactured substances, now being added to or used in the make-up of 'food'.

The ease and apparent flexibility of these additions has made it much easier and more convenient for the purchaser, hence the words 'convenience food'.

This was accepted almost casually over the years, with little if any realisation as to how it was processed or made up, before reaching the shelves of the convenience or food store. There was, and still is, little interest in its consistency. The majority don't know what they are eating.

The unsuspecting public trust the retailer, supplier and manufacturer, as has been done in the past, when the supplier was usually the farmer, who was the natural food producer. Then almost everything was edible and wholesome food.

Only now is it being realised that our bodies cannot cope with much of the processed, additive-laden stuff we are expected to eat.

It is not coincidence that since the upsurge in the use of additives, also the prescribing of chemical drugs or medicines, our hospitals are full and with waiting lists, doctors complain of overwork, with surgeries or health centres often booked out up to four weeks in advance. Despite being told by the medical profession that our dietary habits - the food we eat - are a cause of heart and cancer disease, also much other related illness, they do not appear to have the foresight to warn us of the need to avoid convenience 'foods' which, to put it simply, are almost all of those which contain additives. Verbosity comes again with this quotation. 'Our health is our own responsibility'.

One would imagine that common sense would instil or implant this truism into the minds of many, but when it comes down to how the body is treated by some, 'Common Sense Is Not Very Common'.

Chemical medicines, pills and factory made 'food' additives are now replacing natural nutritious foods.

Modern day medicine treats the symptoms. Seldom if ever is the cause discussed. The notion seems to be that of the need for more pills, more medication, with the underlying problems un-noticed.

Alternative or complimentary therapies have an entirely different approach. Here the idea is to deal with the patient by using, as far as possible, the self-healing abilities of the body, to regulate, control and eradicate the ailment or disease.

To facilitate and assist these marvellous characteristics, a Diet of good food is as medicine. It must be additive free, natural, non-processed, edible and nutritious.

There are thousands of highly beneficial herbal and natural remedies. They are rarely reported on. They cannot be patented. Few stand to make money out of them; neither can the producer finance their promotion. They are all available from the Health Food Store and some Pharmacists.

I COULD BE ACCUSED OF TAUTOLOGY, VERBOSITY OR REPETITION IN COMPILATION OF THIS ENCYCLOPEDIA. WITH OVER 1,000 AILMENTS LISTED AND REFERRED TO, NO APOLOGY IS MADE, AS THE ENDEAVOUR TO PROMOTE THE AWARENESS OF THE NEED FOR NATURAL FOOD AND REMEDIES IS URGED.

Vitamins, Minerals and Food Supplements should not be taken if there is a danger of overtaxing the body, including the stomach. This can happen, with them being of little use, where there is extreme illness, if on an inferior Diet, or if taking an amount of chemical drugs or medicines.

This Encyclopedia gives much advice about the use of natural remedies, including food supplements. There may be some who require further help and guidance. If in doubt ask the Homoeopathic Doctor, Nutritionist or be advised by the Health Food Store Personnel, who are extremely knowledgeable.

The all-too-obvious 'Pills For All Ills' line of thought does not apply to Natural Vitamins, Minerals and Supplements. When using these take what is absolutely necessary, no more.

SEEK OUT AND USE THE NATURAL

Available over the counter from Health Food Stores and some pharmacies, are hundreds of natural remedies, homoeopathic, herbal, plant extracts or minerals from the earth. They are quality ensured, laboratory controlled, packaged and labelled.

WE HAVE THE HEALTH SERVICE WE DESERVE

Almost daily we read or hear of the demands for more finance to pour into the Health, -shall we call it Sickness -Service. The 'Letters to the Editor' columns berate the Government, also the relevant departments, for not doing sufficient to clear the backlog of patients waiting for treatment, through operations or other therapy. People write letters, complain incessantly, moan or find fault. They do not put forward sensible proposals, or set out answers to the problems, except perhaps to ask for more money. They sit back and wait for something to be done. They are blind to the fact that much of the remedy, by way of prevention of disease or sickness, lies in the hands of all. **Their health is their own responsibility.**

Last year, when attending a medical function on the subject of ageism, I was at a table with a group, which included doctors, and brought this responsibility subject up. They were in full agreement when one of them stated, "We know that, but we can't go around telling people this. It would not be politically correct". Again here is another case of not 'Rocking the Boat'.

Hospital treatment is nearly always good, often extremely so. The media highlights complaints about inferior medication or mistakes made in surgery. As is usual we hear little, which is good from that source. Why not give immense credit to the medical profession, including the nursing staff, ambulance crews and others, who do such wonderful work in our hospitals and in treating all who are ill or infirm.

We have a serious alcohol problem and many other points at issue, all of which lead to ill health. Included are fast foods, food and drink additives, which through inferior Diet - coupled with lack of exercise - cause many problems. Much illness can be attributed to the couch potato attitude of television addicts, also the motorcar.

More than one third of children are overweight or obese, with adult obesity also becoming a major health problem. Being overweight, leads to diabetes, which is fast becoming endemic. Figures released about these diseases are alarming. Walks to school are unheard of now, indeed walking any distance is considered a chore by the majority. Some children are now being told that they must not run in the school playground, because of injury fears. **Only in the past 30 years, since the vast eruptions on the market of synthetic drugs and medicines, fast food, food and drink additives, have these and many other health problems escalated. Few realise the dangers of fizzy 'drinks', including 'energy drinks'. All are over-sweetened, being one of the reasons for obesity, diabetes and much illness, major and otherwise.**

Serious exercise is recognised with a shrug of the shoulders, also the cliché: "I must do something about it", seldom followed up. *Turn to Diet, Exercise and Sleep captions in this Guide for advice on how to aid or prevent illness.*

Our mortality rates from some diseases are the highest in Europe. The average exceeded is mostly in relation to cancer, heart and lung disease.

We are told that the Health Service is a shambles. The Government of the day, the various health departments and frequently the doctors, consultants or others are blamed.

The majority have the Health Service they deserve with only themselves responsible for their state of health and all-too-much of the National Health Service problems.

Lifestyle, behavioural attitudes to one's health, including what is put into the most intricate system in the world - our bodies - with overuse of processed foods and drinks, pills, potions and much more which is deleterious, all contribute to ill health.

There is an ingrained line of thought, an attitude, which is entirely, wrong, that: "I'll be all right, there is a tablet or medicine for every ill, the doctor will put me right". Try discussing this topic with somebody who is on medication. The defence or counter will usually be, "I am not like that" or somewhat similar reply. Further questioning will usually lead to the realization that they too can be included amongst the many whom I refer to, believing their health is the responsibility of others, who are very often strangers to them.

Not so many years ago the Health Service could deal adequately with the numbers seeking medical attention. Now things have got out of hand because of the enormous increase of sickness, with ever mounting queues and waiting lists for those seeking treatment. The system is out of control. Many who await treatment have only themselves to blame, because of the manner in which they have mistreated or neglected their bodies. **ILLNESS DOESN'T JUST HAPPEN, THERE'S A REASON.** Too many take risks with their health, going to the edge of the precipice, so to speak. Men are notorious for this attitude, but now we find women equally at fault.

All too easily any one of the hundreds of stoppers of pain, few being cures, can be purchased off the shelf. None are aware of future consequences when taken. There is easy access to the doctor and his prescription pad, which is his cash register, with over-prescribing of much that is unnecessary. Many of these chemicals do more harm than good. Few, if any, doctors will allow a person leave their surgery without prescribing. They should be questioned as to what is in the drugs being stipulated. Are there liable to be side effects or are they safe?

Dr Patrick Wall, who at the time of writing is Acting Health Advisor of the Health Service Executive in Ireland, also being adjunct Professor at UCD centre for food safety, was outspokenly truthful when he said:

"The most amazing thing to me is when people have lost the health and their question is 'Will I have a heart bypass or a stent, chemo or radiotherapy?' Then they will tell you afterwards 'I am walking five miles a day since my bypass - and

I am thinking "Pity you didn't walk one bloody mile before it"
The general idea is that after a bypass or other serious operation one can resume and continue living as before. They do not realise that unless there is a change of attitude to the former way of living, including Diet and Exercise, the treatment will be just temporary. An example of this is that the veins and arteries will again clog up, the reason the bypass was needed.

Cutting out alcohol, giving up smoking, eating vegetables, greens and many other cheap natural foods, to replace the additive-filled processed stuff, leads to better health and a saving financially. The Diet caption in this Guide points all this out with much health-achieving help being given.

What is written in these pages comes from the heart. I have eaten, drank, smoked and done all the wrong things. I ate what was prepared for me. I had faith in those who cooked, just as they trusted the supplier. No thought was given to what was good or what might be bad, what was of nutritive value or otherwise. I was not interested in the make up of food or its constituents. There were no ingredients labels in those days.   Additives, like cigarettes were 'the in thing', an invention that over the years would multiply into an enormous trade. They have grown into a mighty and dominating industry. Much of our food is no longer grown. It is now mostly man and woman made, manufactured.

Looking back, or with hindsight, I realise how ignorant I was about Diet and better health. To my credit I did take exercise, having played competitive games in the past. I felt good but would pay for my unawareness of proper dietary habits. I was not aware of the need for sufficient sleep. Too many act stupidly in relation to their health, just as I did. *The realization came that I had to accept responsibility for my own health. I had to change my lifestyle, my eating and drinking habits. Doing so I was enabled to live without the ten different kinds of medications, which were being prescribed for me. There is now no need for the doctor, except for annual check-up, which all over the age of fifty should have.*

Depending on doctors and the Health Service does not change the lifestyle of those whom they are trying to gratify. Only the person being treated can do this. Very often this change is all that is needed to restore one to better health. I had to find this out the hard way and in doing so have been able to help many, by advising what steps they can take in order to regain better health. It is a fact, that man and woman individually are their own worst enemies at times. Nowhere is this more apparent than when it pertains to their health and how they conduct their lives.

IT MUST BE POINTED OUT AGAIN THAT MOST ARE, AS I WAS, IGNORANT OF WHAT IS IN THE MANUFACTURED, PROCESSED, ADDITIVE-FILLED 'FOODS' AND 'DRINKS' WHICH THEY USE.

Few consumers know anything about the food additives, the E numbers, which are listed on the ingredient labels. This is one of the reasons they do not look at them. They will tell you "I just don't know what they mean". How can they? They do not know where or how to seek information about what the E's stand for, what they are expected to eat. They have no idea what they contain, how they are made up or produced. They know nothing about the hundreds of additives, or thousands of constituents or chemicals, used in the processing or concocting of what is on the shelves, being sold as 'food' and 'drink'. Turn to additives caption

Being interested in the subject for many years, I have made it my duty to ask questions about this, when in the food-store. Whether it is manager, supervisor or other staff, including the checkout cashiers. the reply has always been "I don't know" or words somewhat similar. Very often the answer has been accompanied by a shrug of the shoulders or a shake of the head. Not one person, even in the delicatessen or fast food outlets, had the foggiest idea about the simple information I sought. All are entitled to ask questions about E or other food additives and to be given the answers, just as they would seek information about electrical, clothes, hardware or indeed anything being purchased. With our most important consumer goods, the 'drinks' and 'foods' we are expected to drink and eat, this guidance appears to be irrelevant.

The mighty conglomerates that produce the factory made food, will only do what is absolutely necessary, to keep within the relevant Food Safety Authorities remit. This can also be said about the 'drinks' and 'food' outlets. They will tell the public only what suits, as they advertise and promote their products. They certainly keep all unaware of what is put into the stuff sold as 'foods' and 'drinks'. There will be much blurb on the many overly packaged items. This is aimed at the unwitting, trusting customer, most of whom are very often all too easily taken in, dare one use the word naive. There is a simple way to deal with this. Leave that which is additive filled on the shelves. The resultant improvement in health could be astounding.

There must be huge change in the attitude, with the message being spread, about the need for active and lively exercise, or proper and regular sleep pattern.

The mind set needs to be altered, changed, refocused. Until such time as this is done, the Health Service the majority now deserve will be with us, because of the apparent 'couldn't care less' attitude as to how the remarkable and wondrous human body is treated. It needs care and attention. Only by doing so, thereby having little, if any, need for visiting the doctor, can we expect to have a healthier nation. Then, and only then, will we have the Health Service we deserve?

I REPEAT AND TRY TO IMPRESS UPON ALL THAT EACH AND EVERY-ONE OF US ARE TO A HUGE DEGREE OUR OWN PHYSICIANS.

Balanced Diet, to include natural additive-free food, fibre, fruit and vegetables, combined with exercise, proper sleep pattern, and abstention from smoking and with little or no alcohol is a recipe for good health.

Over 50's should have a medical check-up every 12 months. If on medication tell your doctor if you intend taking food supplements. What you take is your prerogative.

No apology is made for repeating advice about DIET in this Encyclopedia. Over 1000 ailments are listed. The cause of most of them is nearly always improper or inferior diet, especially processed 'foods' and 'drinks' therefore recurrence of theme is necessary.

BEWARE

Quite often in a supermarket, store or shop, which sells miscellaneous goods, in some magazines, and even on market stalls, one sees vitamins, minerals, herbal remedies or supplements, also pharmaceutical drugs and medicines, being advertised or offered for sale. The advertising is often gimmicky, with special offers and cut prices. Some of the manufacturers listed on the containers are unknown, whatever about their reputation. Here are instances bordering on quackery. Reputable manufacturers have their good name to uphold. It is in the interests of all to purchase from a health food shop or pharmacy. Remember it is the health of the partaker, which is of paramount importance. It is number one.

ARE YOU PREPARED TO VOLUNTEER TO HELP
MAKE YOURSELF AND OTHERS HEALTHIER?

Are you prepared to volunteer to make yourself and others stronger and healthier than you have been? Would you like to be trim, fitter than you are, with a better feeling of get up and go?

Would you like help to:
1. Put the medical profession on say, a three-day week! This to include the Pharmaceutical business?
2. Eliminate the waiting time in hospitals, surgeries and other places where there is illness?
3. Save the Government, the tax- payers, much of the billions now being spent on the health service?

Before proceeding to read further please re-read these suggestions or propositions. No doubt you will think that I am daft - foolish in the extreme.
Please read on to discover that I am far from being either. With the aid and cooperation of all, what is written above could easily be achieved. The time put into it by each individual would be minimal. The attitude to change might be difficult, but to see the resultant good health would be as a catalyst, with a huge desire to change the lifestyle.
My request to you, in order to achieve what is set out, is simple and above all enjoyable. Obtain the three books listed below. They are also detailed in the Bibliography section at the end of this Guide. THESE ARE AMONGST THE GREATEST HEALTH ADVICE BOOKS I HAVE EVER READ. The titles do not do justice to the much advice given about simple health facts.

1 **'Your life in your hands, Understanding, Preventing and overcoming Cancer'** by Professor Jane Plant. Published by Virgin Books.
   ISBN 0-7535-0850-8
2 **'The Healthy Heart Programme'** by Dr Richard Fleming with Tom Monte. Published by Michael Joseph an imprint of Penguin Books.
   ISBN 0-718-14593-3.
3 **'Your Body's many cries for Water'** by Dr F Batmanghelidj. Published by Tagman Press. ISBN 1-903571-49-9.

If unable to procure them from your bookshop, these books and much more which gives health and spiritual advice, can be obtained by mail order, to any part of the world from:

For UK:Cygnus, FREEPOST SS1193 LLANGADOG SA19 9ZZ.
Outside UK:Cygnus, P.O. Box 15, LLANDELIO SA19 6YX, UK.

The knowledge and guidance set out in these books, combined with that given in this Encyclopedia, especially what is advised under DIET caption, if accepted and put into practice by all, would mean that what is listed under 1, 2 and 3 could easily be achieved. There would be no extra outlay, with the food and drink bill probably ending up lower than as of now. The books mentioned, which are better than most novels from an enjoyment point of view, would, of course, have to be purchased. Their value would be repaid many times over.

The more who accept what has been written in these invaluable publications, putting it into practice, the quicker the savings in thousands of ways. The health of the population would improve dramatically.

I know a large number of people who have changed to what is recommended in these books. Many I meet or speak with when asked: 'How are you?' reply: 'Thanks to you I feel good' or words to that effect.

If our Government is not prepared to take drastic steps to improve the health of all, also to curb the excessive waste of money squandered by the Health Service, let us take these steps ourselves. Let them (Government) sit back and see the change. They might then get the message.

What is set out in the recommended reading matter is so simple, that it is laughable, proving that our legislators - those who are paid to govern - give little thought to how any improvements can be made within the Health Service

CONTRAINDICATIONS

- Aesculus (Horse Chestnut), Garlic, Ginger or Ginkgo Biloba are not to be used with Aspirin, Warfarin, Anti Clotting or Blood Thinning drugs.
- Agnus Castus must not be taken whilst using oral contraceptives or HRT and not to be taken if progesterone levels high.
- Black Cohosh not to be taken whilst using HRT or oral contraceptives. It should not be taken long-term. Ideal way is seven days on, four days off, for three months, then stop and recommence after 28 days.
- Calcium and Vitamin E to be taken more than three to four hours before or after taking Iron.
- Devil's Claw not to be taken if suffering from Gall Stones or Stomach Ulcers.
- Dong Quai not to be taken if progesterone levels low.
- Echinacea not to be used if with Asthma or Diabetes.
- Ginger not to be taken if Diabetic.
- Ginseng has many contraindications (see Ginseng caption).
- Goldenseal not to be taken if with high blood pressure.
- Iron supplement or calcium must be taken more than three to four hours before or after taking Vitamin E.
- Kelp is not advised for anyone with high blood pressure, kidney disorders or thyroid conditions, unless taken under medical supervision. Certain people may be allergic to Iodine and hence Kelp.
- Valerian must not be taken with anti-depressants or other tranquillisers. The synthetic barbiturates will render them useless.
- Vitamin E should be taken in combination with Vitamin C. The latter taken on its own is all right.

Warning: The dangers of taking alcohol with any form of medication, including the contraceptive pill, cannot be over emphasised. Included with medicines or tablets there is usually an explanatory leaflet. This can include cautions or other vital information relevant to what is prescribed or being taken. Few read these notelets. The warnings should be on the containers or packaging.

SHOULD YOU HAVE A MEDICAL CONDITION, BE ON MEDICATION OR PREGNANT, BEFORE SELF-PRESCRIBING ANY MEDICINE OR SUPPLEMENT, ALWAYS CONSULT A PRACTITIONER, QUALIFIED HERBALIST OR HEALTH FOOD STORE PERSONNEL.

YOU CAN SET YOURSELF UP TO BE SICK, OR YOU CAN CHOOSE TO BE WELL

A VITAMIN

See Vitamins and Minerals Caption.

ABDOMEN - (BLOATED FEELING)

See Flatulence Caption.

ACHING LEGS AND FEET

Take Combination P New Era also Vitamins E and C daily. This is often associated with kidney problems or poor circulation, to be treated accordingly.

ACIDITY – ACID STOMACH

The reason for acidity is usually found in the Diet, with something unnatural being the cause of the acid. Changing to natural foods nearly always eliminates the acidity problem. Slippery Elm, Centaurium, Yarrow, Papaya or Golden Seal are remedies advised. Natural additive free Diet is most important. *Turn to DIET caption.*

ACIDS - FATTY

See Fatty Acids Caption.

ACNE

Vulgaris or Rosacea. I have not seen any remedy to act better, or quicker than a pure wholesome nutritious Diet, assisted by the intake of Brewer's Yeast or Vitamin B Complex. Avoid alcohol and fizzy 'drinks', sugary products and confectionery. The affected person may be allergic to milk or vegetables, such as cabbage, broccoli,

Brussels sprouts or other greens. Other remedies are Echinacea, Blue Flag Root or alternate Pulsatilla with Rhus Tox. Good food and the B complex Vitamin have always given excellent results when prescribed for Acne. *Turn to DIET caption.*

ACUPUNCTURE

Many are turned off because of the thought of needles. This is a wrong attitude. They are so fine that only a very slight tingling sensation is felt. Acupuncture is over 1,000 years in use, being a very good aid for many of today's health problems including anxiety, stress, gynaecological conditions including PMS, nausea and depression. It is a very good help in trying to give up smoking. The addict must co-operate fully, honestly wanting to give up. This is the main reason it does not work for some, as they avail of the treatment, thinking that they need to do nothing, as if it is some kind of a miracle cure. Regularly we read reports of the growing scientific evidence in support of the use of acupuncture, with the World Health Organisation (WHO) having identified up to 50 conditions treatable by this natural remedy. Many doctors are sceptical of the practice as is wont when it comes to simple medication. The proof is there, that acupuncture works extremely well, if the patient is prepared to concur.

ADDICTIVE DRUGS

If trying to withdraw from dependence on synthetic or chemical medicines like Valium, Librium or other addictive drugs it is important to rely on natural unprocessed additive-free foods to build up the necessary systems to improve health generally. Alternatives to these drugs are the natural, non habit-forming, simple remedies, which include Valerian, Skull Cap, Vervain, Passiflora or St. Johns Wort. The latter is obtainable by prescription only in Ireland. I doubt if it is, or will ever be, prescribed by the medical profession. It is too natural. One can go over the border into the Six Counties of Northern Ireland and purchase off-the-shelf, whatever quantity, large or small, one desires.

ADDITIVES IN 'FOODS' AND 'DRINKS'

One has only to read through this Encyclopedia to be enlightened about the overuse of the thousands of substances, many of them factory-made, put into the 'food' we are expected to purchase and eat.

Cheap foods can be, and are, produced by shrewd, astute use of Additives, bulking and other mostly artificial agents, including sweeteners, with poor food or sustenance value, making our health problems worse. They are used to thicken, emulsify, preserve, colour, flavour, sweeten and antioxidise amongst other things. They are used chiefly to cheapen the 'food' and to make it palatable, very acceptable to the taste buds, especially those of our young people. It is not coincidence that we are plagued with allergies, with asthma and other allergy-type ailments becoming almost inherent. ***Does anybody who cares anything about health or Diet ever take the time to read the ingredients labels?*** Some 80 years ago we had less than 50 added ingredients. Most, if not all, were edible examples: being spices, herbs, salt, sugar and water which was probably the first- known addition, also other simple ingredients. ***Today we have well over 5,000 plus, food and drink substances in Additives, with the list being added to regularly. Many of them have almost unpronounceable names. Try reading the synthetic names of some of the additives. Don't think they have all been proven safe, as we have been led to believe. How can anyone tell us that the various combinations as taken into the human body are not part of the cause of ill health.*** Take for instance the essential Amino Acids, which the body cannot make, therefore referred to as essential. We are supposed to obtain these from the food we eat. How can we when many of the chemical or synthetic fillers, bulking or other agents used to cheapen the so called 'food' we are offered, do not contain any of these Amino Acids? Remember they work in conjunction with one another, all being vital to our well-being. There may even be single forms of the acid in some of these synthetic Additives. To take them separately can be dangerous. **Allied to the thousands of chemical medicines, whether pill or potion, being prescribed by the medical profession, also the over 600 non-prescription medication products, many of them poisonous, many of them readily available, off-the-shelf, even from the local filling station, it would appear that our intake is a cocktail of chemicals. Perhaps this is why we are branded as being a sick nation.**

Recently at a supermarket or food store, I picked up a shrink-wrapped packet of bacon, and found it contained: water, salt, lactose, dextrose, sodium tryphosphate, sodium polyphosphate, sodium diphosphate, sodium ascorbate, yeast extract, sodium nitrite, with the smoke being another synthetic item which was made up as a flavouring additive. Here is a typical example of what we are being offered as food. We live in a world where millions starve yet where millions are obese, where there are food shortages and food gluts. We are bombarded with advertisements encouraging us to eat 'foods' that cause illness that we can't afford to treat, with the Health Service in chaos because of the negligence of many. The purveyors of the chemical filled 'foods' get rich, as do the processors and shareholders. We are offered pure and fresh which is often far from being so.

The Additive-laden 'food' and 'drinks' we consume bring much of our present-day illness on. We are told that the 'food' we are offered contains nothing like the goodness of that eaten in the past. How can it when much of the processed products contain Artificial Fillers, Bulking Aids, Preservatives, Salt, Acidifiers, Antioxidants, Stabilizers, Humectants, Raising Agents, Synthetic or factory-made Vitamins and Minerals, Acidity Regulators, Flavour Enhancers, Modifiers, Diluents, Bleaching Agents, Buffers, Antifoaming Agents, Colours, including Azo

dyes, Artificial Sweeteners, Sugar, Bases, Chelation Additives, Emulsifiers, Emulsfying Salts, Excipients, Firming Agents, Gelling Agents, Release Agents, Synergising Agents, Solvents, Glazing Agents, Mineral Hydrocarbons, Gels and Oils? In amongst this lot there are the 5,000 plus 'foods' and 'drinks' substances, which are foisted and forced upon the unsuspecting public.

The EU has issued new guidelines about the safety requirements for artificial smoke, because of fears made known. At the same time we are told that they have ordered a cut in the maximum permitted level of colouring fed to farmed salmon and laying hens. This is used to make the grey flesh of the farmed salmon look pink and more attractive to the eye of the discerning customer. It makes egg yolks more yellow, being detrimental to human eyesight. They do not tell us how these laws will be enforced. It will be impossible to do so. It is almost laughable, if it were not so serious. To add insult to injury they have the audacity to tell us that it is used cosmetically to colour the salmon flesh and the egg yolk, and that the reduced levels will not adversely affect the taste or colour of food. It is ridiculous that a harmful substance should be used in this manner. Why should we, the public, have to accept this dangerous chemical, or any other chemicals being imposed on us? If the lower levels of the chemical will not affect the texture of the food, why use it in the first instance? Those whom we write about, who are responsible for the quality and safety of the food we eat, must take us to be fools, and we are, if we accept any food with colour, Additive or preservative. Again I repeat: 'Read the ingredients label. Leave all which is not natural on the shelf. This is the only way to treat the gigantic, cute, domineering, all-powerful, money-orientated food processors and those who sell the 'food'.

We hear about and also see listed on ingredients labels some of the hundreds of E additives. few know anything about them, what they contain, why they are used. Most people say they do not understand about food and drink additives, including those with the E prefix. How can they when they are not informed? They do not know where to seek explanation or information about these things which they are expected to eat. They place their trust in the manufacturer, producer or retailer. It is very obvious they are not forthcoming with advice, other than to promote the sale of additive filled, so called foods.

It should be mandatory that all food retailers display in a prominent position a list of food and drink additives, including those with E numbers. Set out should be their specific source, function and most importantly their effects, especially on those who are taking prescribed medicines. There are numerous E additives which are detrimental to children's health. Warnings should be given and highlighted.

This is an Encyclopedia about natural health and if you wish to read about something unnatural, which is in hundreds of items sold as food, *see the caption Aspartame.* It is obvious that we are being dictated to by corporate food barons, that we must eat what they process or put on the shelves, most of it unnatural. The adding of the dangerous colour to make the salmon flesh appear pink should make us realise even more that all is not well with our food production. Frequently we have read, or heard, of the dangers of Additives, colours, preservatives and other things that are dangerous which we are expected to purchase as 'food'. Sudan Red colour 1 is one example and there are listed in front of me some 36 Additives that have been withdrawn because of their dangers. How are we to know about the harm, or otherwise, of the other Additives, if we have to wait for long periods of time before minds are made up as to what is safe or what is not? Only by accident in 2005 was it discovered that Sudan Red 1 was in the food chain in Europe where it had been banned in 2003. Its use was prohibited in America many years ago. If it was found to be dangerous in the USA, then why its continued use in Europe? It appears nobody in the food business is to be trusted. *The simple way to avoid these things is to read the ingredients labels and to leave the Additive-filled stuff on the shelves. I do it, many thousands do it and so can you, the reader.* In this Encyclopedia I can only touch on the worrying subject of Additives. Should you wish to know more about them *see Bibliography for details* of the fact giving books *'E For Additives' or 'Not On The Label'.* The former was revised and substantially expanded in 1988. Hundreds of substances, many of them unnatural have since been added. Again few know what is in their make up or what they are purchasing and eating. As already stated most accept what is offered without question. Those who do so are foolish. *Also turn to Processed Foods and Drinks caption*

ADENOIDS

Treatments are Poke Root, Combination Q New Era, Golden Seal or Silica.

ADHD – Attention Deficit Hyperactivity Disorder

This long-winded description can include disruptive, excitable, unruly, bad-tempered, hyperactive children and teenagers, who have behavioural and antisocial problems. As is all too often the case, instead of trying to find the root cause of the problem the easy way out, is that of prescribing drugs. The most common of these is Ritalin, which is a brain drug, a psycho stimulant. It should only be used as a last resort. It may do extreme damage, just as other chemicals can harm the body. It has never been tested as to the long- term affects. *I repeat again and again that where ADHD is diagnosed or appears to be the cause of the person's problems, nothing will remedy it better than change of Diet to pure, natural, foods and drinks, additive-free.*

There is very often a lack of Iron and Zinc in the blood levels of those affected. When blood test has been completed and iron and zinc supplements or tonic given, I have seen a vast improvement in the mental and physical health of those being treated. If there is a major deficiency, the doctor will treat, probably by injection.

There are natural remedies, as listed later, which will also help, but the outstanding natural equivalent of Ritalin can be either Eye Q or Efalex. I have seen these hand, eye and brain co-ordinators used in conjunction with the recommended natural Diet, with excellent results. Like many other so-called medicines, nobody - and I repeat, nobody - can tell us of the long-term consequences of the chemicals being prescribed.

This is mostly a juvenile problem, one I have studied much, to the point where one gets hot under the collar and annoyed. I have seen adults too who had similar symptoms. Here is an example of what a Diet lacking in pure natural nutrition can do to a person. Without a doubt, Diet is the cause of most of the problems of ADHD, call it hyperactivity for convenience. The unnatural colours, additives, preservatives, sugary foods, and the fizzy 'drinks' containing aspartame, and other harmful chemicals, must be avoided. It is a known fact that things like Tartrazine, Aspartame, Saccharin, Caramel, Annatto, Sulphur Dioxide, Sodium Benzoate, not to mention dozens of others, should be avoided. They are detrimental to the hyperactivity disorder. Those who profess to understand the disorder recommend the elimination of certain foods. I have heard of nothing natural, which should be omitted from the Diet. The foods or drinks they refer to, are those with additives.

The answer to this fast-growing and alarming problem lies in the eating and drinking of nutritious, natural, unprocessed foods and liquids, free from what can be called deleterious and harmful substances. Allied to this are the uses of natural Vitamin and Mineral supplements such as a Multivitamin suitable for children under/over 12 respectively. An excellent combination is Kindervital for the under 12's or Floravital for those over that age. Evening Primrose Oil is helpful, as is Udo's Choice Oil. Bach Flower Remedy Impatiens is extremely good. Homeopathy, used in conjunction with natural Diet, has also been a solution. Nux Vomica, when prescribed, is excellent, as is Tuberculin. All of these are over-the-counter natural remedies. Only by trying them can one find what suits best for the problem. *The administering of any supplement or medicine including Ritalin, which I most certainly would not recommend, will be of little use if the pure, natural, additive-free food or drink Diet is not adhered to.* Young people need exercise, they need to burn up, use up excess energy. Persuade them to take up sport, especially team games. Television should not be allowed except for chosen subjects. It helps turn the young into couch potatoes, leading to laziness of mind and body, with resulting health problems.

Explore the alternatives suggested before allowing drugs to be used. This is an ailment, which cannot be described as an illness. *The simple remedy is almost always the use of pure food and drink, free from additives, combined with the natural remedies mentioned. As suggested, see Diet caption and be guided as to what can be extremely beneficial in banishing hyperactivity.*

ADOLESCENT SPOTS

Not to be confused with Acne. Remedy is proper natural Diet, aided by Vitamin B Complex, Echinacea, Calc Sulph and a Multivitamin tablet daily.

AEROPHAGA – (SWALLOWING EXCESS AIR)

If overweight take steps to reduce. Avoid stress. Keep to a natural food Diet, avoiding fats, additives and alcohol, as advocated throughout this Encyclopedia. Eat small meals, chewing the food properly. Rest the stomach every seven or eight days, eating only pureed fruit, natural yoghurt and cooked vegetables. Two excellent homeopathic remedies are Argentum and Lycopodium.

AEROSOLS

Do you use Aerosol containers of anti-perspirants, deodorants and shaving creams? Do you realise what is in the make-up of hair sprays, shower gels, household cleaners and dozens of other fragrant sweet-smelling tins? We have an alarming increase in recent years, since the arrival of Aerosols, of asthma, lung and bronchial disease, skin allergies and cancer. These are just a few of the many health problems, which can be caused by Butane, Isobutane, Stearyl Alcohol, Aluminium Zirconium, Tetrachlorohydrex GLY, Aluminium Chlorohydrate, Disteard Imoniumhectorite, Parfum, and at least another 12 solvents and chemicals used in their make-up and production. They may be potential carcinogens, toxic, neurotoxic or health harming. Do you ever read the warnings or cautions on Aerosol containers? I am not being an alarmist, just giving true facts as is done throughout this Encyclopedia. Use Aerosols at your peril, and that of others. There are many natural products available. One has to search. There should be no need for anything used in Aerosol containers which include any of the chemicals listed here, many of them harmful.

AGEING

You can't stop getting older but you can stop getting old. Age is, or the thoughts of Ageing, are often all in the mind. We are only as old as we feel, which is akin to how we feel. As we get older, exercise seems to become less and less relevant. This is entirely wrong. Those over 50 who exercise regularly enjoy better health, being stronger and fitter in body and mind. Exercise, combined with natural, additive-free food, can work wonders, helping to keep one from ageing.

Diet of pure natural food including fruit and vegetables is the first essential. Don't skip breakfast. Eat Porridge if possible. Take antioxidant supplements, which include Vitamins E, C and A also Selenium and L-cysteine. Rhodolia or Coenzyme Q10 are excellent. Wellman or Wellwoman Multivitamins are recommended, also Pycnogenol. A Calcium/Magnesium/Vitamin D supplement, taken at bedtime, aids bone structure and is very necessary for all over 35, because a deficiency speeds up the Ageing process. Find what suits best and continue to use. Kordel's Prime Time Multivitamin and Mineral Formula is as nutritional insurance for those aged 45 plus. Avoid alcohol, smoking and coffee. Ageing is unavoidable, but you can look younger, feel good, with a zest for living, by changing your Diet and lifestyle. It is never too late to start. *Turn to DIET caption,* also visit the health food shop and seek their advice. There is much to be learned from the personnel. If natural remedies recommended in these pages are not available off the shelf, over the counter, they will order for you. If on medication, or with medical complaint, speak with your doctor before starting on an exercise programme.

Over 50's should have a medical check-up every 12 months. If on medication tell your doctor if you intend taking food supplements. What you take is your prerogative.

AGNUS CASTUS

Health-wise, this is one of a woman's best friends. It is a remedy known for its regulatory action on hormones. Has been proved to be an alternative to HRT. It encourages creation of progesterone and helps reduce oxygen production. Agnus Castus is invaluable for PMS and is also an aid to skin problems. It is used as a remedy for nervous tension, mood swings, depression, insomnia, water retention, breast soreness or pain, also amenorrhoea. This is truly a woman's ally. Not to be taken if progesterone levels are high.

AGORAPHOBIA

This fear of open spaces effects women mostly. It arises from a weakened central nervous system. A Diet, which is purely natural, is recommended. Avoid smoking, alcohol, coffee and strong tea. A good Multivitamin, such as a super one a day-timed release, is an excellent aid to better health, so helping acquire the necessary courage to fight agoraphobia. Other suggested remedies are Sulphur 6C or Aconite 6C. Fish Oil supplements and Udo's Choice Omega Oils have also been a valuable help to eliminate the problem. Pure, natural, additive-free food is as medicine for the problem. *Turn to DIET caption.*

AIR POLLUTION

Cities and towns are apparently the most air-polluted areas. To counter the effect take Hawthorn as an antioxidant, also take Artichoke to aid the liver and digestive system, to help ward off results of chemical pollution, which affect the body.

ALCOHOL

The reader can ask, and rightly so, 'What has Alcohol to do with natural remedies and good health? The answer is nothing, except for the disciplined, who wish to partake of Alcohol as medicine. Small intake is beneficial, or so we are told, but how much can be regarded as small? A glass of red wine is recommended for the heart. A hot whiskey is supposed to be of help when with a cold or chill. Manny Shinwell, late well-known British politician, who lived to be 103, told of how he used to take a tot of whiskey nightly. He did not tell us how big the tot was!

Our Alcohol problem, which is almost out-of-hand, beyond control, is serious. Dependency on Alcohol is a disease, leading to ill health in so many different ways, with kidneys, liver, heart and much of the system being effected. The health and stress problems not only affect the imbiber, destroying organs and emotional well-being, they are also the cause of much distress for family and friends. It is a potential killer and destroyer of health. Much could be written about the evils of Alcohol. Here we can only gloss on it, health-wise.

It is my opinion that there is nothing to be said in favour of Alcohol. It should be avoided. The minuscule benefit, which might or might not be derived from the intake of the highly unnatural, processed, additive and chemical-filled intoxicating liquor, is best forgotten about. *As I have already pointed out in Additives in Food and Drinks caption, we are completely in the dark, kept ignorant, as to what ingredients, chemical and otherwise, are in the many alcoholic drinks so glaringly and prominently advertised.* In early years I learned my lesson about the evils of alcohol, accepting the advice of a close friend and relative, a doctor. He also had a problem in the past, receiving much help from Alcoholics Anonymous, who had helped him and many others. Since those far-off days, I have found that when those who are ill visit me to seek a remedy, one has to ask tactfully if the person is a heavy drinker. Even if it is true, the imbiber will seldom accept the advice that they should give up.

Apart from the time off work, equally as bad if not worse is the relationship of drink to ill health. It always catches up with the drinker. In front of me is a list of various parts of the body, which can be affected by the consuming of Alcohol. No need to list these organs separately. All – yes each and every element, system, the whole structure of the human body, is affected by this evil liquid. Only today, as this Encyclopedia is being written, we are being told that 'Drink-related illnesses are costing our hospitals Billions of pounds annually'. This alone provides sufficient evidence, as if this were needed, to show how detrimental to our health the consuming of Alcohol is. I make no apologies for repeating *'Alcohol' has no benefits whatever, being extremely harmful, even dangerous. Turn to Wine caption.*

ALEXANDER TECHNIQUE THERAPY

This is something, which one could say is a puzzle or an enigma, in that, in studying it one learns nothing new. You already know everything you will learn. I suggested that this was confusing, only to be told: 'You're having your first ALEXANDER experience, you will not progress if you try to learn something new' It is all about discovering what we should not be doing to our bodies and then aiming to stop this.

The idea is to improve posture and gait, simply because so many slouch, are stooped, or sit incorrectly, often moving about in a manner which distorts and does not allow the body to function efficiently. The Therapy has proved to be highly effective for back problems, including lower back pain. For instance, F.M. ALEXANDER, who discovered and promoted the therapy, found that his speech, vocal cords and the throat were highly inefficient because of the way he held his head. His often used expression *'Give nature her opportunity'* is significant in countless ways. Alexander Therapy has an excellent reputation, giving very good results. Practitioners are listed in the Yellow Pages. or log onto www.isatt.net or www.stat.org.uk

ALLERGIC TO GARDEN PLANTS
Take Rhus Tox.

ALLERGIES – FOOD
What is one person's meat may be another person's poison. Much could be written about this all-too-prevalent problem. With Food Allergies the important thing is to find out exactly what to avoid. Here's a prime example of where reading the additive and ingredients list comes into practise. A pure natural Diet is all-important. If you are one who desires better health, the advice given is to abide by the use of natural food and drink. Hay-fever, asthma and eczema Allergies often come from the indoor environment which can include central heating, fitted carpets or soft furnishings, with dust mites or pet allergens. We have become too clean, to the extent that household cleaning products, including aerosols, can cause Allergy. With food Allergy there is the need for elimination Diet to be practiced. This can be done in two stages. 1. Exclude one by one any food, which might be causing the Allergy. 2. If the symptoms disappear then recommence using the eliminated foods, one at a time, to discover which ones produce the Allergy. Here may be found the cause of the problem. Processed additive-laden 'foods' are very often the 'baddies'. A biopsy can be done by visiting an allergist, the difficulty being to find one who can deliver or diagnose properly.

Apart from the food additives, including colour and preservative, other foods which may cause Allergy are: dairy products, including milk and cheese, cereals containing wheat, oats and corn, gluten which is found in grains or cereal such as rye, oats, barley, wheat, including their flours. This is particularly applicable to those with the Allergy known as Coeliac Disease or ailment. Therefore, gluten-filled foods must be avoided, including bread, berried fruit particularly strawberries, seasonings and spices, nuts, casein and other milk-based products, also shellfish, food dressings, citrus fruits and garnishes. Don't become alarmed, as there is much gluten-free food now available, including flour, porridge oats, bread and other edibles.

Exercise regularly. *See Walking and Exercise captions.* This will help in the step towards the easy way of treating Allergies or food intolerances, both of which are linked. *There may even be favourable results before proceeding further, especially if having changed to pure natural Diet as suggested.* Once discovered, the damaging or Allergy-causing food or foods must be eliminated. A worrying problem is that the almost indiscriminate use of antibiotics at some stage in ones life, makes it almost impossible to fight the Allergies. It is quite possible that the immune system or general health of the Allergy-sufferer may be weak or impaired. This must, therefore, be built up to establish better health and resistance. As well as the elimination Diet the following are what the writer has noted as being a big aid in the relief of Allergy or food intolerance: Devils Claw (Pagosid type) 15mg daily of Urtica, up to 600mg daily of Vitamins C Also take Vitamin B complex, including extra Vitamin B5 Pantothenic Acid, Zinc or Echinacea. A proven aid is Acidophilus. Good for the immune system, it helps the body produce the B Vitamins and assists in absorption of food. All are natural, and available from the health food store assistant, who will give much advice about the gluten-free and other foods, which help those with Allergy. These are available in tablets, capsules and powder form, to be taken as directed. If, or when, the Allergy has ceased to exist, it is suggested that a good slow-release Multivitamin be taken daily with the suggested natural Diet being adhered to. *See DIET also COELIAC captions. See Bibliography for details* of helpful books **'Cure Your Allergies'** *also* **'Eat With Joy on Wheat Free, Gluten-Free Diet'**.

ALMONDS

As a snack, for those not allergic to nuts, Almonds are most nutritious. They provide an amount of Vitamin E also the B Vitamins.

ALOE VERA

This has remarkable healing properties, much written about, much advertised. There are many on the market, some being dubious forms of Aloe Vera, even synthetic versions. A Health Food Manufacturers Association (HFA) standard has been introduced. Look for this on the carton or container. There are many nutrients and much goodness in pure Aloe Vera. It contains at least eight of each of the various minerals and vitamins. Use for arthritis, rheumatism, sciatica, irritable bowel syndrome, skin problems, burns and cuts, constipation, also psoriasis. Recommended is the range of Aloe Pura Organic Pure Aloe Vera by Optima Healthcare, which are available as juice, capsules, tablets and gels. Seek further advice from the health food store personnel.

ALTERNATIVE THERAPIES

In today's PILLS FOR ALL ILLS society, the medicinal properties of Alternative Therapies, Herbs, homeopathic and natural remedies, as written about in this Encyclopedia, are not on trial. It is all too much of MODERN MEDICINE, often experimental, which needs severe scrutiny. There are almost 100 complementary or Alternative Therapies listed or practiced. In this book everything written, including that about Alternative Therapies, has been found from experience to be an aid to better health. There are listed in this Encyclopedia only Alternative remedial treatments, which I have seen to be beneficial. The many others not referred to may be all right. This has not been proved to me yet. Just like synthetic or natural remedies, what works for one may not do so for another, so it may be with certain Therapies. *The approach towards treatment, determination and explanation of disease, by conventional as against Alternative natural medicine, is different. Alternative or complementary method of diagnosis is to deal with the patient by using the self-healing and regulating abilities, which are within the body. Modern or conventional medicine is by diagnosis and then treatment, usually by synthetic medicines.* **WHAT A PITY ALL CANNOT BE POSITIVE, COMING TOGETHER AS ONE, CONSIDERING THAT BOTH ARE NECESSARY FOR THE BETTER HEALTH SOUGHT BY SO MANY.** In all situations in life there are imposters or shams, of which there are some in the various Therapies written about. It is imperative when seeking treatment for health problems to find a trustworthy and fully qualified practitioner.

From the results obtained, the relief given, dare I use the word 'cures', Alternative Therapies, have proved very good, especially those listed in this Encyclopedia, under their various captions. One thing about them is that no patient will suffer from barbiturates or other chemical ill or side-effects. When using the word 'cure' as in these writings it must be emphasized that it is illegal for any person unqualified in medicine, synthetic or otherwise to recommend, to offer something as a 'cure', even if it is.

ALZHEIMER'S DISEASE

This disease occurs when the nerve cells in the brain deteriorate over time and the brain shrinks. There are various ways in which this can affect someone, for example severe loss of memory and concentration, with mental ability gradually failing. I make no claims as to natural remedies being of value where this progressive brain deterioration occurs. There is no cure, no turning back the clock. Much, very much, can be done to prevent the disease, and perhaps help the person with Alzheimer's. There is evidence to show that since steps were taken to reduce aluminium levels from Diet and medicines there has been a decline in dementia, including Alzheimer's. Cigarettes, alcohol, coffee and strong tea are to be avoided. A nutritious Diet of natural foods can help slow down the disease, as well as protecting from Alzheimer's. Scientists working on behalf of the Alzheimer's Society have found that a Diet deficient in fruit and vegetables is a prime cause of the disease. *Those with high cholesterol have a high risk, especially for those born with the Alzheimer's gene. Antioxidants are necessary.* Studies find that Vitamins E and C can reduce the risk, being highly protective. A combined antioxidant available from any good health food shop taken with natural food Diet is recommended. *See Diet caption and be guided by the advice which can help and also lead to the prevention of Alzheimer's. Also see Brain Health caption.*

AMENORRHOEA

The holding back or repressing of normal menstrual flow can be distressing. It may be due to being run-down, anaemia, depression, or other health or emotional problems. Natural remedies and supplements, which have helped are Agnus Castus, Black Cohosh or Motherwort. To attain better health and so be rid of problems such as Amenorrhoea a change to natural Diet of pure foods is almost always the best medicine. This can be aided by taking Calcium/Magnesium/Vitamin D and a good slow-release Multivitamin. *Here is where DIET as captioned,* all being natural, is very necessary, because when with better health it is much easier to battle with and fight health and distressing problems, such as Amenorrhoea.

AMNESIA – (Weak Memory)

Treating as Brain Health caption has helped enormously.

ANAEMIA

There are many who from time to time, some quite often, some without realising there is anything wrong, do not have the energy, stamina, get-up-and-go of others. Life to some is an effort. It is as if the body droops. Even the general appearance looks tired, haggard, one could add worn-out. There is often paleness of face, with fingernails white, hair unhealthy or dull, and a feeling of tiredness, with no staying power. This can very often be diagnosed as Anaemia. For some reason or other doctors very often do not appear to pick up this problem unless it is very obvious. There are varying kinds of Anaemia, also many causes, all characterised by haemoglobin levels being low. This is the pigment within the red blood cells. The more complicated or serious types are for the physician to diagnose and treat. However do not be alarmed, because almost all causes of Anaemia are of the simple type. Usually the remedy, so easily and all-too-often prescribed, is Iron. Serious thought must be given to the use of this in the treatment of Anaemia if there is within the system a shortage of hydrochloric acid, which aids digestion. There may be a lack of protein. Being a vegetarian and not taking a Vitamin B12 supplement to counteract the loss of intake, can lead to the serious complaint of pernicious

Anaemia. *See Vegetarian caption.* This too must be treated by a doctor.

Unless there is a loss of blood through accident, internal bleeding, operation or for some other reason the problem can be overcome. The sufferer, who has almost unknowingly been affected, regains a new lease of life and energy. *If in doubt, see your doctor, tell him what you think, ask questions and demand a blood test. This is the simplest and most efficient way to find out if with Anaemia.* If diagnosed with simple Anaemia, you can, if you so wish, turn to natural supplements or remedies. The most important aid to good health is that repeated again and again in this Encyclopedia, which is simple pure natural food untainted by additives or other inedible ingredients. *Turn to DIET caption and be guided by it.* Combine this with an Iron tonic such as Floradix, Vitamin C up to 500mg daily, Vitamin B Complex, which contains Vitamin B12 and Folic Acid. The herb Echinacea, which comes in liquid form, is very useful to help regenerate red blood cells. The Iron tonic suggested is in liquid form, to be taken as instructed on the bottle, being pure and natural. The Vitamin C will assist in absorption of the Iron. These and the supplements mentioned combined with natural Diet will help restore the partaker to normal health, unless there is an underlying or more serious problem.

ANAEMIA - (Pernicious)

This is extremely serious and occurs through lack of Vitamin B12. Can happen to those in mid life 45 – 65 or very often to vegetarians, whose intake of the vitamin is negligible, because of the non-use of meat. Treatment is by doctor, often only by injection of B12 throughout remainder of life. Prevention is by simple natural food Diet and the taking of Vitamin B12 supplement. Taking one tablet daily of Vitamin B Complex will supply the requirement of B12 and other B Vitamins. *See DIET caption.*

ANGINA – (Pectoris)

An attack of Angina comes as a sense of suffocation, sometimes with violent pain in the chest, which is induced by exercise with the victim gasping for air. The heart is one of our most vital organs, a muscular pump to the left of centre of chest. The pain and intense feeling of asphyxiation occurs because the blood supply to the heart is insufficient. The veins and arteries have become lined, one could say clogged-up with furring and fat deposits. This is called Atheroma. This restricts the flow of blood because of the narrowing of the blood course with the heart, the pump so vital to life, being unable to distribute the vital fluid. Often the left arm and the neck are affected by the pain, which is also like a soreness or stiffness. The question I have been asked is: "Why did this happen to me"? The simple answer is because of lifestyle, including Diet of animal fats, processed foods, salt, sugar, lack of exercise, constipation, stress and much else bad for our health. It can be hereditary. This is all the more reason why proper Diet and lifestyle be carefully followed or adhered to. We often hear of hardening of the arteries. Its medical term is atherosclerosis. This is also like atheroma, a blocking of the arteries and blood vessels by cholesterol deposits which hinder the flow of blood. My experience shows that many who have this problem become frightened, believing that they must be extra, ultra careful, resting, taking little exercise and living a restricted life. Angina can be treated to the extent that the ailment will be of little hindrance to mode of living. To help fight or battle the disease means a dramatic change in lifestyle. Again what we eat is all-important. *Turn to caption under DIET,* which explains this. Exercise is equally of value. *It is also important that you speak with your doctor or heart specialist and tell them what natural aids you intend taking. Angina is a serious health problem, where the GP, especially in relation to exercise, must guide you.* At the same time you must not lie down under the problem. The exercise does not have to be strenuous, no need for much other than good, comfortable, footwear and clothing and then walking. This advice to exercise seems ludicrous, as this is what brings on the pain. Gently, gently does it, stopping when the pain comes and then carrying on as stated, gently. The recommended supplements as found under *Diet and Exercise captions,* all combined, will do wonders as you venture slowly, doing more when fitter and able to. *Also see Walking caption.* Be warned not to overdo it. Rest too is necessary. Regular sleep pattern of at least 7-8 hours nightly, with relaxation daily whenever one feels it is needed. A nap, lie down, or siesta in the daytime is like a reviver. The use of supplements and herbal remedies is recommended, provided they are compatible with existing drug treatments. **I have proved, and believe that the arteries can be cleared to a certain extent. To learn about this see both captions 'Heart', also 'Heart Attack, How I Fought It and Now Enjoy Living'.** This can be achieved by carefully putting into practise the advice given. Angina need not be as restrictive as we are led to believe. Those with it can do much to feel good. Be active if at all possible, remembering that slowly and gently one can achieve much.

ANKLES – (Swollen)

Here is a problem, an ailment, which is very prevalent. Little if anything is written about it, or of the causes, or indeed what can be done to avoid, alleviate or treat. Women are effected very much more so than men. Legs become heavy and tired. Being overweight does not help. Try to lose some of the excess if you have a weight problem. Avoid crossing of legs, or wearing of high-heeled shoes, if prone to swollen ankles. Both sexes should avoid smoking because nicotine is very toxic to the circulation, also the drinking of alcohol or coffee. Walking, exercise and climbing of stairs regularly can be beneficial, or do the toe-to-heel seesaw exercise frequently during the day. These suggestions must be combined with eating natural foods as *recommended in the DIET Caption.* Added to this is the taking of antioxidants and food supplements to promote better health. The DIET advice will explain the need for these, also to avoid snacks, sugary foods, cakes, fizzy drinks and chocolate. Take Vitamins E and C also a Multivitamin, which combined with the advice given, should lead to real improvement.

ANOREXIA – (Loss of Appetite)

If not due to a medical or health cause such as liver, kidney, vitamin deficiency, threadworms, stress or other, this may be attributed to a bio-chemical imbalance, a way to bury emotions. Being obsessive and a perfectionist is common amongst those with the problem. It is now usual to treat using counsellors, psychiatrists, psychologists and, of course, the doctor. Often attempts are made to force-feed the patient with processed, additive-filled food or drink, some of it stodgy. The cases the author has dealt with were treated by explaining that one can eat pure natural whole foods, without gaining an ounce of weight and by the intake of Vitamin B Complex, Centaurium, Brewer's Yeast, Vitamin E and a Multivitamin tablet daily. The latter was later alternated every second day with the tonic Floradix. Spirulina capsules are one of the best remedies ever to help correct Anorexic problems as are Kordel's Celery 6000 plus tablets. They should be taken at bedtime. Here is a prime example of where food is your medicine and medicine is your food, by convincing the person that with natural Diet, free from additives, there would be no increase in normal weight. *See Diet and Spirulina captions.*

ANTIBIOTICS

In this synthetic medicine, pills for all ills direction, which the medical profession and the public have taken, we find that antibiotics are certainly not the cure for all ills. The doctors have been warned of the dire consequences of their highly evident overuse. It is admitted openly that prescription control has failed and is out-of- hand. The misuse or abuse of antibiotics can be catastrophic. Like much in our health service, there is nobody at the helm to dictate. I use this strong word, but this is what is needed to curb the all-too-obvious, almost willy-nilly, use of antibiotics. We are told of drug-resistance, a plague of allergies, hear of mothers and young children who have been using these things, probably to excess, and now with all too many and varied ailments and illnesses. Some are niggling, some serious, many to remain with partaker or recipient for the rest of their lives. *A survey carried out showed that at least half of the antibiotics, as used by hospitals and GPs, are unnecessary or improper. For instance, antibiotics should not be used in viral infections. They are being prescribed. They do not work and can even prolong the illness. After all a virus is simple stock and trade medical substitute for: 'I don't know'. All the more reason for non-use of antibiotics in this and other cases.* The public are becoming much more conscious of the over-use of drugs and the resultant side effects. They are turning to natural and alternative remedies, including Homeopathy and herbal treatment. They are visiting the health food shop for advice. As a counter to depression, after use of antibiotics, take Acidophilus and Vitamin B Complex.

ANTIOXIDANTS

These are the compounds or nutrients, which can cope with and control free radicals, which are enemies of our good health. The main antioxidant nutrients are: Vitamins E, C & A (Beta Carotene), also the minerals Zinc, Selenium, Manganese and Copper. Research proves and demonstrates that antioxidants protect against heart disease, premature ageing, cancer, blindness in the elderly, and other health problems. They are beneficial and an aid to treating and slowing down of glaucoma, rheumatoid arthritis, Parkinson's disease and other degenerative diseases. *Here again proper natural Diet is a must for both the health problems mentioned and the proper combining of antioxidants within the system.*

ANUS – (Itching of)

Pileworth or Blue Flag Root taken singly, or combined, can eliminate this problem. Vitamin B Complex is also an excellent remedy.

ANXIETY

There are so many and different, one could add complicated, states of anxiety, that it would be impossible to deal with all in the limited space available. These can be mild or acute. It is often caused by stress, past experiences being resurrected or coming to mind, also other niggling problems. It can lead to an increase in blood pressure, a depleted immune system, with other ailments, which are brought on by Anxiety and worry, much of it - dare one use the word - imaginary. Where the mind and body are in a healthy state, almost all ailments, health problems, even phobias or Anxiety, can be put out of the head. Here, one can turn to the greatest medicine in the world, which is a pure natural Diet of good food. *See DIET caption* and follow the advice given in order to help be free from Anxiety. Calc Phos, Bachs Rescue Remedy and Passiflora are very helpful if Anxious and can be taken with the foods suggested. The whole idea is to build up the immune system. By so doing one can face any crisis in life.

APHONIA – (Loss of voice)

See Laryngitis Caption.

APHRODISIACS

Rhodiola, Damiana or Oysters are recommended. Oysters are the old arousal remedy. Rhodiola is excellent as an aphrodisiac, helping to raise serotonin levels, which leads to better sex attitude. Damiana and Saw Palmetto taken together with

Juniper berries are the most natural Aphrodisiac known. Horny Goat Weed is known as the king of male sexual enhancement and is often used as a remedy for impotence. All remedies, except the oysters, are available from the health food store.

APPETITE – (Loss of)

Usually lost due to or after illness, when feeling low and as a result of emotions. Digestive disorders also lead to loss of appetite. Unless there is some serious underlying problem the appetite can usually be restored by the use and presentation of good tasty, appetising, natural unprocessed foods. To help line the stomach and aid digestion where there is a lack of hydrochloric acid (one of the gastric juices), nutritious home prepared soups, natural yoghurts or tasty milk puddings are an aid. Spirulina is good to help restore appetite. See *DIET caption* for further guidance, where all suggested is natural and wholesome. Very often there is a Zinc deficiency and supplementation is advised. Should appetite-loss persist, treat as serious and seek medical advice.

APPLES

One of our greatest natural remedies, as advised by our ancestors. One cannot eat too much fruit, especially apples. According to recent research they can provide better function of lungs. It has been found that the flavenoids in apples and other solid fruits improve breathing, also chronic cough symptoms found if suffering from emphysema and other bronchial or lung problems. Selenium, taken as a food supplement, either separately or in a Multivitamin tablet, makes an ideal combination with an apple, as it boosts the flavenoids referred to. Apples, including the peel or skin, contain much that is good. *The old adage 'An apple a day helps keep the doctor away' is as true today as ever.*

AROMATHERAPY

This is the controlled application of what are referred to as essential oils, which many believe lead to a state of harmony and a feel-good factor. Those who have visited an Aromatherapist remark on the relief obtained from pains, aches or ailment from which they have suffered. Aromatherapy means using the essential oils to improve health and prevent disease. The oils are administered by massage, inhalation, compressions or baths. The use of aromatic oils in healing is an ancient one. In the move away from synthetic medicines and their dangers, Aromatherapy has become popular, proving to be highly beneficial, often looked upon as a preventative line against illness. It is very important to use only a fully qualified Aromatherapist for treatment.

ARTHRITIS – (Osteo)

Also see Arthritis Diet under next caption

A

Arthritis is one of our most common health complaints. Books, reams of pages and much has been written about this all-too-prevalent disease. For those who suffer from it there is some explanation needed as to the cause or causes. It affects hands, knees, hips and spine. Chrystals of calcium form in the joints, cartilages and synovial fluid. The fluid is like a lubricant, surrounding the joints or bursa, filling the tendon sheath. Arthritis often results in deformed, painful or stiff joints, with movement restricted. It tends to develop in, or after middle age, but recently we find it occurring in young people including children. *When doctors are visited one is treated for Arthritis, just that, Arthritis. Depression, fatigue and much anguish or suffering, which is caused by the sometimes, unbearable pain is not relevant to many of them. The word Diet is seldom mentioned. One will hear little from the medical profession about it.* They don't make any money out of food or the prescribing of it.

DIET IS NUMBER ONE, ALL IMPORTANT, THE ELIXIR IN THE TREATMENT OR PREVENTION OF ARTHRITIS. This is one problem the author writes about with confidence. The very many people who have benefited from advice given, is testimony to the fact that pure, natural foods, along with food supplements and herbal remedies, plus exercise, are the answer to most Arthritis cases. Some who were about to have joint replacements have been able to forego the operation. Wheelchair occupants have returned to gardening. A woman told of how she attended a wedding, which was a week-end affair and went on for some days. Being tempted to forget the Diet prescribed, imbibing unduly, the almost paralysing pains returned. It was over three weeks before she was pain-free, after resuming the advised Diet, which before this lapse she had been adhering to rigidly. This is her story, as told when she referred to the Diet suggested here as *'Being her other Bible'*. Like most sufferers she did not have a 'cure' - only unbelievable relief. The harm, already done, could not be reversed. As used by those who have said: 'Thank You' (or as some reply when I asked how they feel: "Thanks to you I feel good"), there are natural remedies, which can change the lives of many sufferers when used in conjunction with natural food.

Arthritis is not the result of ageing as we have been told in the past. Just as with rheumatoid arthritis, if the immune system is not in a healthy state, then infection in the joints can be extremely harmful. ***Antibiotics are being used indiscriminately, with those being treated at risk of damage to the immune system. Even children are in danger because of their over-use. This is probably the main reason why Arthritis is being diagnosed amongst young people as never before, the other contributory factor being additive filled processed 'foods'.***

If allergic to dairy produce or gluten, as in wheat, grains or other foods, this can be a problem. Stress and worry don't help. Many have found that they are allergic to cow's milk, being intolerant to it. Milk is not the food it used to be. It is hard to digest, may contain traces of pesticides or other contaminants, including animal medicine residues. Fresh milk can now be up to 10 days old when used on its 'sell by date'. This cannot be natural. Now we have foisted on us so-called super milk with added synthetic vitamins. So much for pure, natural fresh milk. If with Allergy one must check for the causes. *See Allergy caption* and follow the elimination Diet as set out.

Some of those given the Arthritis Diet sheet said they could not abide by it. They could not discipline themselves to do so. The many who did all gained immense relief. There were those who did as advised and then returned successfully to some of the foods, which they were asked to omit. Overall the results were exceptional. The writer is convinced that the elimination of the unnatural food additives, taking only pure natural foods, combined with vitamins, minerals and food supplements as suggested, is the answer to the problem of Arthritic pain. Osteo Arthritis occurs in varying forms, therefore, what is good for one by way of food supplement or remedy may not work for another. It is suggested you try out different aids, then keeping to those, which suit best. An example of all this is in the partaking of Devils Claw, Runo or Aloe Vera Joint Complex which contains Glucosamine, where the users found one to be marvellous with the others not giving relief, or vice versa. The remedies which I have seen to give relief and freedom from pain have been selected from some of those used over the past 40 years, are given in order of success: Devils Claw (Pagosid), Runo, Rhus Tox homeopathic remedy 30c, Aloe Vera Joint Complex (ESI Aloe Pura), Joint Ace (Vitabiotics), Wild Yam, Pantothenic Acid. All to be taken as prescribed on labels except Rhus Tox 30c potency, which is to be taken twice daily. *Only use when there is pain.* Some people were able to stop the medication for varying amounts of time when free from discomfort. As an aid to normal metabolism and digestion, also to help alleviate the arthritic pain, twice daily take two teaspoonfuls of Aspells or Martlets Pure Cider Vinegar obtainable from the health food store, mixed with two teaspoonfuls of pure honey in a little warm water. A good, slow release, Multivitamin tablet is a final insurance as it contains vitamins and minerals including Zinc, Copper, Magnesium and other aids to better health. Udo's Choice Oil contains essential fatty acids, being a wonderful help to those with Arthritis. Orange juice mixed with the oil makes it palatable, easier to take. It is best taken just before bedtime. Here one obtains Vitamin D and the equally important Omega oils in a simple emulsified form. The remedies, which suit best, combined with the natural Diet suggested, also the exercise, such as walking, will result in vast improvement and a sense of well being. One needs to be disciplined to be free from arthritic pain. *As mentioned, there is the need for exercise. It is advisable that if with a medical*

problem, a G.P. be consulted before embarking on any kind of serious exertion.
See Exercise caption to learn that one need not be worried about starting any kind

of limber-up, if fit to do so. It can be varied, from doing little, to arduous work-out.
Walking costs nothing, can be very enjoyable and is one of our greatest aids to better
health. Purposely left until last is the advice to take what is both a preventive and
an aid for Arthritis. This is Calcium/Magnesium/Vitamin D supplement, which is
invaluable for bone health, a must, to be taken long term by all over the age of 35,
both male and female. *Also turn to Sleep caption.*

ARTHRITIS DIET

**Everything based on improving or attaining better health included here is to be
used where relevant in conjunction with advice given under** *Diet caption.* **It is
the main caption in this** *Encyclopedia To Good Food, Natural Remedies And
Better Health.* **Many years ago I had an invaluable book, since loaned and not
returned. This happens frequently and can be annoying. It was titled 'The
Arthritics Cookbook' by Dr Colin Dong. It is now out-of-print. From this I
learned much about the vital importance of proper pure food Diet for the
treatment of, or to be free from, the pain of Arthritis. The advice given added to
what I know and have since learned about the disease, is set down in the
captions about Arthritis, both osteo and rheumatoid, also in the Arthritis Diet
described here.**

Drink copious amounts of pure water. Up to eight or 10 glasses daily is as medicine,
being like a lubricant. We do not drink nearly enough water daily. Most people wait
until thirsty. This is wrong. Keep topping up with water. It may sometimes be
necessary to use a filter system, such as 'Simply Water' provide. *See Water caption.*
This will remove the toxic chemical Fluoride, also the horrible Chlorine smell often
prevalent. Tests have shown the filtered water to be extremely pure and natural.
Even a filtered jug will help, but not nearly to the same extent. Listed here are the
various foods and drinks, which over the past 40 years I have found to be, as one
sufferer told me, 'A Second Bible'. It would be impossible to set out the exceptional
results or benefits obtained by adhering to this Diet. Little effort is required to self-
discipline one to be free from Arthritic pain, to be fully mobile, even to avoid
operation for joint replacement.

What To Eat Or Drink

Porridge, muesli, shredded wheat, oat or wheat bran, wholemeal bread, oatmeal,
salads, fresh fish not smoked, vegetables raw or steamed slightly underdone,
sprouted seeds, potatoes, pure natural honey from beekeepers or health food
shops, fruit - avoid citrus, white of egg only, chicken or turkey (free range if
possible), liver, kidney, lamb, beef- these are the only meats allowed - dried fruit
washed and soaked, garlic or garlic supplements, pulses, nuts except peanuts,
homemade or natural soups, weak tea, drink copious amounts of Water. It must be

free from Chlorine and Fluoride. Use butter sparingly. *See Food pyramid* and if everything is natural and additive-free it is good. *See Diet caption* in this Encyclopedia to learn further as to what natural additive-free non- processed foods are available. Visit the health food store to see and ask about their range of foods, spreads and delicacies, all natural.

What Not To Eat Or Drink

Dairy products if allergic to them, otherwise use sparingly, margarine because it contains additives, salt, sugar or any sugary products, meats other than those specified, many others are processed and with additives, pepper, this is one of the biggest triggers of arthritis, white bread, citrus fruit, pastry, cakes, confectionery, biscuits, cookies, sweets, chocolate, anything tinned. *Avoid all foods processed or with colour, additive, preservative or anything unnatural. Read the ingredients label before purchasing foodstuffs.* It is very important to avoid alcohol or fizzy 'drinks' of any kind, also fruit juices made from concentrated juice, coffee or other source of caffeine. Drink weak tea. Pure and natural fruit juice can be obtained at the health food store. Home-juiced fruit is best. Think natural, eat natural, take exercise and have regular sleep pattern. All this will help to conquer the pain which can come from Arthritis.

ARTHRITIS – Rheumatoid

This is an autoimmune disease, one of several where the ailment is caused by inflammation and destroying of tissue by the body's own antibodies. In osteo arthritis there is joint inflammation. In Rheumatoid Arthritis the inflammation is in the lining of the joints. It can occur in any part of the body on either side, including the hands, feet, tendons or spine. It is more prevalent in women, with men being prone to lung problems arising from Rheumatoid Arthritis. It causes pain, tiredness and sometimes loss of appetite. The smaller joints are usually affected. Because of the terrible side- effects, which are encountered where anti-rheumatic drugs are used to repress the condition, including the use of steroid injections, an ever-increasing number of sufferers are turning to alternative, complementary or natural medicine. You will note the word repress is used. This is the cardinal error of the majority of synthetic medicines. Cure is all too often not produced or forthcoming. The resultant side- effects can be debilitating, to say the least.

Those with joint pain naturally associate it with arthritis or rheumatism. There is a vast difference between rheumatoid and osteo arthritis, also there are various other types of arthritis, all of which need somewhat different kinds of treatment. Osteo arthritis is looked upon as being age-related, although this is not strictly true, where like Rheumatoid Arthritis it can occur in early life or at any time. As with almost all illness and health problems, emphasis must be on pure natural Diet, as written about so much in this Encyclopedia. Inferior Diet is the cause of most of our health problems *(see Arthritis Diet as set out in previous caption)*.

In conjunction with the suggested Diet, will only use of some of the alternative supplements, and hopefully find the one most suitable, obtain alleviation or ease? They should be used when partaking of the Arthritis Diet suggested and set out under that caption. Anything mentioned is natural, being available from the health food store.

The herbs Guaiacum and Meadowsweet are very helpful to Rheumatoid Arthritis. Alternate each one by infusing as tea. Place a teaspoonful of the herb in a cup or mug and pour in boiling water. Leave for five minutes before taking. Drink three or four times daily. It may take a little time to become used to drinking these teas, but one soon acquires a taste for them.

Pantothenic acid has been extremely beneficial to the disease. Take 500mg daily for two days, 1000mg daily for seven days and 1500mg daily for 60 days. After this the partaker need only take the daily dosage suggested on container when there is pain and indeed this may be entirely absent. Other beneficial remedies have been:

Two teaspoons of Aspells or Martletts cider vinegar, mixed with two teaspoons of pure honey in a little warm water, taken before meals.

Two Kelp tablets taken daily before morning and evening meals.

One Calcium/Magnesium/Vitamin D tablet daily.

Either Devils Claw or Runo (both have proven results) to be taken only if with pain.

Udo's Choice Oil, which is a blend of omega oils, contains Lecithin and Evening Primrose Oil.

It is a very good source of fatty acids, which are vital to help keep free from arthritis. The easy way to take the oil is on porridge, breakfast cereal or mix with a little fruit juice.

Follow the advice given in Arthritis Diet. It is bewildering that the majority of the medical profession prescribe for illness without mentioning the need for natural Diet, of how factory-made additives can be the cause of the illness.

Very often the intake of unhealthy foods can work against the medicine, with perhaps harmful effects. *To aid sleep see Sleep caption.* The Calcium / Magnesium / Vitamin D tablet, if taken with a spoonful of pure honey and warm milk or water, before bedtime, is a wonderful aid to sleeplessness.

Ayurveda therapy has proved to be of enormous help to many who sufferer from Rheumatoid Arthritis. Qualified therapists are listed in The Yellow Pages.

ASPARTAME

This is a dangerous food additive found in many 'foods' and 'drinks' partaken of regularly. It is a sugar substitute, a sweetener, a drug. As an excito toxin it stimulates the brain to the point of damage. It is now the most consumed synthetic product in use, in fizzy 'drinks', also in certain foods. It is reprehensible that it is used by drug companies in certain of their synthetic medicines. *The United States Food and Drug Administration Toxicologist, Dr Adrian Gross, is on record as stating: "The cancer causing potential of Aspartame is a matter that has been established beyond any reasonable doubt". This product makes one crave carbohydrates, making you eat fat, so gaining weight. It is deadly for diabetics, keeping the blood sugar level unmanageable. It has been linked to memory loss, headaches, skin problems, brain tumours, irregular heartbeat, depression and seizures, amongst many other of the ailments with which we are plagued. It may cause birth defects. We are reliably informed that high levels of Aspartame have being found in brain tumours when removed.*

Here is a classic example of where the powerlessness of Governments is found, when it comes to dealing with the mighty 'food' and 'drinks' industry and their almost indiscriminate uses of some food additives. This is a terrible indictment, which shows what quangos and lobbies can do as they act as bullyboys, in promoting the uses of this and other foods and drinks - additives which may be dangerous to health. Aspartame contains phenylalanine, which is toxic when taken without the other Amino Acids found in protein. This drains or empties serotonin from the system, which is invaluable to the nervous system, causing depression, rage, also violence. **The taking of Aspartame into the body is an obvious reason for the dramatic increase in child hyperactivity or ADHD. Aspartame is found in many fizzy 'drinks', which are the banes of our health, including so called 'energy beverages' for athletes or sports persons. They could better be described as 'calorie dense, sweetened drinks'.** A 500ml bottle of one of these sports drinks, which is constantly advertised, contains more than six teaspoons of sugar. I make no apologies for advising again to read the ingredients labels and to avoid anything unnatural. They should not be allowed in the food, drink and confectionery chain.

ASTHMA

As with many other ailments in the developed world there has been a dramatic increase in the number of people with Asthma, with numbers rising all the time. Much research has been done, with central heating, wall-to-wall carpets, pets and other ideas having been put forward as to why the increase. One of the main causes of this health problem is because of the Diet with which the western world has become obsessed, also the fact that breast-feeding is taboo to so many. Unnatural, processed, fast and other foods containing too much fat, synthetic additives, colour and bulking agents are the order of the day. Add to this the many chemical drugs being prescribed by the medical profession, not to mention those we can all too easily obtain off-the-shelf. Children from birth are now being bombarded with antibiotics and medicines, many of them prescribed unnecessarily. Why did we not have this in the past? Why now? What has happened in our world to bring on all this sickness and ailment despite the seemingly endless new drugs being placed at our disposal? The almost indiscriminate use of aerosols is a leading factor of the much air pollution by which we are surrounded.

Chief antagonist of Asthma is acetylsalicylic acid, known simply as Aspirin. Many drugs contain Aspirin and many doctors are unaware of this when prescribing. There are probably many more of these synthetic mixtures, which are adverse to Asthma. For instance paracetamol, which is an analgesic drug, causes the condition to worsen.

The attitude that Asthma is an incurable disease is wrong. Simply because it has resisted antibiotics and antihistamines does not mean it cannot be banished. I have proved that Diet of pure food as described in DIET caption and the partaking of vitamins, minerals and also food supplements has alleviated and even left the Asthmatic patient free from the ailment. The quickest 'cure', and I use this word without fear of contradiction, has been when those with Asthma have changed home geographically, moving as little as one 100 miles from one area of the country to another. They have never had a recurrence. Add to these the therapy of Buteyko and here we have three entirely natural remedies, all of which have proved exceptional in the treatment of Asthma, allowing sufferers to lead normal lives.

One apple daily and Selenium have been of immense help. Selenium is found in whole grains, meat and sea-food. It is best taken in supplement form to be sure of adequate intake. Apples contain flavanoids, which are unlocked by the Selenium. Also recommended is Galeopsis taken long term. Other aids are Lobelia, Vitamin B6 and Nat Mur. An Antioxidant Complex supplement, which will contain Vitamins A, C and E and other minerals will help boost the immune system. Pure Cider Vinegar as sold by the health food shop has produced some remarkable results. Take two teaspoons of pure Manuka Honey with two teaspoons of Cider Vinegar in some warm water three times daily. Exercise daily, on a regular basis, as suggested in Exercise or Walking captions. This is a must for Asthmatics. The author knows many who are free, with others almost free from Asthma, by practising Yoga. It is a marvellous therapy, teaching correct breathing habits and much more. A high enough recommendation of the goodness of Yoga cannot be made with relation to health and well being of those with Asthma. Partaking of the onion family, including scallions, leeks, chives and especially garlic is recommended for the ailment. The latter is available in odourless form from your health food store. It is one of our greatest health allies. One should not have to be warned of the dangers of smoking, including passive smoke, also the harm of air fresheners and other aerosols as already mentioned. *See Aerosols caption.* Alcohol must be avoided.

See DIET caption to learn about its aid to good health and this includes much, which will help those who suffer from Asthma. It is one of the greatest medicines for the problem.

The therapy of BUTEYKO is an excellent help. It is based on control of Asthma by proper and correct breathing. There are many good reports about its effectiveness and successful results. *See Buteyko caption* also Bibliography section for details of **'Close Your Mouth, Buteyko Clinic Handbook'.**

ATHEROMA

This means that there is an extremely high concentration of fats in the blood, which build up in the arteries, causing blockages, which can lead to thrombosis or strokes. It is often referred to as hardening of the arteries, being sometimes hereditary. The main cause of the trouble is the partaking of excessive animal fats, additive-filled processed and unnatural 'foods' and 'drinks'. Smoking, being overweight, also lack of exercise, are the contributory factors. **I write from experience, being convinced that the arteries can be cleared by the use of pure natural food as recommended under DIET caption, and also by adhering to the advice given under Heart captions.**

ATHEROSCLEROSIS

This disease occurs when plaques of fat adhere to the inner walls of the arteries. Eventually the blood flow is restricted with consequences similar to atheroma. *See Atheroma caption.*

ATHLETES FOOT

This is produced by a fungus or may be a consequence of a skin infection. The chief cause is all-too-often the inadequate drying of the feet, especially between the toes. This should always be done carefully and very thoroughly. I have instructed many, emphasising that this is the main treatment for athlete's foot. In the majority of cases the problem was alleviated. Also advised is to spread a very thin smear of Allergenics Non Steroidal ointment between the effected toes before putting on socks or stockings. The feet, on which we depend so much, very often do not receive the care and attention they deserve. They should be washed at least weekly, unless working in a dirty environment, dried as set out, and treated properly. Further aids are to take Echinacea or Poke Root. If the problem is with fungus take Acidophilus.

ATTENTION DEFICIT HYPERACTIVITY DISORDER

See ADHD Caption.

AYURVEDA THERAPY

This system of Indian medicine goes back to Biblical times. Ayur means 'life'. Veda means 'knowledge'. It is the science of life, with extremely good recommendation from those who have used the Therapy. It deals with every aspect of spiritual, mental and physical health. It has helped with hearing problems, epilepsy, rheumatoid arthritis, allergies, skin problems including eczema, viral infection and heart disease. Therapists are listed in the yellow pages.

B VITAMINS

See Vitamins and Minerals Caption.

BABY FOODS

Next time you purchase baby foods, study the ingredients labels. One well advertised brand shows over 30 ingredients, many of them synthetic or unnatural. Others are somewhat similar. The best before date on some is over 12 months hence. Many baby foods are just like all too much 'foods' on the shelves of the food store or pharmacy. They are overly additive-filled, not being natural. Usually there is an important warning notice printed on. Have you read it? The manufacturers even tell us that breastfeeding is best. *Always read the ingredients labels, at the same time remembering that you are responsible for your health and also that of your child. See Breastfeeding caption.*

BACH FLOWER REMEDIES

The 38 Bach Flower Remedies are medicines for the emotions - simple, natural preparations that are used to treat everyday emotional states such as worry, anxiety and lack of concentration. They are available from the health food store or pharmacies. Dr Edward Bach, a bacteriologist, pathologist and homeopath, whose career took him from University College Hospital to the London homeopathic Hospital and a successful Harley Street Practice, discovered them in the 1930's.

Bach was convinced that the only path to true health was to treat the individual personality, rather than concentrating on the physical symptoms of disease. He found that specially prepared plants could resolve emotional imbalances and that well-balanced people then got better physically, because their bodies were free to heal themselves.

By the time he died in 1936 Dr Bach had discovered 38 remedies, a complete system that could be combined to treat every possible emotional state.

For example, a kind, gentle person who found it hard to say 'No' to other people would be given Centaury, while someone who always tries to hide their worries by making a joke of them would need Agrimony. Both might be suffering from the same physical symptoms, such as insomnia and frequent colds, but the remedies would be different for each person.

When using Bach Flower Remedies it is essential to ignore any physical symptoms or disease. Instead the remedies are selected according to the personality of the person being treated.

The most famous remedy is Rescue Remedy. This is a mix of five remedies - Rock Rose for terror, Clematis for light-headedness, Impatiens for agitation, Cherry Plum for loss of self-control and Star of Bethlehem for shock. Dr Bach selected these five remedies because he felt there would be at least something in the mix that would help anyone going through a crisis.

There are two main ways to take Bach Flower Remedies. One is to take two drops of each selected remedy in a glass of water and sip from this at least four times a day or until the problem has passed. Alternatively the two drops can be put into a clean empty 30ml dropper bottle, which is then topped up with pure water. From this bottle - known as a treatment bottle - four drops are taken four times a day. Kept in the fridge and used regularly, a treatment bottle will last up to three weeks.

The Bach system is as vital today as it was when first discovered. When we feel fulfilled, happy and positive we tend to enjoy better health. We get more out of life and we can give more to our friends and family. But when things happen every now and again we need a little help to stay in balance, to regain control and move forward. This is when the Bach Flower Remedies can help.

Each of these 38 remedies aids a specific problem and really helps resolve emotional fears and traumas and helps one get more out of life.

Agrimony	When you put on a cheerful face to hide problems
Aspen	When you have unexplained fear and worries, are nervous and anxious
Beech	Where you are critical and intolerant of others
Centaury	When you have difficulty in saying no and are anxious to please
Cerato	When you doubt your own ability to judge situations
Cherry Plum	Where there is fear of losing control of your behaviour
Chestnut Bud	Where there is failure to learn from experience, repeating the same mistakes
Chicory	Where one is overly possessive and you expect others to conform to your values
Clematis	Where there is a lack of interest in the present and a tendency to daydream
Crab Apple	Where there is a poor self-image or feeling of embarrassment or shame
Elm	Where overwhelmed or burdened by responsibility

Gentian	Where there is discouragement or despondence
Gorse	Where there is hopelessness and despair, a feeling of pessimism
Heather	Where one is self-absorbed, dislikes being alone and is excessively talkative
Holly	Where there are feelings of extreme jealousy, envy or suspicion
Honeysuckle	When one lives in the past, feels homesick or is nostalgic
Hornbeam	Where there is the Monday morning feeling, doubting your ability to face the day's work
Impatiens	For those who are impatient and easily irritated
Larch	Where there is a lack of self confidence and an inferior feeling
Mimulus	Where there is fear rooted in known causes e.g., spiders, flying, dentist
Mustard	Where one experiences unexplained gloom which comes and goes for no apparent reason
Oak	Where one struggles on though exhausted because of a strong sense of duty
Olive	When you feel exhausted in body and mind
Pine	Where you feel guilt and blame yourself for other peoples mistakes
Red Chestnut	When one is over-anxious or over-concerned for others
Rock Rose	Where you experience terror, frozen in fear and feel helpless, e.g., driving test etc
Rock Water	For those who are inflexible, setting themselves high standards
Scleranthus	For those times of uncertainty and indecision
Star of Bethlehem	For the after effects of shock, grief or fright
Sweet Chestnut	When one is at the limit of endurance and in deep despair
Vervain	When one is over-enthusiastic, argumentative, with fixed principles and ideas
Vine	Where you are strong, filled with a tendency to be domineering or inflexible
Walnut	When one faces major life changes and is in need of protection from the influence of others
Water Violet	Where you prefer to be alone or are proud and aloof - maybe thinking loneliness
White Chestnut	Where there are unwanted thoughts, preoccupations and worries
Wild Oat	Uncertain as to correct path of life, dissatisfied with present lifestyle and cannot decide which way to go

Wild Rose	For feeling of resignation, apathy, lack of interest in the present
Willow	Where there is resentment, have feelings of self pity - "poor me"
Rescue Remedy	A flower combination to help you cope with demanding and stressful situations, Exams, a visit to the dentist, redundancy, any of life's problems
Complete Set	A box containing one of each of the remedies
Rescue Cream	Soothes and restores rough, flaky or chapped skin. Contains a blend of six flower remedies

For more information contact **The Dr Edward Bach Centre, Mount Vernon, Bakers Lane, Sotwell, Oxon OX10 OPZ** or ask at your local health food shop or some pharmacies.

BACKACHE

One of life's most common complaints. Like we do with our body, we take our back and the use of it for granted. How many know how to lift, sit, stand or work properly to keep the back safe? **'A Little Book About Your Back'** as outlined in the Bibliography at the end of Guide gives much information. Back pains can be eased by manipulative treatment such as Osteopathy, Acupuncture or Chiropractic Therapy.

Rucksacks and children's schoolbags are often ill fitting with little thought given to their design. They are all too often over filled. Parents seldom realise the burden of the school bag. This can lead to back problems in later life. There are many forms of Backache, the most common of which is lower Back pain, which could be prostate problem. Because of wrong method of lifting or as a result of accident there may be vertebrae or disc complication. *See under caption for specific remedies; sciatica, osteoporosis, rheumatism, arthritis, lumbago, fibrositis, lower Back pain, etc.* **It is not widely realised that some suffer Back pain because of defective thrombin in the blood, an enzyme which helps clear fibrin, which repairs damaged tissue. Ask your doctor to do a blood test, explaining why you are making the request.** Relief of certain Backache is gained by taking Runo, Devils Claw (Pagosid), Combination G (New Era) or Wild Yam. The Alexander Technique Therapy has proved to be excellent, with many favourable reports of Back problems being put right. *See Alexander Technique caption.*

BAD BREATH

See Hallitosis Caption.

BALANCED DIET

How often do we hear of this? The majority understand this as being a Balanced Diet of any foods, additive-filled or otherwise. This is wrong. Only a Balanced Diet of pure natural additive-free food can be nourishing. *See DIET caption* to be guided about natural foods which go to make up Balanced Diet.

BANANAS

They are full of goodness, one of our best snack foods, also a good source of potassium, magnesium and phosphorous. In the stomach they act as a buffer, neutralising excess hydrochloric acid. The taste, aroma and satisfying hunger qualities are the Banana's main attractions.   There is much which can be written about their health-giving benefits.

BARLEY WATER

A kidney tonic, being a healthy invigorating drink. To five cups of water add half cup of pearl Barley, quarter stick of cinnamon, a little ground ginger and simmer for 20 minutes. When cool, strain, add fresh lemon juice, and sweeten, if so desired, with pure honey and drink once or twice daily. Will keep for five days in refrigerator. Barley Water drinks bought off the shelf in the supermarket are mostly with additives and are not natural.   If with additives leave on the shelf.   Read the ingredients labels.

BATES METHOD FOR BETTER EYESIGHT

This is based on vision education. It means much more than just eye exercises, as one learns to use the eyes and brain in different ways, to improve the way we see. It was developed out of the work of Dr W.H. Bates (1860-1931). The Bates method incorporates a range of practises based on the twin principles of relaxation and movement, to normalise the relationship between eyes and brain, so improving function and condition. Many of those sufficiently disciplined to follow the simple advice given have been able to leave their glasses aside. See Bibliography for book details or contact **The Bates Association, P.O. Box 25, Shoreham-by-Sea, West Sussex, BN43 6ZF UK. Visit the website www.seeing.org**

BATH - (Hot)

Before entering a Bath or shower, some look forward to and like to enter when it is extremely hot. This can be harmful to the system and the skin. Better to enter when it is reasonably warm and then run the hot water to increase the temperature.

BED

How many give thought to the most important aid to proper and good sleep? Do they replace the Bed within the time stipulated by the manufacturer? It is advisable to turn the mattress regularly to prevent the interior springs remaining uncoiled.

The Bed should be a place of precious relaxation, preferably not too hard as orthopaedic beds are, unless with back problems and for which the latter type of Bed is recommended. Normally it should be neither too hard nor too soft. Do your pillows feel comfortable? Like synthetic food fillers not being good, so with the pillows! The feather pillow as of old is still the most comfortable, as it fills in between head and shoulders when resting on it. A comfortable Bed leads to good and restful sleep which is as medicine to the body.

BED SORES

They usually occur because of a lack of Vitamin C, also a Zinc deficiency, in the system. Allergenics Non Steroidal ointment has helped enormously. Change the patient's position frequently. Keep risk regions dry such as heels, elbows, hips and shoulders.

BED WETTING – (Children)

This is sometimes hereditary. It also occurs because of lack of love in the home, insecurity, family disputes or school worries, resulting in it being a psychological problem. It can also be as a result of food allergy. *The majority of Bed wetters over the age of five do not have the capacity to control their bladder during sleep. In this case it is necessary to reduce the intake of liquid for three or four hours before bedtime.* The following have been found to help solve the problem: KaliPhos and Nat Mur alternated daily or Cranesbill, Plantago or Causticium have also been good. I have seen two things which stop the Bed-wetting. Protein is needed to help level off the blood sugar during sleep, to allow for proper brain function. Before Bedtime give natural cereals, pulses or nuts. Pure additive-free peanut butter from the health food shop is a source. The other remedy is an old one handed down over the years, simply a piece of raw potato eaten last thing at night. I can testify that it has worked for any child for whom I have prescribed it . During the daytime, children whether thirsty or not, should be given plenty of water to drink. As well as being good for the child this helps enlarge the bladder. It is another aid to solving the Bed wetting problem.

BEE STINGS

Apply Bicarbonate of soda mixed to a paste or malt vinegar applied neat. Remove sting as quickly as possible by rubbing out, not pulling out.

BELCHING

Treat as Flatulence Caption.

BELLS PALSY

Pure natural Diet as with most ailments is all-important. *See DIET caption.* Vitamin

E taken as 100iu for 30 days then 200iu taken for 30 days and 400iu daily long-term is excellent aid to recovery. Also of benefit are Echinacea, Black Cohosh or Combination A, New Era. Black Cohosh should not be taken long term.

BETA CAROTENE

This is an antioxidant, a preventative and fighter of diseases, an immune booster. It is claimed that a Diet rich in Beta Carotene is an insurance against certain types of cancer also prostate and cardiovascular disease. A Beta Carotene Combination supplement is the best source, to be used alongside pure natural balanced Diet from which Beta Carotene should come in the first instance.

BIBLE

The Book is the biggest seller in the world. Don't ignore it. It gives sound advice, including that regarding health. Proverbs 25:27, tells us 'It is not good to eat much sweet things'. This is a warning to all as we eat the additive filled, sugarised, junk food on offer. 1 Corinthians 6:19 warns us to 'Look after our bodies'. Sleep, of which many leave themselves short, costs nothing. There is much free to aid all of us. The Bible is a mine of spiritual wealth, including advice on health. Genesis 1:29 says 'Behold I have given you every herb bearing seed upon the earth'.

BILBERRIES

Good for healthy vision and eye disorders. They help circulation and varicose veins. Excellent for haemorrhoids during pregnancy. When taking in supplement form use same strength at all times.

BILIOUSNESS

Occurs usually as nausea and belching. May be due to constipation or acidity associated with bad Diet or alcohol. Milk thistle, Combination S New Era or Blue Flagroot are remedies. Proper Diet is important. *Turn to DIET caption.*

BIOMAGNETIC THERAPY

See Magnetic Therapy Caption.

BIOSTRATH

See Tonics Caption.

BLACK COHOSH

This is a herbal remedy used mainly to treat pre-menstrual symptoms, also difficult or painful menstruation. It may also be used to help with menopause problems including hot flushes and mood swings, cramps, low back pain and tinnitus - *see relevant captions.* Usually it has to be taken for four weeks before results are seen.

Stop the use during pregnancy or breast-feeding. Do not take Black Cohosh long term.

BLADDER INFECTION

For mild infections take Pure Cranberry Juice and Vitamin C together or take Cranberry Supplement capsule. Most juices in supermarkets or convenience stores are not pure juice. The health food store will supply Pure Cranberry Juice.

BLEEDING GUMS

See Periodontal Disease Caption.

BLEPHARITIS

See Eyes Caption.

BLOATED FEELING

See Flatulence Caption.

BLOOD – (Impure)

Pure natural Diet is number one remedy. *See DIET caption.* Blood Tonics are Floradix, Silica, Echinacea, or Combination D New Era. *Also turn to Nettles caption.*

BLOOD PRESSURE – (High) – (Hypertension)

I have seen many restore their Blood Pressure to normal, including myself, by using natural methods. Of utmost importance is the Diet, which must be of pure natural foods. Avoid alcohol, smoking, including passive, also salt and sugar. We obtain far too much of the latter, with them being almost impossible to avoid. Everything mentioned in this Guide is natural, available from a good health food shop or some chemists. They may be taken with anything prescribed by the doctor, unless otherwise stated. *Tell them what you are taking or intend to take. They will know little or nothing about them, unless familiar with natural remedies, or additive free food, which is highly unlikely.* Combined with the Diet recommended in this Guide take Hawthorn, Rutin, Vitamins C and E, Lecithin Granules, Zinc with Copper tablet combined, Calcium with Magnesium tablet combined also garlic. If, like myself, you cannot digest raw garlic, then take an odourless one a day Garlic capsule or tablet, which gives all the goodness of this invaluable root. The Vitamins C and E are extremely good antioxidants, working in tandem. In order to be assimilated into the system, take one Vitamin E capsule 100iu for 30 days, then 200iu for following 30 days and one 400iu or 500iu thereafter daily. To learn about the goodness of the other suggested remedies turn to the relevant captions. *Also see Heart captions.*

If overweight steps should be taken to lose some of the excess. The Zinc will be an aid for this, also Dandelion and Helix Slim. The latter two are herbal aids to help control weight when used in conjunction with the natural Diet repeatedly advocated, prescribed and written about in this Guide. Exercise is vital. *If with health problem or on medication be advised by your doctor before serious exertion.* The exercise suggested is walking, which can be to your own pace according to how energetic you feel. *See Exercise caption.* Relax, enjoy yourself, at the same time helping to normalise the blood pressure. *Read fully the DIET caption,* which describes how natural food is one of the best medicines for blood pressure, whether high or low.

BLOOD PRESSURE – (Low) – (Hypotension)

Unless there is an underlying problem or blood loss due to accident, internal bleeding or other ailment Low Blood Pressure can be corrected. It is all too often caused by debility of the systems. Antidepressants must be avoided. The root cause must be treated and if nothing serious found then the natural good food Diet mentioned, also some vitamins and food supplements, should help to correct. From your health food store can be obtained Prickly Ash Bark, Vitamin B12 also Kordel's Celery Seed 6,000 plus, which are all excellent remedies for the ailment when taken with additive free, nutritious food. Avoid smoking and alcohol, being guided by the Dietary advice. Take exercise such as walking. *See Walking also Exercise captions.* If on medication be advised by your doctor. Tell him what you are taking or intend to take. George Bernard Shaw had Low Blood Pressure, but this did not stop him in his pursuits and work. People with Low Blood Pressure usually have long lives. *See DIET caption.*

BLOOD SHOT EYES

See Eyes Caption

BLOOD SUGAR LOW

See Hypoglycaemia Caption

BODY ODOUR

Often occurs because personal hygiene is not on the list of the perspirer, resulting in stale sweat, which when mixed with or added to fresh perspiration makes the odour objectionable. Deodorants, some of which carry warnings, are not recommended to solve the problem. It can be as a result of over-active sweat glands or improper functioning of bowels or kidneys. Almost always a change of Diet to pure natural foods can be the answer, also the addition of some Vitamins, Minerals or Food supplements. *See DIET caption.* Take Silica, Zinc, Vitamin B Complex or Wild Yam, all in tablet form from your health food shop. Bath or shower regularly.

BODY WARMTH

Here are two words which mean snug, cosy, comfortable, warm body and more. They mean better health. Thousands of times I've given advice to those, who particularly in Winter time, appear to almost traipse about, often with silk stockings, open toed light sandals, flimsy clothes, with little if any underwear and complaining about the cold. They are often with coughs, colds or other avoidable illness. Men are equally at fault. One must be alert to the change of seasons. Be practical, wear warm clothing, including heavy stockings or tights. Women and children are the chief rule breakers regarding the wearing of thin clothes. Children can only be guided by the parent or guardian. Warmth is almost as important as food. Frequently the lightly clad people referred to venture out from their centrally heated homes, to be met by the elements of our Winters. This is highly detrimental to their health. The wearing of hats or caps is laughed at -. 80% of our body heat escapes through our heads. There is much evidence that keeping warm, keeps one healthy. The doctors could very often prescribe warm headgear or clothes, but then there is nothing to be gained monetary- wise, except by prescribing antibiotics or other synthetic pills or potions.

BOILS

They occur because of blood impurity, usually as a result of bad Diet, which should be corrected. Floradix or Biostrath Elixir are good tonics and blood purifiers, as are Silica, Echninacea or Garlic capsules or tablets. This is one ailment where detoxing is recommended by the intake of natural foods. Drink copious amounts of water. *See DIET also Nettles captions.*

BOLDO

This is an excellent remedy for water retention syndrome.

BONE HEALTH INCLUDING BRITTLE BONES

In the body, of which the Bones are the framework or skeleton, there are over 200 in number. Unless Bone problems are due to infection, such as TB or other ailment, the health of our Bones is not helped by inferior Diet of processed or fast foods. It is not helped in our damp and wet climate where we do not take proper steps to protect the joints. Disorders of the Bones, especially the joints, are widespread today. The chief protector or aid to Bone health is a balance of Calcium, Magnesium and Vitamin D. The natural remedies circle has impressed this on us for many years. Only recently has it dawned on the medical profession that Calcium is a must. Only some of them now prescribe it. All over the age of 35 should take Calcium/Magnesium/Vitamin D supplement, Ostron or Bone Nutrient Complex tablet. Activjuice, which is high in Glucosamine content, is a well know natural aid to better bone health. Equally important is natural DIET also body warmth as mentioned. *See also Osteoporosis and Body Warmth captions.*

BOWEL SYNDROME – (Irritable)

See Irritable Bowel Syndrome Caption

BRAIN HEALTH – (Including Weak Memory)

To those worrying about weak memory, being forgetful, with memory loss, including being unable to remember names, mislaying things and not being able to remember where left, it must be said 'Don't find fault, find a remedy'. Most important for both the health of the Brain and the body is pure natural additive-free food and drink. Exercise of both mind and body is very important. Keep the Brain active and enjoyably employed. Read books including puzzle books, write letters or do crosswords, even if left unfinished. Don't bother about newspapers or the television as they only depress. Joining voluntary organisations enables one to meet others, helping to make friends. Take up a hobby. Keeping active, keeps the Brain active. Take each day as it comes, doing just one thing at a time. ***Allowing your mind to fill up or to become cluttered, feeling that you should be doing many things, is an extremely bad mental habit. This way of thinking only hinders the marvellous element which is the Brain. Relax body and mind regularly. Sit down, visualise things unrelated to every day life. Think of friends, places to visit and the things you must do which are enjoyable. Relaxing the mind regularly helps sharpen the Brainpower.***

Don't try to store everything in the Brain. Keep a diary or carry a notebook or pad, writing things down which you feel should be remembered. These are aids to your mind or memory. I am an old person in years, being young in body and mind, using a battery-operated pocket memo. This is simply because a pen or even the notebook could all too frequently not be found, especially when away from home. Previous to this I always used a notebook   Now there is no excuse for taxing the Brain with reminders, many of them often trivial. *Research tells us that older people have more than sufficient Brainpower for memory. They do not use it properly, filling it up with much thoughts or ideas which are wholly unnecessary.* It is not what comes to mind, it is how we insist on thinking about it, how we sort out the necessary from the inessential. This I have proved to be precious advice over the years, as was the advice to use a diary and later the pocket memo. First thing in the morning I always read yesterday's diary page and clear the pocket memo. It does much good, because it creates a chuckle or a laugh, as one looks at all the things written and undone, now of no importance, far different from how it appeared the previous day. The problems of yesterday left undone, not crossed out, appear as irrelevant or unimportant. The unnecessary and, at the time often worrying, ideas were not stored in the Brain, it being therefore unburdened.

The need for a balanced Diet of pure additive-free food is repeated. Equally important is the necessity to avoid Fluoridated or Chlorinated water. Here can be one of the main reasons for Brain deterioration. Fluoride is a noxious and toxic substance that should not be in our water. Turn to both Fluoride and Water captions.

Following are excellent supplements to keep the Brain healthy, which when added to the natural Diet suggested, make an enormous contribution to the Brain including the memory: Lecithin granules, Udo's Choice Oil to obtain the necessary Omega Oils, Vitamin B Complex, Lemon Balm either taken fresh or as Melissa herb tablet or tea. Rhodolia is a great aid to memory and concentration, as also are Rosemary or Ginkgo Biloba. The latter is not to be taken with blood thinning medication such as aspirin or warfarin. All these aids to Brain memory and general health can be obtained at your health food shop. *See Exercise and DIET captions.*

BRAN

See Fibre Caption.

BREAD

All too often taken for granted, accepted without question, as to goodness, purity, sustenance, or otherwise. The additive-filled Bread of today is not what it should be. Much could be written about the subject. This is a Guide where one can only dwell fleetingly on Bread. *White Bread which was accepted as good food because of the ingredients, also the method of baking up to about 30 years ago, is now processed, factory-made, with flour treatment agents, so called improvers, ascorbic acid, bleaching and other additives. It is now mostly made by what is known as the Chorley Wood Bread Process, one of the modern over-processing, fast food methods of producing cheaper 'food'. Where it took hours to ferment and knead the dough it is now done by electrically operated high-speed mixers, which agitate the mix for only a few minutes. Low protein, soft or finer flour, with more added water and, of course, the extra additives, some of them synthetic, are the recipe for fast Bread.* This is one of the main reasons why in recent years we hear the call for a return to the use of bran in our Diet. The Bread we are now offered is all too often just processed, additive-filled, part-baked dough. Some of it is of inferior quality with little if any nutrition. An example of this is in the 'Bread' very often used as a loss leader in the food shop. It could often be said to resemble eating cotton wool. *Nothing could be more tempting than the aroma of home-baked wholemeal Bread.* It is highly recommended for its starch, fibre and much other nutritional goodness. At the same time there are many nutritious Breads, especially wholemeal, to be found in some outlets, including the health food shop. One must search for them. *Again the advice is: "Read the ingredients label. Leave that which is additive filled on the shelf".*

BREAKFAST

Read the Diet caption to be guided by what is partly repeated here. **Breakfast is the most important meal of the day and should not be skipped.** It should be of natural, unprocessed, additive-free, non-sugarised cereals. Of the over 80 breakfast 'cereals' counted, as being offered for sale, many in psychedelic-coloured packaging, which are over refined, treated and altered, there are only two which have nothing added, nothing taken away. Some are with added synthetic vitamins and minerals, which when processed and heated are of little value. Others are just fillers, being sugarised, having being made acceptable to the palate or taste buds, especially that of our young people. The two referred to as being natural are Shredded Wheat, which is slightly processed and Porridge Oats. The latter is pure food, unadulterated. Added to the cereal can be oat or wheat bran, wheat germ, sunflower seeds or linseed. One can also partake of pure fruit juice, fruit or bread, especially if it is wholemeal. In the health food store are fruit spreads or jams, which are sweetened with fruit juice - no added sugar. Sugar should be avoided. No apology is made for repeating the advice to read under DIET to learn of the value of a proper nutritious Breakfast.

BREASTS – (Sore & tender)

May be a hormonal problem. Recommended is what is often referred to as a woman's best friend, Agnus Castus, also Evening Primrose Oil. Ask for high strength EPO.

BREASTFEEDING

Until recently the media and the medical profession, including the maternity fraternity would have us believe that Breastfeeding, which has always been and still is the natural way to feed a baby, is not correct, being frowned upon. To those interested in the natural way, with all things being additive-free and good for the health of the child, Breastfeeding has always been accepted as the best method. Breastfed first and then on to natural foods. The up-to-date, state-of-the-art, relatively cheap liquidiser makes it ever so much easier to produce natural vegetable and fruit-based, highly acceptable, nutritious meals, when breastfeeding weaning time comes.

UNICEF has got it right as they tell us **"Imagine that the world had invented a new dream product to feed and immunise everyone born on earth. Imagine also that it was available everywhere, required no storage or delivery – and helped mothers to plan their families and reduce risk of cancer. Then imagine that the world refused to use it. After a century of unprecedented discovery and invention, even as scientists discover life itself, this scenario is not alas a fiction. The dream product is human**

breast milk, available to us all at birth and yet we are not using it."
Despite the Health sectors advice to Breastfeed, it is being ignored, with the information not reaching or being conveniently ignored by many, including the disadvantaged. Those in the low income or social class bracket are the least likely to breastfeed.

Research shows that infants who are breastfed may be at a lower risk of being overweight or obese later in life. Other benefits include prevention of allergies, infections, including the mother's risk of breast cancer being lowered. Breastfed milk is free. When a mother is properly nourished there is no doubt that Breastfeeding is best, also her baby should not require supplements for at least six months. The child's digestive system and kidneys are unable to cope with solid food, including cereals before the age of four months at least, and these should be introduced gradually. Many are not aware of the dangers of feeding solids too soon to a baby. The bowels are not strong enough to accept this type of food. The solids of pure natural edible nourishment should be introduced very slowly in liquidised form, with the weaning from milk done equally so. Feeding with solids too early in life can lead to colon inflammation which is colitis, also bowel and other stomach problems in later years. When weaning, a good natural remedy to discourage suckling is to apply Aloe Vera Juice to the nipples.

A well-known liquid baby food, taken from the shelf in a supermarket, gives a sell by date of over 12 months hence. The ingredients label shows over 30 additives, amongst them being Citric acid, Calcium hydroxide, Potassium hydroxide, Tri calcium phosphate, Tri sodium citrate, Sodium chloride, Choline chloride, Taurine, Zinc sulphate, Copper gluconate, Manganese sulphate, Potassium iodide, Sodium selinite. One must ask the question: 'Why the need for all this in a baby food? Do any mothers read the ingredients label of what they purchase off the shelf? Reading this list must be sufficient proof that where it is at all possible breastfed is best.'

BREATH – (Bad)

See Hallitosis Caption.

BREATHING

Many people unknowingly breathe incorrectly. Proper Breathing techniques help to promote better health, often giving one a relaxed feeling. It is good for relief of stress, also to ease pain, including menstrual pain, even hot flushes. Do you ever Breathe deeply and fully, filling the lungs, extending the chest? If posture is not correct, neither is Breathing. Proper Breathing technique is essential for avoidance and relief of asthma attacks. For all who wish to learn about and improve their Breathing with resultant good feeling Yoga is recommended as is the wonderful therapy of Buteyko. This is an invaluable aid for asthma. It could not be more natural. *See Buteyko also Asthma and Yoga captions.*

BREATHLESSNESS

This must not be accepted as normal, unless after exercise, when powers of recovery come into practise. If with feeling of Breathlessness or with tightness in the chest requires examination by your doctor. If the difficulty to breathe is distressing the underlying cause must be found in order to treat. It is associated with heart disease especially angina, farmers lung, emphysema or bronchitis. For those other than with heart or angina disease, relief has been obtained by use of Lobelia tablets also Combination J New Era.

BREWER'S YEAST

This is a rich source of Vitamin B Complex also RNA and DNA, the nucleic acids which are so necessary for cell growth. Dried yeast is high in the acid content. To help banish acne, itch and other skin problems, including dermatitis, it is excellent. Brewer's Yeast is very good for the treatment of eczema. Many do not know about the goodness of Vitamin B Complex for the treatment of skin diseases. Brewer's Yeast contains this vitamin in quantity.

BRITTLE BONES

See Bone Health also Osteoporosis Captions.

BRITTLE NAILS

See Nails Caption.

BROCCOLI

Broccoli is one of our greatest medicines as food. *See Fruit and Vegetables caption.*

BRONCHITIS

There are two kinds of Bronchitis, chronic and acute. With the latter there is usually a yellow/green phlegm, a bad cough often painful, a raw throat and wheezing, also breathlessness. One may feel ill for up to 10 days. The cough may persist for longer. Often chronic Bronchitis can result from repeated attacks of acute Bronchitis, smoking, dust or other air pollutants. It occurs often in the elderly. Being run down, lack of exercise, inhalation of nicotine, improper breathing, impure air, all lead to Bronchitis. *It often occurs or develops after a cold or flu. Avoid polluted air, keep wrapped up for body warmth, stop smoking, try losing weight where necessary.* With acute Bronchitis, treating with antibiotics will not help as it is seldom caused by bacterial infection. See your doctor and discuss, also remembering that there are many things natural you can do to help relieve Bronchitis and obtain better health. The immune system must be built up. Here is an example of where proper nutritious food aided by food Supplements and Vitamins would have helped prevent the Bronchitis. Similarly it can help to alleviate the problem. *Let good food be your medicine and medicine be your food.* Added to this are the taking of excellent restoratives such as a Multivitamin tablet, Lobelia, Cider vinegar and Manuka honey, two teaspoons of each in a little warm water three times daily, Garlic capsules, Echinacea, Thyme drops or Iceland Moss. Everything mentioned can be obtained from your health food store. If the advice about natural food Diet is followed there can be vast Bronchial health improvement.

BRUISES

Arnica is excellent. Not to be used on open wounds. Other aids are Echinacea liquid or Elder.

BRUISING EASILY

Can be put down to lack of Vitamin K which comes from natural foods, especially green vegetables, including cauliflower, broccoli and cabbage. Meat, including pigs or lambs liver, is high in this vitamin. Inferior Diet leads to Bruising easily. This occurs quite often in the elderly, also being a side effect where there is weight loss. Even a small bump will cause Bruising. Apparently the capillaries, which have become lazy, do not maintain their stability in either the elderly or those who are overweight. Take a good Multivitamin tablet also extra Vitamins E and C, not more than 500mg daily of the latter, to help avoid Bruising.

BUERGERS DISEASE

Although a serious condition, natural remedies have been of much help. Unless the person ceases smoking, there is little hope of success of any treatment. I have noted where sufferers gave up smoking, took the advice given, and within six months came off the doctor's medication. They continued with Dietary food supplements and vitamin advice, being restored to good health. It is usually men who are affected. The suggested treatment, which can be taken in conjunction with whatever your doctor prescribes, is the all important natural Diet, to which is added Vitamin E to be taken as 100iu daily for 30 days then 400iu or 500iu daily to be taken thereafter. Vitamin C should also be taken because both vitamins work in conjunction with one another. Also recommended are Brewer's Yeast, Calcium/Magnesium, Lecithin granules and Hawthorn. Take gentle exercise. Any exercise possible would be of help, even down to sitting on a chair and swinging the legs when unable to do more. *When feeling unwell it is advisable to speak with your doctor regarding exercise before taking it up.*

BULIMIA

This eating disorder is usually a problem of teenagers or those in their 20's. Can be traced sometimes to Zinc deficiency or may be endorphin related. There are many symptoms. Where excitable the person should be given Valerian also Skull Cap, the latter being an aid to stress, fear and anxiety, which are some of the causes of Bulimia. There may also be an imbalance of hormones. Sometimes it can be traced to food allergy. Very often with the aid of proper natural additive free Diet, also the use of food supplements, Bulimia can be conquered. Some recover of their own accord even if they receive no treatment. What is suggested will speed the alleviation and a return to normal health. The natural Diet is the most important aid or medicine. I have found that Spirulina when taken or given on retiring to bed can be the answer to Bulimia. Also recommended is the taking of a Multivitamin tablet, Zinc or Brewer's Yeast. All are available from your health food store. *See DIET caption for some excellent advice, also Allergies caption.*

B

BUNION
To relieve pain take Mag Phos. Rings are available to place around the Bunion, helping to prevent further inflammation or swelling. Where skin is broken seek medical help. Applying Manuka Honey will help the healing process.

BURNS AND SCALDS
For minor Burns or Scalds use pure honey such as Manuka, which has marvellous healing properties. Always keep a jar in the medicine cabinet. Smear it over the Burn or Scald; there is no need to cover it. Take a Multivitamin tablet, Nat Mur tissue salts or Echinacea to aid the healing process.

BUTEYKO Breathing method for asthmatics
Professor Buteyko's radical method of treating asthma cannot be sufficiently praised. It teaches how 'asthma can be cured by learning how to breath properly'. From my experience of its use I firmly believe this statement to be true. I cannot understand why it is not widely publicised. Scientific trials show results that within three months there were:
70% less symptoms - coughing, breathlessness, wheezing;
90% less need for reliever medication;
49% less need for preventer medication;
(Results are based on scientific trials of Buteyko breathing at The Mater Hospital, Brisbane in 1995). *See Bibliography for details* of the book *'Close Your Mouth'* by Patrick McKeown which is a guide to the Buteyko method.

BURSITIS
Also referred to as housemaids knee or tennis elbow. Take Prickly Ash Bark, Calc Fluor or Wild Yam, Magnesium or Zinc. If there is no improvement it may be due to arthritis or rheumatism and should be treated as such.

BUTTER

When we visit the supermarket and view the shelves at the Butter section, there are also innumerable brands of so-called Butter substitutes, low fat greases, margarines and other similar-type spreads, many being well presented in Butter-shaped packaging. **If only the discerning purchasers would take time to read and study the ingredients label and then try to understand about some or all of them, much would be left on the shelves.** Only Butter is pure and natural. Use sparingly. There is little if anything injurious to our good health in pure Butter. This cannot be said about the so-called substitutes or spreads. Most of these are artificial, containing hydrogenated oils and fats, both animal and vegetable, being refined, processed, denatured, or adulterated. They contain an amount of water, up to 20 percent in some instances, salt, preservative, emulsifiers, flavourings, colouring also synthetic vitamins, with other additives to give them the creamy palatable texture.

The question can be asked "Why is margarine bought in such quantity?" The manufacturers at your expense and mine have the money to advertise. They are not worried about the health of the nation. They are only concerned about the bottom line – their turnover and resultant profit.

One of the results of huge promotion by the 'food' conglomerates is that purchasers are often brainwashed by the incessant advertising of spreads, which are supposedly low in fats. The ingredients are not mentioned. Too often we hear of the virtues of margarine being low fat. The manufacturers, also the purveyors, should be honest and tell the unwitting user about some of the ingredients. We should learn to read the ingredients labels. At least they print these on the packaging, knowing that the majority do not look at them. The discerning should leave these spreads on the shelves, buying pure natural Butter instead. Butter when used sparingly gives us little fat and remember we do need some in our intake of food. When used to excess certainly it provides us with an excess, as does margarine. Butter is pure and natural. Margarine is not. *See Margarine caption.*

BUZZING – (in ears)

See Tinnitus Caption.

EXERCISE IS TO THE BODY WHAT READING IS TO THE MIND
(APOLOGIES TO R. STEELE)

C VITAMIN

See Vitamins and Minerals Caption.

CAFFEINE

Over many years I have accumulated a bulging file on this regulated drug. Here is one subject where everything that is written about the addictive and harmful substance is discreditable. Not one good word health wise has been or can be said about it, except by the infamous 'soft drink' producers and the coffee sellers. It is a health hazard, retarding sleep, causing anxiety, irritability, leading to high blood pressure and other ailments, many of them serious. It is an addictive drug. Having had a Coke, have you ever wondered why very soon afterwards you crave another? There have been calls for the addition of caffeine to fizzy 'drinks' to be banned. The 'food' and 'drinks' industry is too powerful to allow this happen. My lone voice says: "Leave anything which contains caffeine on the shelf". Will my voice be heard above that of the mighty multi-Billion monied caffeine providers of coffee, fizzy 'drinks' and other items, which contain it? Again the health of the nation will suffer while they make their millions. Taking caffeinated or fizzy 'drinks', also alcohol, shows the disregard many have for the intricate system, which is the human body. When with illness the many referred to, who abuse their physique, have only themselves to blame. They do not realise this, all too often blaming the Health Service for their plight.

CALCIUM

See Vitamins and Minerals Caption.

CALC FLUOR, CALC PHOS, CALC SULPH

See Tissue Salts caption to learn about these excellent homeopathic remedies so easily obtained. When used singly or in combination they are invaluable as corrective treatment for many of our present-day ailments and illness.

CANCER

The word Cancer should strictly speaking be used to describe malignant tumours (tumours which can spread), as opposed to benign tumours (tumours which

A to Z Guide to Good Food and Natural Over the Counter Remedies • 69

cannot spread). Much is said or written about Cancers of which there are many types. We are reliably informed that between a third and a half of some Cancers are caused by improper or unnatural Diet. Here is irrefutable evidence, if this is needed, that there is something radically wrong with what we eat and drink, what is in our food chain. One of the chief causes of Cancer is smoking.

Good health is the birthright of every human being, but the modern way of life makes it almost impossible to reach and continue without self-discipline. We must, therefore, control our bad eating and drinking habits, also our lifestyle or mode of living. With Cancer all forms of therapy should be considered, then the person decides which route to take. Listen to all who offer advice, then be guided by what is best. In addition to conventional medicine the treatment of bladder, breast and colon Cancer has been helped by the use of Vitamins C and E. Vitamin C has also proved beneficial for other Cancers, as has Selenium and Co Enzyme Q10. The brown rice Diet for Cancer has received much praise. Put into a pan a cup of brown rice, mixed with a cup of water and place on gas mark 4 or 180C until all of the water has been absorbed, when it will be ready to eat. I have heard much about the excellent results obtained in the treatment of Cancer by the use of juiced carrots, grapes and pure honey. A woman told of how she treated herself over 10 years ago, maintaining the Diet saved her life. To help regain strength let pure food be your medicine and medicine be your food. The book *'Your Life in Your Hands', Understanding, Preventing and Overcoming Cancer* by Professor Jane Plant gives invaluable information on the subject. See Bibliography for details. Its title should be sufficient recommendation. It is written by a doctor, who is also a scientist, who had cancer, now free from it for several years.

In this book Doctor Plant highlights the value of natural food, as written about under DIET caption in this Guide.

CANDIDOSIS – (candidiasis)

This infection occurs where Candida Albicans, a yeast like micro organism, becomes rampant due to the overuse of antibiotics, impaired immune system, the pill or where the friendly bacteria is out of control. Often brought on by infection, stress or worry, with the main cause being nutritional deficiency due to inferior Diet. *Turn to DIET caption* for the main remedy, which is pure natural food. Take Acidophilus or Acidophilus powder. Health Food Store personnel will advise when you purchase the remedy. Avoid yeast and milk products until free from Candida. *Also see Thrush Vaginal and Thrush of Mouth captions.*

CARABUNCLES

See Boils Caption.

CARDIOMYOPATHY

It is not widely known that a voluntary support group under the aegis of Cardiomyopathy (UK) and the Irish Heart Foundation assists patients and their families. *Web pages are www.irishheart.ie and www.cardiomyopathy.org*

CAR/MOTION SICKNESS

See Travel Ailments Caption

CATARACTS

See Eyes Caption

CATARRH

Deep breathing exercises help to dispel and keep one clear of Catarrh. An excellent remedy is two or three teaspoons of Cider Vinegar with two teaspoons of pure Honey in some warm water, taken three times daily. Some prefer to take it between meals. Potters Catarrh Mixture, Plantago, Garlic oil capsules or Combination Q New Era, are also recommended.

CELERY SEEDS

They are a simple aid for cystitis, rheumatoid arthritis, gout, menopause and also high blood pressure. Crush or grind the seeds before infusing and make as tea, using two teaspoonfuls placed in a cup, on to which boiling water is poured. Stand for 5/10 minutes and drink. Celery seeds contain much goodness and can be obtained from the herbalist or Health Food store. Kordel's Celery 6000 plus tablets are an easy way of obtaining the goodness of Celery Seeds.

CELLULITE

This usually appears as dimpled, orange peel like skin, on thighs, legs and bottom. Inferior Diet and lifestyle are the main causes. Over 70% of women have it, whether slim or rotund. Natural pure food Diet is the chief remedy, as is the necessity for intake of fluids and the need to improve the circulation. *See DIET caption.* Regular exercise is equally important. The major creams advertised are a waste of money without exercise, intake of proper Diet and liquids. Take Lecithin granules also Vitamins C & B Complex.. The advice given, coupled with what is written about Diet, will help solve the problem. You will read of where it is necessary to drink eight or more glasses of water daily. This can work wonders for health, vitality, skin and the elimination of Cellulite. Few realise the necessity to drink copious amounts of pure water, which acts as both lubricant and medicine. *Turn to Water caption.*

Oatmeal also Breakfast Captions.

CHANGE OF LIFE
See Menopause Caption.

CHAPPED HANDS
See Hands Captions.

CHAPPED LIPS
See Lips Caption

CHESTINESS
See Respiratory Health Caption

CHICKEN POX
Take plenty of fluids. Keep cool to avoid itching. Take Rhus Tox when with infection. Calendula cream or Allergenic Non Steroidal cream helps to heal. Manuka honey spread on the spots is a natural healer, with marks seldom left.

CHILBLAINS
Often due to a calcium deficiency. Tissue salts almost always solve the problem. Calc Phos is principal remedy or Combination G New Era. If broken use Kali Sulph. If cracked use Calc Fluor.

CHILD AILMENTS
- Bad Tempered - Kali Phos
- Screaming in sleep - Kali Phos or Nat Phos
- Teething - Camomile or Combination R New Era
- Hyperactive - *See ADHD caption.*

See under various children's ailment captions for other remedies.

CHILDREN AND TEENAGER'S HEALTH
Much can be written on the subject of children's health. How much of it will be observed or put into practise is something to be hoped for. *Everything written in this Guide is from experience and also from the heart, being put down as has been observed in everyday life. The advice given is built around that experience. Medical advice is not being replaced. What is suggested is complementary. If you or your children are worried about ailment or particular health problem, it is*

recommended that you see a doctor.

Remedies for Children and Teenager's ailments or illness are to be found under the many captions listed in this Encyclopedia. If in any doubt as to their suitability or remedial goodness, speak with and be guided by the Health Food Store personnel who should be familiar with all of the natural remedies recommended.

C

The pressures, peer pressure, influences, almost coercion, being put on some of our young people today is, to my mind, asking too much at times. With the focus on higher education, much is expected from students, who in some instances are being pushed beyond the limit. Some parents fail to realise that their sons and daughters are perhaps not academic material, not being that way minded. Thought should be given to them putting their hands instead of their heads to use, maybe taking up a trade or other way of living. Some of our finest businessmen did not even finish college. The exam papers being set by third level academics are extreme. Again the question can be asked: 'Is there a need for this in order to make a living? Is there a need for all this pressure to attain results?' When I was a boy there were happy times, despite strict discipline and little money. There were no pressures as we have now. This included what I ate. Whatever was put on the table had to be accepted whether I liked it or not. There was no: 'I don't like this, I don't like that'.

It has served me well. We heard little about children's ailments such as depression, learning difficulties, mood swings, obesity, ADHD, asthma, digestive disorders including Crohn's or Coeliac disease and many more of the huge health problems with which our youth are plagued today. The only vaccination given was for smallpox, diphtheria or polio. We heard nothing and knew little; neither did our parents, about vitamins and minerals, synthetic medicines or the modern-day 'foods', over-processed, additive-laden, and all so attractive to the eye and the palate. We ate plain natural, healthy food and drank pure water. We consumed little alcohol or fizzy 'drinks', chocolate, sweets, confectionery or other sugarised products. Orange or lemonade we shared from the bottle with our friends. From a bar of chocolate we got one or perhaps two squares, just as we were given one or two sweets from the bag. *Today eating one or two bars of chocolate or the full bag of sweets is the norm. There is a need to re-emphasise the dangers of excess sugar, sweeteners or fatty foods such as chips and crisps. We are what we eat, drink and exercise. This includes those of all ages. See SUGAR caption.*

There is much wrong with the state of children's health. The retort might be: "We are more aware of children's health". We are not. What I have just written is all too true. We have a problem, one of our own making, because we accept what the moguls in the food and drug industries present us with. We do not fight back and refuse to accept their fare. All too few parents are unaware of the goodness, the nutrition of pure, wholesome, natural unadulterated food. **The ingredients labels are seldom if ever read. These show what is in the 'food' which children eat. Much of it is factory-made, of little nutritional value and does not deserve to be called food. Here is one of the main reasons for ill health amongst young and those not so young. Lack of exercise must also be included, also the need for sufficient and proper sleep pattern. Many know little if anything about natural or alternative remedies, which are available for children.**

Too much reliance is placed on synthetic medication. 'If the kids are ill the doctor will cure them' is often the attitude. The pills for all ills idea, prevails. It is a fact that more children are having learning problems, with behavioural attitudes very prevalent. Alcohol abuse is up and on the increase, with even seven year olds drinking. Synthetic pills, potions and so-called medicines, some of them dangerous, are prescribed willy nilly, with the long-term consequences in most cases unknown. Could these be the cause of so much of our present-day malady or disease, especially amongst our children and young people? Our immune systems are being damaged or destroyed without thought given to the consequences. *Parents buy chemical remedies off-the-shelf in their local store, often being administered with no thought given to long-term harm created. The majority of these synthetic so-called remedies are not even cures, being just temporary stoppers of the problem. How many are aware that children must not take aspirin or aspirin-based medicines, of which there are many? They can be dangerous. I do not have to defend myself when I promote these theories. Questions can be asked such as: "Why are so many children frequently stressed, being prescribed habit forming amphetamines"; "Why so much autism, which has more than tripled in the past 15 years"; "Why so many children with ADHD".*

Do you know what ADHD stands for? For those who do not, please read the caption under ADHD. It stands for Attention Deficit Hypersensitivity Disorder. Still further questions to be asked. "Why such a big word or description"? Because it covers a multitude of problems all associated with ADHD. Included are: inability to concentrate, mood swings, fatigue, depression, digestive problems, dyslexia, emotional troubles, hyperactivity and much more. Dozens of other questions could be added about our *Children and Teenager's Health.* Many simple answers are to be found under the various headings in this guide. *Here is one time where the children cannot be blamed, with the foundation for some of the problems for later life being laid down before the child is born. Pre-natal influence is one of these problems, as the mother-to-be listens to much modern jargon and meddle poured out by the many professional, semi-professional and other do-gooders who give the impression of knowing it all. Breastfeeding went out of the equation, very often on the advice of these people.* Now it is being advised as they realise they were wrong.

Until recently much of the prepared, one might say fast 'food', baby 'foods' were in tins. Despite being told for many years that this was not right they eventually relented and changed to jars and plastic containers, when it was proved to them that much of the little good in the product was being destroyed, especially Vitamin B1 so necessary for nerve function. Processed 'foods' for the young are of little or no use, sustenance- wise. They are of less value to infants, many of them being unnatural. *See Baby Foods caption.* Provided the food the mother is eating is pure and natural, then nothing better can be found for a baby when weaned. Simply mince or liquidise. Do not add sugar or salt. You know then that it is nutritious.

A survey carried out by the Consumer's Association magazine **'Which'** found that 40% of 420 baby food products tested contained sugar, sweetened fruit juice or both and 60% of all breakfast products had sugar added, despite Government advice that baby foods should contain little or no sugar.

Children of all ages are notorious for ignoring any good natural food, including vegetables, salads, even meat, put before them. They think they can exist on cakes, sweets, crisps, sugary 'foods' or fizzy 'drinks'. They are not aware of the unhealthy consequences. If they are not disciplined in this respect it can lead to all sorts of health problems, physically and mentally. The health and future well-being of the child is the responsibility of the parent or guardian. Children have to learn about the taste of good food from the mother or guardian. They will be guided and governed by the eating habits, the example set. A major fault in today's upbringing of children is that parents allow themselves to be dictated to, especially when food is the issue. Vegetables are a prime example of refusal to eat, with much time spent trying to convince young people of their goodness and the necessity to eat them. Kids who don't like vegetables will usually eat one - pot cooked dishes, such as casseroles or stews. The vegetables can even be liquidised to put in with the meat. Meals such as casseroles or stews are full of nutrition.

Most of the children and teenagers minor ailments or illnesses, as set out under the various captions in this Guide, can be treated by the use of certain alternative, homeopathic or herbal remedies. Ask your local health food store assistant, homeopathic doctor or trained herbalist for advice. You will be surprised how helpful they can be. Read the labels or instructions carefully. Tell your doctor what you are doing or intend to do. Unless with serious illness many of the natural remedies can be taken in conjunction with those prescribed by your GP. Think natural whether for food or remedy. **The emphasis throughout this Guide is on Diet, Exercise and Sleep. Turn to and read these captions because they are of vital importance to the health and vitality of all, especially children and teenagers.**

Our young people in some instances take up sport or other form of exercise. All too many do not, some having become lazy, being described as couch potatoes. In the past we walked and ran much, including to school. We had chores and work set out for us. Pocket money had to be earned, as jobs were provided or set out. With the advent of the motorcar, also the modern conveniences at hand, the chores of bygone days are no more. Television is now one of our greatest health hazards. In many homes it is never switched off. *The necessity for exercise, also sufficient and proper sleep pattern cannot be underlined or highlighted sufficiently.* Just as the parents or guardians of our youth must teach and educate about pure natural additive and sugar- free foods and drinks, so also must be dictated, arranged and organised the need to participate in sport, exercise, training or work-out. There is an amount of discipline required but it can be as fun, also being highly beneficial and healthy.

CHIPS AND CRISPS

Potatoes are an excellent source of pure food when boiled in jackets, mashed or baked. They are fat-free, being a source of Vitamin C also containing other edible nutritives. Like much health advice given which was not correct, we were told of the dangers of potatoes with regard to overweight problems. We are now informed that this advice was wrong. The only potatoes to be avoided are Chips, Crisps or roast potatoes, which are usually saturated with oils, being a danger to good health. Pure oils are best, but we are advised not to use pure virgin cold pressed oils for deep fat frying. Almost all Chips commercially sold, are cooked in cheap oils, much of it used and reused, leading to hydrogenation or inferior oil. The processors will resort to unacceptable methods of reducing the quality and, therefore, the price. The writer has evidence and experience of this. Crisps are equally as harmful as the Chips referred to. Like the fast foods as written about by Eric Schlosser in his hard-hitting best seller **'Fast Food Nation',** they are best left on the shelf. They are certainly of little, if any nutritional benefit, usually containing exorbitant amounts of salt, with a big question mark over some of the other ingredients. Up to 30% of fats are in most Crisps, all processed, having been overheated. Crisps are only a harmful filler with no food content. Avoid them even when hungry. *See the two captions Cooking Oils also Cooking Oils, How They Are Produced.*

CHIROPRACTIC

This is a form of manipulation where the Chiropractor diagnoses and treats bones, joints, muscles including the spine, thereby helping to bring relief, improving the health of the various organs and the nervous system. It is one of the largest branches of alternative therapies practised, being hugely successful. The British Medical Journal, not tending to praise anything alternative, reports that a study found that patients who received Chiropractic treatment for lower back pain improved 70% more than those on hospital treatment.

CHLORINE

Drinking water is now treated in many areas by disinfecting with the toxic and foul smelling Chlorine. This is one of the basic materials of the chemical industry. The E.U. has issued a warning about its use, stating that it is cancer linked. The dangers to health are ignored, the warning falling on seemingly deaf ears of those who supposedly govern. *Turn to Water also Fluoride captions.*

CHOLESTEROL

To control to safe levels be guided by *High Blood Pressure caption* in this Guide. Managing Cholesterol, blood pressure and circulation, with resultant general feeling of well-being, can be attained by disciplining oneself with regard to proper Diet and lifestyle. Diet is number one. If you are a smoker and cannot or will not give up, then advice, other than to give up, will not solve your problem. *Exercise is very important. Before taking it up, if you have been inactive or with serious health problem, speak with your doctor. Reading the Diet and Exercise captions* has helped many with high Cholesterol and blood pressure also with varicose veins and other circulatory problems, allied to cardiovascular disease, which have been normalised, with the patient returning to extraordinary better health. *Even those with serious heart problems have benefited enormously by the advice given under Blood Pressure - high, Exercise, Heart and DIET captions.*

CHRONIC FATIGUE SYNDROME

Also known as ME which means Myalgic Encephalomyelitis. Fatigue can be caused by many ailments or conditions, especially if with autoimmune problems. With M.E., which is extreme fatigue and which has become increasingly common, there is no apparent cause to be found. It often comes on after influenza, occurring mostly in women, especially young academics or students. It is linked to the behaviour of the immune system, which can go awry unless kept in a healthy state. *Much success has come through the use of the HAY DIET, which is described under separate caption, and fully in the books as listed in Bibliography.* Supplement with a good Multivitamin, Echinacea, Garlic capsules also Udo's choice oil and Spirulina. I have seen sufferers recover 90% in a few weeks, with return to good health within 4/6 months, where Hay Diet was followed diligently. It is difficult, with some not having either the energy or inclination to follow through the instructions devotedly. Those who have returned to good health agree that the discipline to follow the guidance was certainly worth it. Recently I had telephone calls from two mothers to thank me for recommending the Hay Diet. One said it was the answer to her prayers.

CIDER VINEGAR AND HONEY

Here is one of nature's greatest aids to better health, to relieve niggling and what could be regarded as minor ailments, which to the sick or suffering are major. Try telling of its curative properties to all in the medical line of business, including the doctors and pharmacists, and they will probably laugh at you. Recently I saw Aspell's Cider Vinegar on the shelf in a chemist's shop. People ask for it or it would not be stocked. Much has been written and said about the goodness of Cider Vinegar, but this seems only to reach those who are interested in natural health, also natural remedies. It is used by many in the treatment of animals. ***Throughout this Guide Cider Vinegar is mentioned many times and the following are some of the illnesses or ailments for which it has been found beneficial: arthritis, asthma, digestive disturbances, flu, colds, catarrh, sore throat, general health and well-being, hay fever, heart including blood pressure, laryngitis, to restore the voice quickly, rheumatism and slimming. It is best obtained from the health food store as pure Cider Vinegar made by Aspells, Martletts, Whiteways or Applefords. The usual way to take Cider Vinegar is by mixing two teaspoons in warm water, adding two teaspoons of natural Honey as sold by the bee keeper or the health food shop.*** Some find it difficult or impossible to take. If so try taking one teaspoon of Cider Vinegar to two teaspoons of Honey, increasing to two teaspoons of Cider Vinegar later. Others, especially children, have no difficulty. Some of the brands of Cider Vinegar mentioned are easier to take than others. Find the one most suitable. It can also be bought as a prepared mixture. The health food store or book shop stock or can obtain books on the subject of Cider Vinegar and Honey. *See Bibliography for further information*

CINNAMON GROUND

To help regulate blood sugar, take half teaspoon of Ground Cinnamon twice daily. Place on breakfast cereal, such as porridge or take in liquid form by mixing with milk or tepid water.

CIRCULATION – (Poor)

Treat as High Blood Pressure Caption

CLAUDICATION

Treat as High Blood Pressure Caption.

CLAUSTROPHOBIA

Treat as Anxiety and Agoraphobia Captions.

COD LIVER OIL

Udo's Choice Oil or other properly proportioned Omega oils, of which there are some, have made inroads into the sales of Cod Liver Oil. The latter is an age-old remedy, still excellent as fish oil. The taking of Cod Liver Oil has proved to be highly beneficial for nails, hair and skin health. It is an aid to the heart, veins and arteries, helps prevent night blindness, being a good dietary aid. For those who find it difficult to digest try taking it when retiring to bed or if this is difficult put in a screw top jar with pure orange juice. Shake well and drink. Manuka Honey when mixed with Cod Liver Oil and smeared over psoriasis of skin has ended the problem for some sufferers. After the descaling it must be continued for some time to eliminate the redness. Cod Liver Oil contains Omega 3 only. This is necessary in a proper balance with Omega 6. Udo's Choice Oil has the correct proportion of Omega 3, 6 and Fatty Acid Oils, being an invaluable aid to better health. *See Udo's Choice Oil caption.*

COELIAC DISEASE

This is an inability to digest gluten, which is a protein found in wheat, oats, rye and barley. It must be managed carefully through the Diet and once organised, knowing what to avoid, it becomes quite easy as a natural way of living, in more respects than one. One of the chief reasons for occurrence is too early introduction of solids, such as cereals, to a baby's Diet. Early weaning, which is all too common, can lead to this. Visit an Allergist, it may entail a biopsy, or you can as with an allergy, omit all foods, which contain gluten or dairy products, then gradually reintroduce to your Diet one item at a time. Wheat intolerance is the most common. There are many gluten free flours, breakfast cereals and breads available, also other gluten free foods. Oats is the least likely to be problematic. If in good health, which comes through partaking of pure natural food Diet, the digestive tract should begin healing once the gluten is removed from the Diet. One must be vigilant as gluten is in hundreds of foods like packet soups, gravy, pastas and also much of the over-processed 'foods' we are offered. Think and eat natural. There are many natural aids to recovery, all gluten free. Include in the Diet natural additive-free yoghurt, bananas and other fruit and vegetables, especially broccoli. Raw carrot juice is excellent. Aids to proper Diet are Vitamins A and B Complex, also Calcium and Magnesium. Visit your health food shop and be surprised by both the knowledge which they offer and the range of gluten free foods available. Also recommended is the book '**Eat With Joy on Gluten Free Diet**' as listed in the bibliography. This has been a wonderful help to many with Coeliac disease and stomach problems. *See Allergy also DIET captions.* Natural Foods are Pure Foods.

COFFEE

The growers of Coffee are being disgracefully exploited, with families being forced out of their only chance of a livelihood in some Third World countries. It is a fact that Coffee prices paid to the producer are at an all-time low, at the same time prices have risen exorbitantly on the Coffee markets of the Western world, with the usual propaganda about crop failures. At one end of the world people purchase the beverage-making Coffee beans in various forms, especially granules, not realising that the producers are being screwed beyond acceptable limits by the giant, powerful, money-orientated purveyors. Many of the Coffee farmers are on the breadline, impoverished, while we again contribute handsomely to the outlandish profits of the 'food' and 'drinks' industry. Only those who promote or have vested interests can say anything good about Coffee. Like caffeine, there is nothing commendable to be said or written about it, as the masses continue to drink the highly caffeinated Coffee or fizzy 'drinks', very often to excess, when it becomes drug-like. The drinker becomes dependant upon it without realising that it can be a health hazard, leading to headaches, constricting of blood vessels, reducing absorption of minerals, especially Iron, also causing imbalance of Calcium. It is a stimulant, therefore best avoided. *See Caffeine caption.*

COLD – (Common)

Over the years I have accumulated bulging files on sniffles, sneezing and runny noses. They mean nothing, because prevention is the all-important remedy. My close relative, a doctor, from whom was learned so much about natural Diet and living, once told me: "I treat many for colds and they usually last 7/10 days. If I don't treat them they last 7/10 days". It is enough to make all realise that the many chemicals and drugs advertised and prescribed for colds are a waste of money, with some probably doing harm in the long-term, especially to the immune system. When with cold it should not be suppressed, because it is 'caught', as we say when our inner system has been neglected, defensively. Have you ever noticed how much better the feeling is some 7-10 days after the cold has cleared, when the virus has been eliminated from the system, if in reasonable health beforehand? Those enjoying reasonably good health, especially when partaking of natural Diet of pure additive-free foods, aided by a tonic or food supplement, are much less likely to suffer from colds. Tonics such as Floradix, Floravital, Biostrath, Salusan or a good Multivitamin tablet are a safeguard, just as they will help to build the system after a cold. Echinaceaforce is one of the best natural cold preventions or remedies known. October onwards demands good food, warm clothing, also a tonic or Echinaceaforce. The modern processed additive-filled Diet is the cause of much of the niggling illness and ailment we are plagued with as our bodies and immune system receive little benefit from this kind of 'food'. Good food is as medicine, helping to prevent colds and flu. *See Body Warmth and DIET captions.*

COLD SORES

See Lips Caption

COLITIS

Probably the most common of all bowel complaints, being extremely difficult to diagnose, as there are many common conditions which produce similar symptoms. Those with lactose intolerance (dairy product allergy) are often incorrectly diagnosed as having colitis. Invariably brought on by bland, detrimental, shall one say useless Diet, also by worry, anxiety, severe stress or more especially where antibiotics have been used, all too often overused or prescribed. Avoid smoking and alcohol. Pure natural unadulterated Diet of good food is the important remedy. Aids for the problem are fruit and raw vegetable juices or purees, eggs, fish, liver, liquidised soups, steamed foods, including garlic and celery. Avoid coffee, fibre, hot or cold drinks, as medium warmth for food and drink is best. If allergic to dairy products, including cows milk, they must be omitted. Porridge, which is a smooth fibre, is acceptable. Some patients have also been able to take a tablespoon of bran and similar amount of wheat germ. Food supplements, as an aid to rebuilding the system or preventing complications, are Vitamins C & A, also Zinc and an Amino Acid Complex tablet. Manuka honey, also Acidophilus have proved highly beneficial.

COLITIS – (Ulcerative)

Diet must be gluten free and should for 7-10 days consist of fluids and liquidised food, with nothing solid. Take nutritious soups, liquidised fruits, carrot juice and slippery elm. Slowly get on to more varied natural foods, including steamed fish and vegetables, plain natural yoghurt, low-fat cheese and mashed potato. Supplement with Manuka Honey, Wild Yam, Tormentil long term, Vitamin A up to 10,000iu daily, Vitamin B Complex, plus extra Vitamins B 12, and C. Tormentil taken long-term is both a remedy and a preventative.

CONFECTIONERY

In the past Confectionery was regarded as cake, often referred to by past generations as sweet cake. A second slice or helping would be discouraged or perhaps refused. Today many hundreds of items could be labelled Confectionery because of the high concentration or prevalence of sugar or other sweeteners. They are almost all highly processed, containing dubious food additives, being unnatural. From a health aspect there is nothing good to write about Confectionery. It should be avoided as far as possible. Much confectionery is, like many breakfast cereals, ice cream and sweets, laced with sugars, artificial sweetners, including aspartame, additives, hydrogenated fats and salt. I would not allow my dog to eat some of them. There are so many things, which can be classified as Confectionery that real discipline is needed to avoid them. *See Sugar caption.*

CONJUNCTIVITIS

See Eyes Caption.

CONSTIPATION

Much is suffered, written and said about this often, serious problem. There are many reasons why one can be Constipated. No two people are affected in the same manner. What brings relief to one is often of no help to another. It is often due to lack of exercise, overuse of laxatives, bad Diet, stress, or there may be underlying conditions. As a natural remedy unprocessed wheat bran taken as four or five dessertspoons every four or five days on porridge at breakfast time has proved a very good aid. Other natural laxatives are one teaspoon or more of Flaxseed or Psyillium Husks. Udo's Choice Oil or Black Strap Molasses are other remedies as is Bioforce Bowel Essence. Exercise and proper natural DIET go side-by-side to help eradicate the problem. Increase the intake of fluids. Drink up to eight glasses of water daily. It is a great body lubricant, being as medicine to the system. Everything mentioned is natural, being available in the health food store or from pure water supply. It is not advisable to use the so easily obtained chemical laxatives on a long-term basis. They can do irreversible damage. Think natural. *Some worry unduly about Constipation. The fact that one does not defecate daily does not mean there is a problem. I have yet to see or use anything better than four or five dessertspoons of bran every four or five days or when necessary, which may even be every two or three weeks.*

CONTRACEPTIVE PILL

The use of the hormone oestrogen, progesterone, synthetic Pill leads to a drain from the body of essential vitamins and minerals. To counter this it is very important to keep to a purely natural nutritious Diet. *See DIET caption* and be guided about where it may be necessary to take certain supplements. The use of the pill leads to Zinc deficiency. Ensure that the intake is brought up to the R.D.A., which is obtained in a 15mg Zinc/Copper combination tablet such as Quest brand. Visit the health food shop and be advised. Because of its steroidal content the Contraceptive Pill can interfere with the bowel, making it extremely difficult to diagnose what the stomach problem is. Similarly where there is an allergy it can be triggered off to the extent that it is almost impossible to treat. Alcohol should not be taken if on medication and this includes the Contraceptive Pill. The short or long-term consequences are unknown.

CONTRAINDICATIONS

See introductory pages of the Guide, under Contraindications heading, to learn about the inadvisability of mixing or using certain vitamins, minerals and chemical medicines.

COOKING

Cookery lessons in early life are an excellent recipe for a healthy lifestyle. Getting children to eat well begins in the kitchen. They will appreciate good nutritious additive-free food when they see pure ingredients being prepared and cooked. Cooking food is not time consuming as is generally thought. Purchase a simple cookery book. Once organised and started it is a good hobby. I can vouch for this. *See Diet caption and get started.* You will never regret taking up cooking which, with the pure ingredients so easily obtained is another step to better health. It can be fun, especially if done with others or family members. Allow the young to experiment and then enjoy what has been cooked or made up. Think natural and use natural ingredients.

COOKING OILS

There are certain oils which are health-giving, being aids to well-being. Included are fish and omega Oils. Cooking Oils are in an entirely different category, with all-too-much being anything but healthy. Many of these oils, obtainable off-the-shelf from the supermarket or food store, are over-refined, having been heated in the processing. They are not easily ingested into the system. Don't mind the label, which like many food descriptions, almost brainwashes the customer, so finding another, which does not understand the health implications. Many fried oils are a danger to our health, therefore what has been fried contains an amount of bad oil and is also to be avoided. Commercial users, who are cost conscious, invariably purchase the cheapest cooking or frying oils. This is injurious to health, as also is the constant overuse of the oils, which are often strained, added to and reused. Pure virgin Oils, which are unrefined and unprocessed, are the only pure cooking Oils which can be recommended. In the countries where Olive Oil is easily available and looked upon as being the best Oil to use, the incidence of heart disease is relatively low. Be Oil wise. *Think natural,* Pure Virgin Olive Oil is best. Always store the Oil in an airtight container in a cool dark place. Exposure to light and air can destroy the Vitamin E and other antioxidants within. Cold Pressed Virgin Olive Oil must not be used for deep fat frying. *See Cooking Oils, How They Are Produced caption, which includes a chart setting out how they are processed. Study the difference in the make-up of refined and unrefined oils. One does not have to look further to realise that processed oils are inferior.* The health food store can supply pure virgin unprocessed Oils such as Safflower Oil, Sunflower, Linseed and others, including cold pressed Olive Oils.

COOKING OILS. HOW THEY ARE PRODUCED

The accompanying chart sets out how the many Oils we see on supermarket and food store shelves are produced. Study the production methods to note the processing, bleaching, deodorizing, injection methods, degumming, pressing, heating, crushing and much else that goes into making Cooking Oils which are anything but natural. The lard and dripping used in bygone days for cooking purposes and which many have decried, was natural. Note the small amount of work necessary to produce pure Oils as shown in that section.

HOW COOKING OILS ARE PRODUCED

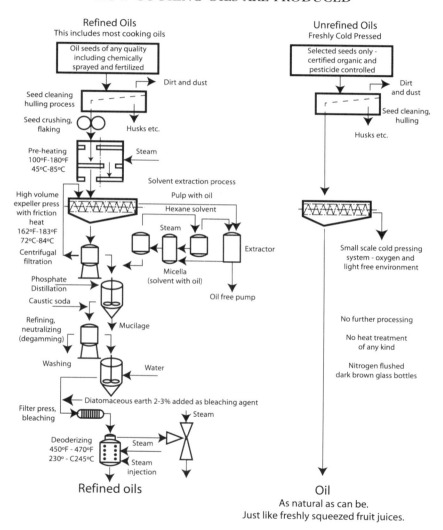

CORONARY HEART DISEASE

See Heart Captions.

COSMETICS

Skin care is a multi-Billion-money industry. It has been shown that as much as 20% of chemicals used in their manufacture and make-up are known to be harmful. This is certainly not helpful to those with sensitive or other skin problems. This guide is about natural health including the skin. Like food additives being dangerous, so also are many cosmetic additives. There are very good natural cosmetics and skin care aids such as Allergenics, Aveda, Anika, Jason, Tisserand, Dead Sea Magik and others. Long-term use of Silica, Cod Liver Oil, Udo's Choice Oil or Perfectil can provide radiant beauty to skin, hair and nails. They are purely natural and highly recommended. Everything mentioned is available from your health food store, some chemists or health & beauty outlets. *See Skin Care caption.*

COUGHS

Much is written about this subject. There are many and varied kinds of coughs from the delicate, or often affective habitual dry cough, to the very serious type. They are caused by irritation to the mucous membranes of the respiratory tract or airways. It becomes extremely troublesome when uncontrollable, when the tickling-like sensation cannot be stopped, being like a relief valve, necessary to bodily function. It should not be repressed as too often happens with chemical medicinal drugs. There are many natural remedies which can be used to gain relief. Potters Vegetable Cough Remover is to me the elixir of cough removers. All natural medicinal liquids should be well shaken before taking the recommended amount. Being natural they do not have a suspension agent or preservatives. There are other natural treatments such as Manuka Honey mixed with Blackstrap Molasses in warm water, Echinacea, Angelica, Thyme or Horehound.

- **Ferr Phos or Slippery Elm are soothers for dry coughs.**
- **Kali Mur for stubborn white phlegm.**

Coughs usually come with or after colds. A tonic is often needed to restore to better health. *See Tonic caption.*

CRACKED HANDS

See Hands Caption.

CRACKED LIPS

See Lips Caption.

CRACKS AT CORNER OF MOUTH

See Mouth Caption.

CRAMP ABDOMINAL

See Stomach Caption.

CRAMP IN LEGS

See Legs Caption.

CRANBERRY JUICE

Pure Cranberry Juice is an excellent remedy where there is urinary infection. As a remedy for minor kidney infections it is very good. I have seen Cystitis banished when pure Juice or Cranberries have been taken. Most Juices are made up from concentrated Juice, having been diluted, often with additives. Pure natural Cranberry Juice is available from the health food store. Cranberries liquidised, mixed with natural yoghurt and pure honey can be used as an after lunch or dinner sweet. *See Kidney caption.*

CRATAEGUS

See Hawthorn Caption.

'CREAM'

This is now available complete with 'food' additives mixed in, all propelled from an aerosol type container. The chemical propellant, which is also in the so-called 'cream', dispenses the stuff on to the food offered. I was in a hotel kitchen recently, doing some research about 'food' and the use of microwaves. I witnessed the shooting out of this extremely white 'cream' as it was put on plates for four ladies who had ordered afternoon tea. On each plate there was a heated scone, done in the microwave, with a little square plastic container of additive-filled jam. Reading the large lettering on the container gave one the impression that it was pure cream. Reading the ingredients label told an entirely different story. The mind boggles at the thought of using this mixture, which is sold as 'cream'. It is not surprising that many are sick.

CROHN'S DISEASE

This is a distressing exasperating bowel and digestive problem. It can be extremely painful, with diarrhoea, tired and lethargic feeling, which leads to significant loss of weight. Often incorrectly diagnosed as Irritable Bowel Syndrome or other bowel disorder. Recently it has been discovered that it occurs because of abnormal or transformed genes. This may explain why there are so many varying symptoms, why it is almost always hereditary, being so difficult to identify. It is associated with weak immune system. Proper Diet is necessary. Avoid roughage, using porridge and Slippery Elm to replace it. Drink copious amounts of pure chemical-free water, up to eight or 10 glasses daily. Carragheen Moss (Irish Moss) also Slippery Elm, made as gruel, are good aids to the stomach and bowels. Avoid cabbage, broccoli, brussels sprouts, bananas, cows milk, onions and swede. Eat only pure natural additive-free foods. A gluten and or dairy-free Diet has been beneficial for many with Crohn's Disease.

Food supplements, which have helped to restore health to the immune system also to banish the diarrhoea and pain, are Tormentil and Calamus aided by Vitamin B12, Udo's Choice Oil and a natural Multivitamin tablet. As stated, proper natural Diet, excluding the foods mentioned, is extremely important. *See DIET caption.*

CUTS

Minor cuts can be treated after washing and drying by applying:

- **Honey, pure and natural, such as the excellent Manuka type, which will help draw out any foreign bodies.**
- **Tea Tree Oil diluted or Allergenic ointment, both of which assist to halt infection.**
- **Powdered Ferr Phos which will help dry cuts quickly, as well as being a healer. Leaving cuts, particularly if they are minor, uncovered, usually leads to quicker healing.**

CYSTITIS

This is a bacterial infection of the bladder, with women much more prone than men. Hormonal changes are often responsible. Caffeine, sugar and additives as in fizzy 'drinks' and foods are enemies of the urine tract. Deodorants, soaps, tampons, washing powders and other modern so-called hygienic aids are often the cause of the problem. The best remedies, which I have prescribed, are D-mannose or pure (not made from concentrate) Cranberry Juice and Dolomite. Take tablets of the latter several times daily. Other remedies which have helped banish the Cystitis are Echinacea, which both boosts immunity and clears infection also the homeopathic remedy Cantharis or Kordel's Celery Seed 6,000 plus. All suggested are natural, therefore with no side effects. Where Cystitis is more serious, perhaps with bleeding, it is imperative to seek medical aid.

THERE PROBABLY HAS NEVER BEEN A PERIOD, IN THE HISTORY OF MANKIND WHEN THE VALUE OF PURE FOODS AND ADDITIVE - FREE NUTRITIONAL DIET WAS MORE ESSENTIAL THAN NOW.

D VITAMIN

See Vitamins and Minerals Caption.

DAIRY FREE DIET

Some opt for this kind of Diet, for others it is a necessity. Allergy to milk can cause diarrhoea, bloating, stomach pains, lethargy, headaches and other ailments. It can be traced by allergy test or simply by omitting all milk and other dairy products, including butter, yoghurt, cream, cheese and even margarine. These can be in other food products including dried foods, such as packet sauces, soups, confectionery etc. of which there is now a vast range. Leave out of Diet for seven to 10 days, replacing them one by one to find the culprits. Goat's milk can often be used safely. Dairy free alternatives are soya and rice milk, also milk free cheese and pure yoghurt. Visit your health food store and see their range of alternatives, plus other aids, when on Dairy Free Diet. Number one is a need for Calcium/Magnesium/Vitamin D combined supplement, to ensure proper intake of calcium, to help ward off brittle bone disease/osteoporosis. *See DIET also Allergies captions* and be guided by the advice given.

DVT

See Deep Vein Thrombosis Caption.

DAIRY PRODUCTS

As food sustenance, all dairy products, especially milk, are excellent when used in moderation in a proper balanced Diet of nutritious food. Hard cheeses are best avoided. A small number are allergic to dairy products and must, therefore, take steps to eliminate the cause. Being allergic to dairy products and being intolerant to lactose or milk sugar can be two different things. Many have lactose intolerance, being with little of the enzyme lactate and don't know, often being diagnosed with colitis or other bowel problem. *See Lactose Intolerance caption.*
Milk is a complete food for the young at start of life and helps lay the foundation for later health. It contains the very necessary vitamins, minerals, calcium, protein, carbohydrates, fat and much more. Low fat or

non- fat types of milk, natural yoghurt and soft cheeses have the same nutrients as full or half fat varieties. Many perceive milk as fattening, often cutting down, as they try to lose weight. They are wrong, because as well as being highly ineffective, they are losing out on the important calcium needed for strong bones and prevention of osteoporosis, also missing out on fibre and other valuable aids to good health. The only worrying thing which often occurs to me is that milk when purchased is very often in a polythene container, also that the sell-by-date can be up to 10 days hence, not being like the fresh milk purchased in a glass bottle in days past. We are now offered super milk, which contains synthetic, factory-made vitamins and minerals. The latest fad, where additives now appear in milk, is that of flavours. Another instance of processed drinks, which should be pure and natural, but are not. Is this because so much of what we are offered as 'food' is 'foodless'? *The health experts, who push Fluoride on us, against the wills of the majority, are now in cahoots with the chemical industry as they put forward the idea of fluoridated milk. What a disaster this would be! Milk is either pure milk or it is not milk.* Why mess around with one of the few products still offered as pure sustenance? Leave milk-additive free. Butter is pure and healthy when used sparingly, containing no additives as in processed unnatural margarine. *See Butter caption.*

DANDRUFF

See Hair Caption.

DEAFNESS

A certain amount can be done to help eliminate some of the impediment. I have seen those who did nothing for years, then seeking advice, finding that the hearing could be vastly improved. There are various types of Deafness such as:

- Conductive, which may be due to inner or outer ear infection, earwax or perhaps after a cold or as glue ear.
- Perceptive Deafness, which can come from noisy workplace, overloud music in confined spaces, side effects of antibiotics or from Meniere's disease.
- Presbyacusias Deafness, which occurs with age.
  See a specialist and like many who have been prevailed upon to do so you may be surprised at the outcome. Ayurveda treatment by qualified practitioner has often resulted in better hearing, giving extremely good results. If with a hearing aid keep it in proper working order by regularly renewing batteries and servicing. An inefficient aid can make the Deafness very much worse, then often leading to stress, depression or other nerve and health problems. *Turn to Ears, Hearing also Ayurveda therapy captions.*

DEBILITY

See Rundown Caption.

DEEP VEIN THROMBOSIS (DVT)

This occurs where there is impaired circulation with sluggish blood flow. If the legs are swollen and sensitive seek medical attention, because the problem can become very serious. It is now heard of frequently, often occurring when flying at altitude or soon afterwards. It is not only flying which puts one at risk, it is also common after operations or if injured. Pregnant women are more at risk, also those who take birth control pill. Sitting in a confined position for journeys of over two hours duration can bring on the problem. To help prevent DVT if travelling by car, make frequent stops and take exercise. If travelling by plane, train or coach drink lots of water, move about, and walk in the aisle, moving the legs, ankles, arms, hands and fingers, also flexing the toes and feet by way of exercise to assist blood circulation. The juice of a lemon mixed with water, taken every two hours, helps enormously. Avoid tea, coffee and alcohol. Try not to sleep in the all-to-often-cramped space. Do not cross the legs. Vitamins A, C and E are an aid to better circulation and avoidance of DVT, if taken for some days previous to and on day of travel. *Where relevant, turn to Travel and Holiday Health caption.*

DEMENTIA

There are two types, Degenerating Dementia (Alzheimer's Disease) and Vascular Dementia. Common in old age, although it can occur earlier. In almost all cases Dementia is progressive and irreversible, therefore prevention must be in the minds of all, although much can be done to help to halt or slow the progress of the disease. Smoking is a major brain, mind and body enemy. Nutritious, properly balanced Diet of natural additive-free food and drink is one of the keys to brain health. Research has recently shown that drinking up to two glasses of red wine daily, particularly Chilean or Californian Merlot, helps in the prevention of Alzheimer's and Dementia, but more important still is the fact that blood pressure- lowering therapy reduced the risk considerably, also helping to slow the deterioration. High blood pressure is a major risk factor for stroke, which in turn is a risk factor for Dementia. *See Blood Pressure, Alzheimer's, Brain Health and DIET captions.*

DEPRESSION

There are over 2,000 ailments listed, including many minor ones, in files and papers, which I have accumulated, with which our bodies can be affected. Very often we think we have huge problems until we hear those of others, then realizing that ours are minor compared to theirs. There are certain complaints one could describe as puzzling. One of these is Depression. To some it comes almost overnight. With others it is a slow on-coming ailment or problem. *Long-term Depression drains your energy, distorts the mind, causes much distress and affects those around you. Although the sufferer does not realize it, poor health or debility is almost always the cause of it.* This, allied to stress, loneliness, fear or phobia - call them emotional problems - all add up to that Depressed, lonely, fatigued, no get-up-and-go feeling. We have to listen daily to the doom mongers, as we are blitzed or harassed with newspaper stories, on the hour or even half hour radio or TV bulletins. All seems to be bad news, an amount of it about foreign countries that is of no interest to us, as we endeavour to cope with our problems in life.

If we live in a climate of depression it is not surprising that we attract into our own lives concepts that effect our own emotions. If we are in good health, these things do not seem to affect us; we just shrug them off and press on with living. *The writer has seen many rid themselves of depression, negative attitudes, emotional and other such problems. They are now able to bear the stress of modern-day living, because they accept it and live the simple advice given. Stress, anxiety and depression are all similar.* Being prescribed tranquillisers and other synthetic medicines, including the tablet Prozac, only make things prolonged, or worse, especially when the patient tries to give these drugs up. **Sadly there is within our community a strong feeling that the doctor can provide pills for all ills. The majority are just stopgaps, having no curative properties. Anti-depressants are certainly not the answers. They cause side effects, conceal or mask the affects, very often leading to addiction.** In these islands the weather, especially in the Wintertime, can be depressing. Even so it is always much better outside, than when looking out through a window. Many do not realise this, especially those who are suffering from what is another form of depression called S.A.D.S. (Seasonal Affective Disorder). It occurs because of a lack of light, daylight, sunshine, or brightness of the day in the person's lifestyle. As with any form of depression, stress or emotional problem, it is essential that as well as diet being number one, so also is the taking of exercise, including breathing exercises, preferably outside, in fresh air and daylight. *What easier, cheaper, better way of taking this than by walking? It has helped many to overcome depression, and associated ailments. Turn to the caption on Walking. It is simple and instructive. If on medication, or with serious health problem, speak with your doctor before taking up any form of strenuous exercise. Turn to S.A.D.S. caption.*

Do not allow yourself to bottle up feelings. Confide in a close friend or relative. Talk is cheap but it is good to do so. Keep the brain active by reading or doing puzzles such as crosswords. Avoid alcohol, smoking and passive smoke. Write letters. This is a wonderful way to express oneself. It is really therapeutic.

Thomas Bartram, the well-known herbalist, founder of Gerard House natural remedies, author of several health books, including his **'Encyclopedia Of Herbal Medicine'** also Editor of the quarterly magazine **'Grace'** devoted to nature's way of living, gives us this valuable advice about Depression. *He tells us about: "The happiness all are striving for as they charge along, as if it were at the end of the road or tunnel. It is all around and about us. No need to search for it. It is with us, in what we do and say, in how we treat our friends, approach our work, how we live our lives". His words as taken from the wonderful 'Grace' magazine include: "Have you considered the role of Diet on the way you feel? Happiness is to do with feelings. Feelings are much influenced by what goes into the body".* Have fresh green vegetables, fresh fruits and wholegrain cereals. One of the most common causes of Depression, the opposite of happiness, is the continued use of coffee. There are various good teas available. Drink it weak. Aromatherapy is growing in popularity. Spoil yourself. An essential oil may cheer and enhance a feeling of well- being, especially lavender oil. It is a gentle nerve sedative; it is a great calmer-down. Walk every day of your life, stride out in obvious enjoyment. Walking is the most natural means of relaxation. Press arches of feet on a tennis ball to stimulate aqua pressure points. In breathing there is an art. Do you enjoy it? Try standing before an open window and breath deeply. Feel air enter every corner of your lungs. This is my way of thinking and doing.

Turn to the Diet caption because I am convinced that with proper nutritious food, also with addition of some food supplements, including the excellent Rhodolia, also Udos's Choice Oil, eliminating smoking and alcohol, one can feel so much better that no problem is too big to overcome. Skullcap, Damiana or Valerian are extremely good remedies and aids, all natural, with no side effects, being non addictive. Too many either dwell on the past, or worse still, worry about the future. Forget this. Look after your health. Yesterday is gone. Tomorrow is another day. Live for today. You are very often surrounded by this happiness that so many strive for. Just seek it. Live your life one day at a time and be happy, remembering that pure unadulterated food is like medicine, as is exercise and a proper and regular sleep pattern.

DEPRESSION POST NATAL

See Post Natal Depression caption.

DERMATITIS

This word covers a range of skin problems including certain allergies. Detergents, cement, mineral or hydrocarbon oils, solvents, garden plants, certain kinds of clothing, jewellery and much more can be the reason. It is essential that the cause be diagnosed before treating. Nutritious Diet of natural foods when supplemented by Vitamins E, C and B complex, or a Multivitamin tablet, help to ward off Dermatitis. Lack of B Vitamins is often found in those with the problem, hence the need for Vitamin B Complex. Allergenics ointment and cream is 100 per cent natural, derived from non-chemical ingredients, being non steroidal and suitable for all skin types. All Allergenics products are dermatological tested, so each product is safe to use on Dermatitis. They have proved to be exceptionally good for skin problems. *Turn to DIET caption, which can also be as medicine to the body.*

DETOXING

This subject has only become noteworthy in recent years. Previous to this, when Detoxing was mentioned, it referred to the drying-out of a person suffering from alcoholism. Of Detoxing it can honestly be said, that I have seen come - and just as quickly go - over the years, fads in the pursuit of a healthier lifestyle. Almost all were just a money making gimmick. Short-term Detox can do more harm than good.

Why did we not have need for Detox until recent years? I will tell you. We ate pure unadulterated, additive-free food, including vegetables, fruit, fresh fish and meat, with little processed. **Junk and fast 'foods' were out.** If you feel you must Detox then do so, at the same time taking Detoxia or Spirulina, which are an advance support while you spring-clean your body. Detoxing should not be commenced if with illness, stressed, depressed, feeling lethargic or rundown. To Detox long-term, with resultant better health, energy and vitality, including good skin, nails and hair, *turn to DIET caption* and be guided by the advice given. Good food is the best Detoxant known. There'll be no need for Detox later if this is adhered to. Eat regular meals, taking time to eat and chew properly. Don't skip meals. Breakfast is the most important one. Juice, fresh fruits and vegetables are excellent detoxers. *Study the Food Pyramid caption to be guided further, also see Slimming caption.*

DEVILS CLAW

Here is a herb, a plant, which gets it name from the large claw-like fruit or tuber it produces. *It can be placed in the top category as a herbal remedy, taking its place alongside or even above many of the best chemical medicines manufactured. Its anti-inflammatory and pain-relieving properties have been proved. There are no known side effects.* It should not be used during pregnancy or if with duodenal or gastric ulcer. Devil's Claw has proved excellent for the relief of rheumatism, arthritis, gout, sciatica, back pain, lumbago and neuralgia, also as a mild liver tonic, detoxant and diuretic. I have found Pagosid brand to be extremely good.

DHOBIES ITCH

Usually affects men in Summer or hot weather. Avoid tight man-made clothing, wearing cotton next to skin. Wash and dry the affected area before applying diluted tea tree oil two or three times daily. Take Vitamin B Complex as prescribed on label.

DIABETES

Drugs and natural remedies can work together to aid the health of the diabetic. The incidence of Diabetes, we are told, is becoming endemic, also that new drugs to treat other illnesses carry a greater risk of Diabetes.

There is a definite link between vaccines, such as used for whooping cough, and the maintaining of normal levels of glucose in the blood. In the United States, where vaccines are grossly overused, there are 20 million Americans with Diabetes. Many Diabetic foods have been condemned as unsuitable, with misleading information on the food labels. Smoking, sugar and sugary products, being overweight and alcohol are enemies of Diabetes and better health. *Diabetes in middle age is becoming an ever-increasing health problem. However, by following a healthy, natural, unprocessed food-eating plan, staying at a normal weight, exercising regularly and with proper sleep pattern, it can be prevented and certainly helps enormously if with the disease.*

Visit you health food shop and seek advice about natural foods and other edibles suitable for diabetics, such as Meridian sugarless spreads, also much more. The addition of Vitamin E and Lecithin granules to the Diet has enabled doctors to cut down on insulin, as well as improving the health of the Diabetic. I have seen many good results in the past where the affected person changed to natural foods. Exercise is of vital importance. It need not be strenuous. *See- Exercise and Walking captions.*

A half-teaspoon of ground cinnamon, twice daily, taken with liquids or on breakfast cereal, helps regulate the blood sugar. Following the **HAY DIET**, using only natural additive free foods, has helped enormously, even to becoming insulin-free. It is my belief that this is the greatest Diet ever devised. It is health giving and helps one attain normal weight. Some use natural food, gluten free, in conjunction with the Hay Diet, which is referred to under caption in this Guide. *If with Diabetes be guided and advised at all times by your doctor. What is suggested or recommended here is entirely natural, food based. All have a right to the best advice and treatment available. It need not necessarily be based on drugs or synthetic medicines.*

DIARRHOEA

The first thing to determine with Diarrhoea is why is it occurring? It can be due to different diagnoses (i.e., where signs and symptoms are shared by several ailments) such as gastroenteritis, colitis, salmonella poisoning, Crohn's disease or other bowel problems. Manuka honey in tepid water prevents dehydration, often being a lifesaver. Aloe Vera has proved an excellent remedy, others being New Era Combination S, Ferr Phos or Tormentil. Two teaspoons of Manuka honey every hour for four or five hours is a good bowel or stomach medicine. Drink plenty of fluids, preferably tepid water. If Diarrhoea persists for more than 48 hours seek medical advice.

DIET

This Encyclopedia is written to help those who wish to, or those interested in feeling well, to learn about natural foods, also to help choose natural over the counter remedies, including vitamins, minerals, food supplements also herbal or homeopathic remedies. ***The biggest single factor, which is the cause of ill health, is DIET. It is also the greatest remedy. It should be one of the uppermost concerns of all, both young and old.***

In many instances where there is illness, or if feeling unwell, a simple change to natural food and drinks can be excellent medicine and may not necessitate the use of Supplements

There is a difference between Diet and dieting. They are entirely different subjects. Those not aware of this might be misled, not understanding about the pure natural Diet as written about. Dieting is about losing weight, slimming or trying to lose weight. I don't like the word slimming because it can lead to major health problems if done to excess. The Diet written about here will help decrease the weight, especially if the partaker exercises daily and fairly rigorously. ***Before embarking on any exercise routine and if with a medical condition, it is vitally important to speak with your doctor and be advised.***

A regular pattern of sleep is extremely important for good health. Like good food, sufficient and regular sleep is as medicine.

Like those within the medical profession, I cannot understand why so many are turning to the high protein Diets as written by, shall we call them 'celebrities'. In the long-term these so- called Diets or dieting can only do harm, serious harm, to the health of those who take them up.

What you eat is of major importance to your health. It often means only a simple or small change of choice of food, from where one is partaking of something where there is a deficiency of minerals, vitamins, or other sustenance required to keep the body systems healthy. Carbohydrates, fats and proteins may be out of balance. Simple, natural, additive-free foods, as written about here, also where necessary, some food supplements, vitamins, or minerals, as described later, will help to provide suitable nutrition to enable one to attain better health.

Grains, fruits and vegetables should be the foundation for your Diet, including super foods such as Brown Rice, Beans, Peas, Lentils, Oats, Wholemeal Pasta, Baked Potatoes, Bananas, Nuts and Seeds (except peanuts). *Study the Food Pyramid caption.*

If you are interested in losing weight, you will gain an amount of knowledge by reading about the DIET urged. You can improve your health and vitality immensely by following this advice, also that under Exercise, Sleep, Detoxing and Slimming captions.

Obesity is, we are told, much more prevalent amongst the lower income group. It is increasing at an alarming rate. Is this because the unwary, those who know little or nothing about the excessive use of food additives, purchase these cheaper processed products, because the incentive is in the pricing, the saving of money? Cheaper 'foods' are mostly additive-filled, with little nutritives. Bulking agents and other fillers make the so-called 'food' cut-price. We are what we eat; we are what we partake of. Few give thought to what goes into the body. They would not put inferior fuel in the tank of their cars. Cheap ' food' can prove to be very expensive.

The human body is far more intricate than any internal combustion engine, consisting of glands, systems, joints, bones, flushing methods, filters, the senses, also hundreds of other intricate or fascinating attributes or facets. The human body is taken for granted by many who do not care about how it is treated. The human body is supernatural, a marvel, and a wonder unparalleled. It has wonderful healing, restorative and renewal properties, if helped. This help is usually sought when illness occurs, much of it through our negligence; therefore we seek a cure from the doctor. Sad to relate, more often than not it is not just a cure, being merely a stopper of pain. The sufferer or patient will not be questioned as to DIET, what is being put into the body.

Our whole bodily system is taken for granted. We do not stop to think that here is something we cannot replace, cannot obtain spare parts for, should look after, and take care of. All should be extremely alert to the dangers of smoking, alcohol and synthetic chemicals, whether as food additives, or avoidable pills or potions. There are well over 5.000 substances in food-additives now, compared to approximately 50 some 70 years ago. They are being added to daily as further factory-made 'food' ingredients are formulated. Much of them are of no value to our health. As set out in this Encyclopedia the greatest medicine is DIET, just pure, natural, unadulterated food, combined with food supplements, also with vitamins or minerals, if or where necessary. These will provide suitable and excellent nutrition to enable one attain better health. Good food and good mood go together.

It can be repeated again and again, we are responsible for our own health, also where relevant that of our families. Very often we have only ourselves to blame, being our own worst enemies.

Obesity, as already mentioned, is becoming a worrying problem from a health point of view. It is widespread in America and we are fast catching up. One might be sued if names are mentioned, but the fast 'foods', fizzy 'drinks', fries, the grease-ridden, sugarised trash which we are offered, should be and must be, shunned. It is taking a long time to get the message across about the dangers of this, or the need for an additive or chemical-free Diet. The majority do not appear to be interested, trusting the manufacturers and retailers as has been done in the past. Poor eating habits are amongst the chief causes of obesity.

Only today as I walked in a small town, the fast-food shop could be likened to a beehive, except for the type of stuff being sold. Literally dozens of uniformed students, many of them pale-faced, some unhealthy-looking, queued for and purchased a dole- out of chips with light brown liquid, which made the whole thing look most unappetising. This was served on blue paper mache trays. To those used to other than the type of 'food' described, there were approximately two or three mouthfuls. Almost all had an aluminium can or plastic bottle containing a fizzy 'drink'. Further on at the filling station, two young children emerged with two small white bread rolls, in which could be seen a thin slice of ham. Also in their grasp each had a bottle of a supposedly 'energy filling drink', which contained Aspartame, and other chemical-additives. The onus must be on the parents or those responsible for the youth to stop this kind of eating and drinking. We cannot function properly and that includes mentally, physically and socially, if not taking proper nourishment. *To read about the dangers of sugar, so grossly over used now, turn to Sugar caption also Fizzy Drinks caption.*

Amongst the authors and scribes, especially the media, we have the do-gooders, the advisors, also psychiatrists, psychologists, counsellors and those who seldom give us good news. Only this week, during course of conversation with 12 students who sought advice about exercise, including the benefits of Yoga, the writer introduced the subject of Diet, suggesting correct or better eating habits. One who had been advised to use only margarine instead of butter, when questioned as to whom gave the advice replied: 'One of the experts who visited the college'. There is no person who can claim to be an expert. My advice to these young people and to you the reader is: 'If it is natural it is good'. Margarine is not natural. Read the ingredients label. It contains additives. Butter is pure butter. Smeared on bread or used sparingly there is no harm in it. Frequently these 'experts' we hear about are proved wrong. *See Margarine also Butter captions.*

EAT A PROPER-BALANCED DIET. How often have we heard this advice? It is a hackneyed phrase, but oh so true, except that only a minority accept the advice or ask the question: 'A balanced diet of what?' I could name a varied number of 'foods', which, if taken over a period, would give a balanced Diet of much alien to the health of the consumer, with little nutrients. Having a balanced Diet, which gives daily benefit, requires thought, preparation and perhaps advice. Once on the right track all comes naturally, in every sense of the word. The advice is in this caption about DIET, including PROPER-BALANCED DIET of nutritious health-giving foods

Set out on page 99 is an easy-to-understand guide to healthy eating, which can be of much help to those who seek advice about good food.

Instead of jams or marmalades, unless they are free from sugar or artificial sweeteners and with high fruit content, use sugar-free spreads from the health food store, some supermarkets or food stores. Meridian or Whole Earth products are brand names to look for. They are high in fruit content, being sweetened and thickened with pure fruit juice, equally as cheap as some jams. Here's another case of bureaucracy gone mad, where full of fruit- only spreads, including Seville orange marmalades, also raspberry, strawberry, cherry and other fruits, cannot be labelled as jam or marmalades, because they are not made up with sugar. They are called SPREADS.

Drink pure water between meals. We are advised to drink up to eight glasses daily. Very important is a glass or similar measure of tepid water first thing before breakfast. This acts like a cleanser. Often we are told not to drink with meals. This is discretionary. *Turn to Water Caption.*

Use the twice-weekly rule of
1. Meat or Poultry   2. Fish   3. Eggs   4. Cheese.

Eat foods from each group, except fish, no more than twice weekly. Fish should be eaten as often as possible, being extremely good food, especially oily fish. *Turn to Fish and Fish Oils caption for further guidance.*

Eat salads regularly. Some say: 'Ob, I don't like salads'. This is often because they look on it as bit of lettuce, a tomato with perhaps a slice of ham. This is not a salad. Included in a nice salad can be nutritious edibles such as lettuce, tomato, peppers - both red or yellow, beetroot, onions, garlic, chives, parsley, dandelion or other herbs, sliced banana or apple, grated raw carrot, celery, chopped mixed nuts (not peanuts), or sprouted seeds as grown on a window ledge. Pure virgin Olive Oil or homemade French dressing can be used, or use natural additive- free salad dressings or spreads as sold by health food shops. Meridian or

What The Food Groups Contain and How Much Of Each Should Be Eaten					
Food Groups	Bread Cereal Potatoes	Fruit Vegetables	Milk Dairy Foods	Meat Fish	Foods containing fats or sugars
Which Foods are included	Breads, Rice, Oats, Maize, Millet, Rye and other Grains, Pasta, Noodles, Potatoes, Plantains, yams, bananas & Tomatoes	Fresh & Frozen Fruit & Vegetables Salads, Beans, Lentils, Pure Fruit Juice, Dried Fruits, Vegetables which can be eaten cooked or raw. Sprouted seeds and pulses	Milk, Cheeses, Natural Yoghurt, Soya and Rice Milks.	Beef, Pork, Mutton, Lamb, Liver & Kidney, Free Range Chicken and Turkey, Fish and Eggs	Butter, Margarine, Oils, Mayonnaise, & oily salad dressings, Crisps, savoury snacks, Biscuits, Cakes & Puddings, Ice-cream, Chocolate & Sweets, Sugar Sweetened Drinks.
Advice	Eat plenty of these foods. They should form one third of the diet	Eat at least five portions a day of these foods; they should form one third of the diet	Eat or Drink moderate amounts	Eat moderate amounts of all foods in this group	Use only pure Oils & Butter. Avoid fatty or sweet foods, fizzy drinks & margarines.
Comments	Choose whole grain varieties. These starchy foods provide energy & fibre. Starchy foods are filling & can reduce desire for fatty or sweet foods	Fruit and vegetables are a major source of vitamins, minerals, dietary fibre and other metabolically active compounds.	Choose lower fat products when possible. They usually contain comparable amounts of B Vitamins & Calcium, but may be lower in Vitamins A & D. Use butter sparingly. Avoid margarine.	Use lean meat, removing the fat. Skin poultry. Eat fish, especially oily fish twice weekly. Beans & Lentils are a rich source of B Vitamins, dietary fibre & metabolically active plant compounds.	Don't eat crisps, cakes, biscuits, confectionary or sweets. Omit sugary products and savoury snacks. Note the advice about Oils, Butter, fizzy 'drinks' and alcohol as captioned in this Encyclopedia.

Ballymaloe brand dressings are delicious. Homemade Florida cocktail is very nutritious. Include chopped apple, celery, broken walnuts, raisins or sultanas, with a natural dressing. Who said they did not like salads? They are natural, health giving and full of goodness. Side salads in small portions are ideal to add to most meals, being an extremely healthy food, an excellent digestive aid.

The need to eat fruit is emphasized over and over in this Encyclopedia. The proof is there that it is health giving. In France, where the amount of fat consumed is equal to, or more than is taken here, the incidence of heart or circulatory problems is very much lower. They have a high intake of fruit. One cannot eat sufficient fruit. *Turn to Fruit and Vegetable caption.*

There should be a liquidizer in every kitchen, just as there should be a pressure cooker. With the aid of the former, very nice drinks and purees can be produced. A little imagination can work wonders. Fruit, to which is added pure fruit juice or water, can be mixed in. Raw vegetables can be eaten when pureed, with salad or main meal. Experiment, and continue to eat what you like best. Make sure you keep the recipe. If I make something enjoyable, all-too-often it cannot be produced again. Frequently I make a puree of fruit and vegetable mix. Use more fruit, any fruit will do. This makes for a nice blend, helping to neutralize the vegetable taste. It is purely natural, simply good.

A good quality, modern-type pressure cooker is a valuable asset in the kitchen, and is also an addition from a health perception. It enables one to produce healthy meals, in a fraction of the time normally taken. Pulses, brown rice, or other edibles, which need soaking overnight, can be cooked instantly. Quick cooking in a minimum of water helps retain the vitamins and goodness. Full meals can be cooked in one pan or pot. Only one cooking utensil to wash up! With the Prestige pressure cooker comes a good-user guide. Read the instructions carefully before using, or better still, have someone explain how to use, and perhaps show you what to do. There are recipe books for pressure cookers, also instructions in the booklet provided. All this helps one to make simple, delicious, nutritious meals with little delay.

Fresh fruit salads are easy to make up. Avoid tinned fruit, or anything tinned, as they usually contain additives, such as preservatives. Select the fruit, wash and rinse, then cut up or slice, mix together and add pure fruit juice to sweeten. Equally good for this purpose is tepid water, into which is mixed some pure, natural honey, which when dissolved and mixed with the fruit, helps to provide a good health-giving dessert. Off the shelf fruit juices are mostly made up from concentrated fruit juice, with most to be avoided. Use the liquidiser or a juicer to make pure natural juice, into which the whole fruit can easily be incorporated, with little waste. Pure natural, full-fruit juices are available from the health food store. *Much sold as pure is not pure!*

Sugar and salt are to be avoided as much as possible. There is no need for a saltcellar or container on the table. We will not be short of either as they are impossible to avoid in the Diet of today, being grossly overused, both enemies of good health. Our system needs salt, but only very sparingly. *Turn to Salt caption.*

Breakfast cereals are a prime example of excessive use of additives. ***It must be repeated, highlighted or underlined that breakfast is the most important meal of the day. A good nutritious breakfast sets one up for the hours ahead.*** Smokers tend not to eat at breakfast time, to the further detriment of their health. Over 80 different packaged cereals have been counted on the shelves in the supermarket. One well-advertised, processed product shows over 30 ingredients on the label, much of them synthetic. There are only two cereals - I repeat two - which have nothing added, nothing taken away. They are Shredded Wheat, which is slightly processed, and a wonderful cereal, also Porridge Oats which is the oat kernel rolled. ***There is no more natural food than the oat. It is not processed, sweetened, or made tasty when sold as porridge oats. Many, especially the young people, will not accept porridge when made in its natural state. It has not been refined or treated. It has not been made to suit the taste buds, by the addition of sugar or other ingredients. Pure, natural honey when added to porridge gives it a unique sweetness, with both oats and honey being second to none as a start to the day.*** Try getting used to porridge without sweetener. It is easy, especially if you equate it to good health. Oats, whether as flakes, flour, pinhead, or oat bran - provided they have not been processed, coated or treated in any way, just natural - contain a balance of carbohydrates, Vitamin B Complex, Calcium, Potassium, Magnesium, also other nutrients. These are all highly beneficial for a healthy system, including the control of cholesterol and blood pressure. *Turn to Oats and Oatmeal caption.*

Prunes being eaten or the drinking of prune juice is almost frowned upon, being for some reason viewed with disfavor, often regarded as a joke. This is a wrong outlook. Here is a natural way to keep the bowels free and to obtain the mineral; Iron, so necessary to our well-being. Constipation is the affliction of many, resulting in headaches, lethargy, bloated feeling and other uncomfortable effects. It certainly does not help the blood pressure or circulation. Always wash prunes before steeping overnight in boiling water, even if the instructions tell you they are ready to eat. The water or juice when cold is equally good. Three or four juicy prunes at breakfast-time are a tonic. *A simple solution for constipation is to mix three or four dessertspoons of natural wheat bran with breakfast cereal, to be taken every four or five days or as required.* Soaked overnight with dessertspoonful of linseed, there is no better natural laxative.

Eat wholemeal bread. Many of the white breads have had much of the goodness removed, being only a filler, often with many additives. Avoid the cheap brands as sold in the supermarket, almost always as a loss leader. Read the ingredients labels as already harped about in this Encyclopedia. Home-baked bread is best, especially the wholemeal loaf. *Turn to Bread caption.*

Eat fish. Any fish is good except that in sealed plastic packaging or artificially smoked fish. The fake colour or smoke is unacceptable as it is often overused, therefore being a danger to health. Fresh fish is a must in our Diet. In Finland and Greenland it has been found, that despite their high-fat Diet, there is low incidence of heart disease because studies have confirmed the effective merit of fish oils, as well as finding other health benefits. Much could be written about the goodness of fish in relation to DIET. ***There is a big question mark hanging over the once all-supreme salmon. It is now farmed, being reared in cages, fed with artificial chemicals, including a toxic colouring agent, which makes the grey flesh of the battery-reared salmon turn pink, in order to make it acceptable to the purchaser. It is not natural.*** So, therefore, where there is doubt, omit salmon from the menu, unless you are sure of its origin. Before purchasing fish from the food store look at the ingredients label. Some packaged fish contains additives. *See Fish and Fish Oils also Salmon captions.*

Of meats, liver is an exceptionally good source of Vitamin B and other vitamins, being very nutritious. Be guided by the advice given of eating meat and poultry no more than twice weekly. Meat boiled in a pressure cooker can be thickened to make broth, soups or stews. Stews, with vegetables added, are a welcome Winter warmer. Be extremely choosy when buying white meat. Most birds, including chickens and turkeys, are reared intensively. Notice the bones in that of the confined bird. There is usually brown staining at the joints when the meat has been removed after cooking. This is where the salmonella occurs. Demand and try to procure free-range. Similarly with eggs, there is a noticeable difference of the yolks of eggs from the birds which roam freely, and those, which have been cooped up. *Turn to Meat caption.*

Dispense with the frying pan. Grill, poach or steam instead. I repeat the advice to steam vegetables. Do not boil them.

Much of the cooking oils on display are over-processed, not being beneficial. Pure virgin, first-pressed oils, as sold in the health food shop and some food stores, are pure. There you will find a selection of sunflower, safflower and others, including pure olive oil. This is the oil of oils. In countries where olive oil is used chiefly, the incidence of heart disease is comparatively low. For cooking and salads it is the best of all the oils. Olive oil must not be used in the deep fat fryer. If interested in better health one will not use this method of cooking. *Turn to both captions, Cooking Oils, also Cooking Oils – How They Are Produced.*

Microwave food is to be avoided. We had to wait a long time to be told of the fatal consequences of smoking. No doubt some day we will be told of the effects of microwaving. Scientists are studying the uses of microwaves and there is

controversy, with politics now entering the debate of what appears to be a contentious issue. This is not being alarmist. The American Institute of Science Journal prints the disturbing story. As with all foods, drinks or whatever we partake of, IF IN DOUBT LEAVE OUT and this includes the use of the Microwave oven. *Turn to Microwave caption*

For those who live on their own, or those who maintain they have not the time to cook, there is no excuse for not eating natural additive-free foods as suggested in this Encyclopedia. They are available. One just has to search for them, then when found, becoming aware of how simple it will be to obtain them. Visit your health food store and be surprised at the nutritious fare available. Some of our supermarkets now have a health food section as well as a range of natural or additive-free foods. The best place to seek advice about natural foods is from the health food shop. An example of all this is to be found amongst the 'Meridian' brand of foods of which there is a good range of products. As their slogan implies: *'Naturally different, naturally better'*. Select from their Tahini, Sesame, and Organic cooking sauces, including Sweet and Sour also Balti. There are Rogan Josh, Tikka Masala, Pasta and Soya Sauces, organic Salad Dressings, pure Fruit Juices, Chutneys, Pickles, Ketchup, Malt Extract, also Fruit spreads. These can be used in combination with the many other pure natural foods available, all additive-free. ***By following the advice given, turning to natural food Diet, with necessary food supplements, gives one the courage, the extra zest to tackle something new, including cooking. Time can be found to do the simple things required to attain good health.***

Soups, all pure and natural, can be made with the aid of that health asset, the liquidizer. Space does not permit me to give recipes. The advice is to refer to a good simple cookbook. Soups can be made up in whatever quantity or portions desired. They can then be frozen in the chosen amounts, according to the number being catered for, whether one or more, to be used as and when required. The writer knew nothing about cooking, other than to boil an egg, or make wholemeal bread, before being given a cookery book, and told to get started. Very soon the making of soup, or whatever one decides upon, comes natural in more than one definition. There is only natural goodness in what is suggested. ***Recently when reading the ingredients lists on 'soups', more especially the dried packet sort, some of them well-advertised brands, they contained lists of fillers, additives and other agents, which were deplorable. The word 'soup' was an incorrect description. The person who accompanied me described it as 'trash'. There is no doubt that many food processors make good food bad. Here is another example of food additives at their worst.*** *See Soups caption.*

Milk puddings, made with natural ingredients, are filling and nutritious. Flaked or ground Brown Rice, Sago, Tapioca, also whole wheat Macaroni can all be purchased in the health food store. The flaked or ground brown rice is easier to cook than whole brown. The latter is best steeped over night in boiling water. Strain the water, add milk or water and cook. Whole or flaked brown rice has not been de-husked to make it white. It contains much goodness, being an invaluable food, unlike white rice.

If allergic to certain foods, as some are, the advice is to eliminate them one by one from your Diet, and see how you feel. After a week or two they can be reintroduced, again one by one. You will then find out which food or foods you are sensitive to, these to be avoided. Those mostly correlated with allergy are: citrus fruits, dairy products including milk, also yeast, wheat and eggs. *Turn to Allergy caption* if with this problem.

Apart from: *'Food being your medicine or medicine being the food you eat',* there is often a need for vitamins, minerals or food supplements. Much of our food, especially the processed and additive-filled 'foods' on offer are highly deficient. It is not unusual to see synthetic vitamins and minerals being listed as ingredients alongside artificial fillers and bulking agents. This is further proof, as if this is needed, that the 'food' offered is often foodless. Even some of the natural foods are low in goodness.

Tests carried out in recent years by soil analysts show a marked depletion of certain minerals, which were there in abundance in the past. This may be due to modern farming methods or environmental factors, which are now beyond our control, including the overuse of artificial fertilizers. For example the amount of Selenium, which the soil contained, has diminished alarmingly. Selenium is an essential mineral and nutrient in the fight against cancer, also being good for eye health and to relieve lupus syndrome. Taken in conjunction with Vitamins E & C it is an excellent antioxidant formula. This is another food supplement, which is obtainable from the health food store. *No supplements will take the place of processed, additive-filled food. They are excellent when accompanying natural and pure foods.*

Our health can be damaged, or at risk, from the overuse of antibiotics, the toxic residue of chemicals, including synthetic medicines partaken of, the air we sometimes have to breath, with a question mark regarding the overuse of many food additives.

As pointed out already, the human body is a complex mechanism, which requires a varied intake of good foods and liquid, which should contain essentials, including vitamins, minerals, fatty acids and pure goodness. All must be natural. All-too-often we appear not to be getting these necessities. They regulate the health of bones, muscles, blood and fluid flow; keep the systems and metabolism normal - also much, much more. Amongst other aggravations are: stress, which increases cellular activity; anxiety and tension, which are allied to stress; insufficient sleep; irregular meals; and the pace of modern-day living. They all combine to deplete the body of many of the minerals and vitamins so necessary to ensure good health. *It is therefore often very important to add supplements. If doing so make certain to purchase the natural product, as sold by the health food outlet. Many chemists have now decided that they should be stockiest of the natural remedies. They have condescended to turn to the natural. It is almost unbelievable. They just had to; as they could no longer resist the call for alternative, non-habit forming, no side effect remedies. Most annoying to the discerning, is the matter of display by the pharmacist, of natural remedies, including herbal, homeopathic, or food supplements. Being eager to promote and sell their high-profit synthetic products, as made by the giant drug companies, certain of these and other chemicals medicines or tablets are cunningly placed in with the natural product. All-too-often they speak with those who seek an aid to better health, at the same time recommending their chemical medication. Be discretionary. Support your health food shop to be sure you are being sold natural remedies or products.*

Unless one is ill and requires a particular remedy, there are various combined or multivitamin tablets or medicines available. If with a problem which requires a particular remedy, look under that caption in this Encyclopedia to find out what is suggested. Where it is possible, add to whatever other supplement is decided on as being suitable. *Under Vitamin and Minerals caption,* the résumé and descriptions cover almost all vitamins and minerals.

Where one is concerned with obtaining better health, when combining proper Diet as written about with vitamins and minerals, it is suggested to use and alternate a herbal tonic such as Salusan, Floradix, Floravital or Bio Strath. *Also see Nettles caption.* Kindervital is a very good tonic or pick-me-up for children. They must be stored in the fridge because there are no preservatives in them. The following week take a Multivitamin as appropriate and continue to rotate weekly. Learn all you can about natural remedies, and you will be surprised how easy it is to be knowledgeable. Ask questions, especially in your health food shop. Study the RDA (Recommended Daily Allowance) advice on the box or container. This always errs extremely on the safe side. We now find that much higher RDA levels have been recommended or suggested. *Repeated again is the advice to speak with and question the health food personnel. They are extremely enlightened about health problems.*

Where there is a need for extra, such as Calcium/Magnesium, both work together, so necessary to prevent osteoporosis, for bone, teeth, muscle and nerve health, then take as required to obtain the correct amount. All over the age of 35 should take this supplement. Calcium/Magnesium/Vitamin D tablet taken with a little water at night-time is better than any sleeping pill, being natural and health giving to the body, including the bones.

Iron helps to correct and prevent anaemia, also to remove blood impurities. Care is needed here because too much can be dangerous. Better less Iron than more.
Folic Acid helps prevent Spina Bifida. Sufficient Folic Acid should be in a Multivitamin tablet. It is a must, before, during and after pregnancy. Pregnacare Multivitamin, which contains Folic Acid, is highly recommended for before and after conception.

Take Zinc/Copper, with the two working in tandem, for prostate, skin and hair health. Every cell in the body needs Zinc. It works in conjunction with Copper and is very necessary for the immune system, supporting the body's natural defences. All over the age of thirty-five should take this mineral, because the body does not make Zinc when one gets older.

Lecithin, which is a soya-based product, is highly recommended for circulation, heart, brain, memory, liver and nervous system. It is essential for every cell in the body. It is an aid to gall bladder function, also helping to break down the fats in foods eaten. It is best taken as instructions on label, on porridge or cereal. It is not recommended in its dry state. Few know about the excellent health-giving properties of Lecithin. *See Lecithin caption.*

Vitamin A is good for vision, especially night vision. Benefits bone and skin health, being an antioxidant, an aid for sexual functioning and reproduction. A Multivitamin tablet will usually supply the Recommended Daily Allowance.

Vitamin B Complex is invaluable for so much that is good health. It is certainly Complex in many ways. Here is one Vitamin, which can be taken above the RDA. Vitamin B Complex has an excellent safety record. Nicotinic Acid, part of the complex, taken in excessive amounts is harmful to the liver. As made up in Vitamin B Complex as sold in the health food store, there is no danger. It is harmful only if taken separately over and above the RDA. Some of the main aids of Vitamin B Complex are to red blood cell formation, female reproduction, protein and amino acid metabolism, neuro transmitters, digestive system, liver, healthy eyes, skin, hair and nails, growth and repair of body tissues, appetite and very much more. It gives R.D.A. of Vitamin B 12.

Vitamins C and E are antioxidants which work extremely well together as free radical scavengers, good for maintaining and helping to control cholesterol and blood pressure levels, for mental health, immune system, energy production and much more. Vitamins C and E are, to me, two of our greatest health-promoting and protective agents. In order to allow for proper absorption by the system, it is advisable, when taking Vitamin E to always start by taking 100iu's for 30 days, then

200iu's for the following 30 days and then 400 or 500iu's daily thereafter long-term. IU is a unit of measurement used to determine the amount of Vitamin E per capsule. One cannot over-emphasise the good of Vitamin E. It should be remembered that Vitamin E and C work better when combined.

Calcium and Vitamin E must not be taken with Iron. They must be taken four hours apart. When taking certain Vitamins the urine will be yellow or green in colour. This is nothing to worry about.

All vitamins, minerals or food supplements should be taken with food, unless instructed otherwise.

One of our greatest aids to good health is Garlic, which can be described as herb or vegetable. It's something, which has universal recognition. How often have I been told: 'I cannot take it' or 'I don't like the smell' or 'I don't like it, I've never tried it'. Read on, because many are not aware that apart from being available in any good vegetable shop or supermarket, as root or clove, Garlic is one of the most popular off-the-shelf tablets or capsules sold in the health food store and now by chemists. They are odour controlled, just one a day. Many pages could be written about the all-round goodness of garlic. It is our greatest health-giving root. Here is a medicine, a food, which should be used daily. It is recognised as a support for mind and body. The oil it contains is highly effective against respiratory problems, such as those brought on by influenza, colds, bronchitis and catarrh, also as an aid to relieve whooping cough. It is a lung tonic also good to aid digestive problems. It aids the circulation and heart. Garlic could be said to be the ideal 'cure all' *See Garlic caption.*

Sprouted Seeds and Pulses are extremely good health-giving foods. *See Sprouting caption.* Their goodness cannot be highlighted sufficiently.

Having read this caption on DIET, hopefully you have learned the need for pure natural unadulterated food, with so many other suggestions, in order to improve health and remain healthy. There are many like myself who practise what is written here. Most of them have little if any illness, seldom having to visit the doctor. Perhaps this is why the medical profession do not recommend natural Diet or anything natural.

I repeat: "I am convinced that much of the additive-filled stuff we are expected to accept as 'food' and 'drink', combined with the pills or medicines so readily available on prescription, or off-the-shelf, are the main causes of much of the illness and ailments with which we are plagued. Much of the synthetic drugs and the chemicals in the food chain can harm our body systems and health, as highlighted in this Encyclopedia. A natural food Diet, combined with supplements where necessary, allied to exercise and regular sleep pattern, is the keystone, the foundation to better health and well-being".

I have purposely left until the end of this caption to tell you what I believe to be probably the greatest Diet ever devised. This is the HAY DIET, which is explained under caption in this Encyclopedia. If I needed to use a SLIMMING DIET this would be the weight-watching guide for me. Those who have used it to enable them lose weight swear by it. It can be of extreme benefit to health of body and mind. *See HAY DIET caption.*

DIETING

Many thousands of books and much else have been written about Diet and Dieting. There is a difference. Diet is what you eat. Dieting is very much about what not to eat. *Over the years we've heard of the many slimming diets including: Zone, Atkins, Herbalife, Pritikan, Jenny Craig, Scarsdale, the Fruit Only, Vegetable, Soup, Grape and countless others. Many are contradictory. Like pop stars they have their time, then being forgotten about. All have made good money for the originator.* Jason Vale, author of 'Slim 4 Life', says: "Dieting can have a negative effect on the figure, starving the body and so making you fatter". How many realise this? Imagine a Diet of jelly, pork burgers, strawberry shake and other additive-filled foods as championed by one best selling prime mover. In this and many others the idiocy of such drivel, containing ill-advised views, is lamentable.

Good health must come first, before accepting the much-hyped foolish opinions of those whose interests are purely monetary. The best-sellers list shows up the gullibility of all-too-many that purchase the publications about Slimming and Dieting.

One of the oldest methods of losing weight, also being extremely health giving, is that of eating half a grapefruit twice daily. Recent research tells us what was known well over a century ago, that grapefruit is a good slimming aid. *See Grapefruit caption.*

There is no quick-fix remedy, no magical results. A huge amount of the advice given for these fad Diets can be harmful to health.

The Atkins Diet is an example of all that is wrong in what can rightly be referred to as the slimming industry. Many including Dietetic and Nutrition Associations, also those who liase with them, have condemned this promotion of red meat and saturated fats in what is a low carbohydrate diet, which is so serious that the Food Standards Agency thought fit to issue a warning against it. The gurus behind the Atkins Diet then had the nerve, call it shamelessness, to suddenly warn Dieters to limit their intake of the meat and saturated fat which they have recommended. The latter contains the waxy substance cholesterol, which raising its levels in the blood, leads to heart disease and obesity. *How can these people change their minds, then get away with it, after lining the bookshelves with their best-selling, questionable, or open to doubt publications, which are varying. Consider the millions made at the expense of those who have been all-too-easily taken in, with the health of many being jeopardised. It must be added that the reply from Atkins tells us that they wanted the health experts to: "Feel comfortable with this Diet". What about the partakers? All this, over 12 years from the time of launching the Diet. What about all those who have put their invaluable health at stake throughout this time? To the writer, whose ideas and proof of good health by actual Diet are at the opposite end of the scale to Atkins, 'this is an indictable offence'.*

Willpower in this kind of scenario only produces short-term change, at a cost, health- wise, as it creates constant stress, not having dealt with the root cause of the problem. The change is not natural, so eventually one gives up, goes off the 'Diet', stops exercising, loses interest, reverting to the old ways.

As they get older, many can look back on the attempts made to have a curvaceous figure, the realization of the foolish thoughts, also the time and money put into something, which did not work. ***Few realize that there are those - thin or fat, buxom or rotund, with large bony frame or petite skeleton, where it is impossible to attain what to their mind is par excellence, better than all others. Do you who seek this skinniness, realize that apart from being extremely obese, hardly anybody is interested in how you appear? Most men will tell you they like a healthy, jolly, well-rounded woman, happy, relaxed and with a sense of humour.***

Proper nutritious, additive-free food and drinks, as set out in DIET caption of this Encyclopedia, added to Exercise and proper Sleep pattern, also captioned, will provide the partaker with a healthy body and resultant well-being. Proportion your body and your Diet by thinking, eating and drinking natural. As an insurance against increased weight one can add two teaspoons of each Cider vinegar (Aspells) and pure Honey mixed with tepid water. Also take Helix Slim (Bioforce), Kelp tablets, Lecithin granules and a good natural Multivitamin tablet. Visit your health food shop, ask questions, be advised about all the natural products available, none of which will increase weight, many doing the opposite. *See Diet, Slimming also Detoxing captions.*

DIGESTIVE PROBLEMS

Digestion begins in the mouth with the food being ground by the teeth. *Many do not take time over their food, not sitting comfortably, relaxing, eating slowly and deliberately, and chewing every mouthful properly. Otherwise than this, plays havoc with the digestive system. As with their bodies, the majority takes the digestive system for granted.* The food enters through a tube to the body, which factory-wise processes it, from where the nutrients are transferred or carried to the relevant systems. Space in this Encyclopedia, with its many captions, does not permit further description of this wonderful mechanism, which is all too often subjected to abuse and neglect.

To be free from digestive problems, a proper Diet of natural nutritious additive free food, as under DIET caption, is important, being the foundation for better health. Eat regular meals. Breakfast is not to be skipped. Avoid foods that cause allergic reaction such as dairy products, packaged meat, which usually contains additives, also coffee, alcohol, vinegar, spices, fried foods and anything containing fibre which must be avoided until one gets the digestive system back to normal. Food supplements, which aid the system are: Enzyme Digest, Lecithin granules, Vitamin B Complex, Iceland Moss, Charcoal, Molkosan, Slippery Elm or Royal Jelly. Some with milk allergy may still take milk by using Lactase. Most digestive problems are listed under their various headings such as constipation, indigestion, diarrhoea, loss of appetite, gastritis etc. As advised proper Diet of natural foods is the important medicine and if one eats pure foods daily there will be little or no indigestion with no need for remedy, synthetic or other.

DIVERTICULOSIS, DIVERTICULITIS

These are colon problems with both being treated as one. The former is milder and with no inflammation, which if not diagnosed early on leads to the latter. This ailment can be helped enormously by proper nutritious Diet of natural non-processed foods, aided by food supplements and herbal remedies. This may appear somewhat contradictory, simply because the non-use of fibre or roughage over a period of time has caused the problem. The medical profession will say that fibre must not be taken until such time as the inflammation has been overcome. Doctor George Thosteson, a medical journalist, is in agreement with many natural therapists when he writes: *"It was formerly assumed that roughage should be kept to a minimum in the diet of diverticulitis. Now it appears that this is not the wisest course. Patients are better-off with a moderate amount of bulk, since there is less stress when the colon is comfortably full"*

Avoid bran, taking fine oatmeal porridge instead, which can be as softish. To help alleviate and banish the diverticulitis take Slippery Elm, Manuka honey, oatmeal porridge as soft fibre, mashed banana, pureed steamed carrots, swede and boiled potato. Food supplements and natural aids are: Udo's Choice Oil, Fennel, Tormintil, Vitamin B Complex, and Folic Acid. Only when the inflammation has been eliminated can a slow return be made to full Diet. It is sometimes necessary to eliminate milk and other dairy products or even glutenous foods such as wheat and other grain products. With discipline and caution one can live with diverticulitis, often finally eliminating it. Improper Diet and extremely hot food and drink are often the cause of the problem in the first instance therefore extra vigilance is needed. *See DIET also Allergy captions.*

DIZZINESS

Here is one of the leading complaints for which doctor's advice is sought. It is an inner ear problem, with no easy diagnosis as to why affected. Often occurs on jumping out of bed, walking, or when you stand up quickly, resulting in brief drop in amount of blood flowing to the brain. Other causes are: low blood sugar, anaemia, stress, and tiredness, being over-warm or poor circulation. A half-teaspoon of ground Cinnamon twice daily helps regulate blood sugar. Other natural aids are Floradix or Floravital tonic, Ginkgo Biloba or Vitamin B Complex. Shiatsu therapy has proved to be an excellent remedy. If the dizziness persists see your doctor, as there may be circulatory or other problems to be treated accordingly.

DOCTORS AND GP'S

The use of conventional or synthetic medicine has almost got out of hand. Where the doctor was the family doctor, just that, without the lure of big money and modern day management, with resultant pressures, almost all had this quiet, shall we call it bedside manner? Today the practitioner is not alone pressurised, besieged by his patients, but also by so many in the drug industry that have vested interests. Public bodies, health boards, research laboratories, the drug companies and many others allied to medicine now aim at directing their lives. The evidence of suicide is high amongst the medical profession. They too should be told to slow down to make life easier for themselves. It is extremely difficult to do so when the vast monetary rewards beckon.

What a pity the natural and the synthetic cannot come together to practise their medicinal knowledge and skills. To most of the medical profession anything natural is anathema. As my doctor friend told me: "We were taught nothing about natural Diet or remedies or indeed any kind of Diet". I have much respect for the medical profession especially my good doctor friends. There is a 'BUT'. Many of them adopt this superior, defensive, almost arrogant, 'Holier than thou attitude', with little time for the patient. The bedside manner practiced in days past is almost gone from the hurried life lived by the profession, as they charge headlong in the pursuit of financial gain, often giving little time to the patient. *As well as doctors being taught nothing about the greatest medicine known, a Diet of pure natural food and drink, neither are they trained about what it feels like to be a patient, something they should b~*   *v aware of. They are seldom receptive to ideas from circle. This is particularly so with regard to anything* ctors in the surgery or health centre, with their quick-fire for the prescription pad - their cash till – before even person.   Many who visit are not physically ill, requiring id, including reassurance. Some are afraid of the doctor, who visitor is seldom given the opportunity to discuss the health *y patients know more about what is wrong than the*

practitioner does. It is time most doctors and GPs took stock of themselves and began listening more to their patients. ***They need to look into the mind as if it were a mirror.*** This is what the alternative therapist does.

The medical profession, the pharmacist, also the high-flying multimillion drug industry, should remember that modern chemical synthetic medicine only came into being a little over a century ago.

The over-prescribing of antibiotics has at last been admitted to. It has also been admitted that much of what is turned out by the pharmaceutical conglomerates is of little use. Despite all this, it is prescribed almost willy-nilly. It must be repeated and the message got across that the immune system of many people is being destroyed. It cannot be replaced.

Admittedly it is not all the fault of the learned GP, because often the patient has no idea what is wrong and cannot or will not explain. ***Those who seek treatment should be more open with their practitioner, giving all the facts and truthful answers to the questions asked. In many instances the knowledgeable doctor, who knows best and suggests that the infection or ailment will clear up, is coerced or forced by the parent or other, insisting on a prescription for antibiotics to treat themselves or the person they accompany. Many think there is a pill for all illness, not realizing the harm of antibiotics or the long- term consequences of synthetic medicine.*** At the same time the patient, the customer, who is responsible for keeping the doctor in a job, should assert the right to proper treatment, being in no awe of the person they are seeking advice from. Ask questions, refuse to be fobbed off, demand answers to help solve the problem. The GP will have all the more respect for you as he realizes your earnestness. Very often a simple blood test gives the answer regarding much of the ailments so prevalent. Few would even think of demanding that this be done.

We always seem to hear criticism about our health service. Much of this could be avoided if only we were more careful about what we eat and drink, including the use of synthetic medicines and pills, all too easily available, also the need to take exercise and maintain a proper sleep pattern. Seldom do we hear of the good being done by the medical profession, especially our surgeons, specialists, nurses and all those at the hub of what is being done to correct the diseases brought upon those who have, in most cases, only themselves to blame.

Speaking with a doctor friend recently we talked about how the older person, would seek help for an ailment, mental or physical. Time will be spent, with diagnosis made and advice given, including prescribing of what is thought to be the necessary aid to better health. The patient, whether because of age or other quirk, is not for changing and does nothing to change the habits or lifestyle, conveying the medicines home and then refusing to take them. Both of us agreed that: 'There are none so blind as those with vision who cannot see.'

Those who have had reason to visit a doctor have told much of what I relate here, to me over the years. The majority were women who were afraid of the GP, not being prepared to stand up to those by whom they felt intimidated. A little niceness goes a long way to helping, especially if feeling unwell, whether mentally or physically.

Figures reveal that Irish doctors received over €6 million for treating 40,000 'ghost' patients. The majority of them were dead. Here is an 'indictable offence' with no action being taken. Their Trade Union, the autocratic Medical Organisation, has refused to repay the monies. If this were done by a layperson, prosecution would probably follow.

Two elderly women were with me recently. Both told of how they enjoyed good health through exercise and partaking of natural foods. One asked me: "What is the difference between the doctor and God". I replied that I did not know. The second lady raised her voice to reply: "God does not think he is a doctor, but many doctors think they are God"

DOG

My greatest aid to physical fitness and to discipline me to take regular, by this I mean daily exercise, is the Dog. Here is a friend, one who does not answer me back, who looks me straight in the eyes, who understands my language, including the word 'walkies'. Owning a Dog has many advantages and good features. You cannot avoid the daily walk for several reasons, chief of which is a sad or bored look in the eyes, or the fierce bark. Look after your friend and his trust and devotion, allied to the exercise, will repay you richly.

DRINKING CONTAINER

Always drinking from the same glass, cup or mug helps to prevent the spread of cold, 'flu or other germs.

DROPSY

See Oedema Caption.

DROWSINESS

Mentioned here, with a word of advice, from one who has often been effected. If driving, stop and have a wash with cold water. Breathe deeply for several minutes. If it occurs later be warned, pull off the road and have a rest. Sometimes 10 or 15 minutes are sufficient. Do not persevere hoping it will go away. **Remember lives can be at stake.** Many who feel drowsy at work, while driving, or at other times, will not admit to a lack of sleep, where the pattern of it is often bad. Insufficient and improper sequence of sleep is detrimental to health and concentration. *Turn to Sleep caption.*

DRUG THERAPY

The medical profession freely admits that there is an over-reliance on drug therapy, with far too much dependency. *We are informed, that fewer than half the patients prescribed some of the most expensive drugs, derive no benefit from them.* The excuse put forward is that the genes in the patient interfere with the medicine, and this is why it does not work. This comes from one of the Chief Executives of a multi-national drug company. He has been honest enough to inform us. Then we find others of his medical profession colleagues who are openly critical of this person who has told us the truth. *Nowhere do they stand up and tell us either the short or the long-term effects of these unnatural drugs or medicines. It is obvious that the main objective of all this is money for all concerned. All too often the health of the prescribee, yes that of the nation, is irrelevant. We are entitled to ask: "Is the relationship between the drug companies and the medical profession too cosy?"* We hear of new guidelines, but like many of the new rules and laws enacted, who will police them? THE MERRY-GO-ROUND WILL CONTINUE. If only the medical profession were taught much about pure natural additive-free food and Diet there would be less need for medicine, especially the off-the- shelf, prescription-free chemicals, the majority of which can often be harmful to that intricate system, which is the human body. The Pharmaceutical Society openly admits that there is abuse and misuse of over the counter drugs. Codeine is mentioned also antihistamine containing products and analgesics. To police the matter would be difficult, one could add impossible. *Turn to the 'Food', 'Drinks', Pharmaceutical Drugs and Health Service Merry-go-Round chapter in opening pages of this Encyclopedia.*

DRY MOUTH

See Mouth Caption.

DRY SKIN

See Skin Caption.

DUODENAL ULCERS

See Ulcers Caption.

D.V.T.

See Deep Vein Thrombosis Caption.

DYSLEXIA

There is much misunderstanding about this learning problem, which often results in students and those who are affected, not making it known that they have a difficulty. They have a different way of learning, therefore there is a need for a different method of teaching and appraisal. Studies show that males are affected up to four times more than females. Dyslexia is seldom a sign of low intelligence. A homeopathic doctor told me that the problem could be overcome by introducing the HAY DIET and that he had obtained excellent results through its use. I have also spoken with students and their parents who acknowledged the good health regained through use of the Hay Diet for Dyslexia treatment. Supplement this by adding a children's Multivitamin, because children have a need for valuable nutrients such as Vitamins C & E also Calcium, Iron and Zinc. Also suggested is Udo's Choice Oil, which is a blend of Omega Oils, adding with Lecithin Granules to cereals or porridge. All foods should be pure, natural and non- processed. Lecithin is an excellent brain food, having many other health-giving properties. *Turn to Brain Health caption.*

DYSMENORRHOEA

See Menstruation Caption.

DYSPEPSIA

See Indigestion Caption.

DYSPNOEA

See Breathlessness Caption.

DYSURIA

See Urinary Problems Caption.

E VITAMIN

See Vitamins and Minerals caption

EARS

During the lifetime of a person various Ear problems arise. Two things, which are vital for Ear health, also better hearing, are often ignored. One is the need to periodically have the Ears examined for wax and to have it removed, if present. Many have continued through life with what was a hearing problem, which could so easily have been put right. Number two is seldom taken into account and that is Diet. Inferior Diet is the major reason for heart and circulation problems. Hearing loss and inner ear symptoms are often a lead up to heart disease, which includes arteriosclerosis. Seldom will a doctor diagnose this, and even if it were, one doubts if a change to pure natural nutritious food would be prescribed. *See DIET caption and be guided by the advice given.* Suggested remedies for ear troubles are:

- Earache with burning throbbing sensation: Ferr Phos.
- Earache with noise in head: Kali Phos.
- Earache in children: Alternate Kali Sulph with Calc Phos or take Pulsatilla tablets or tincture.
- Catarrh in middle ear: Plantago or Ferr Phos.
- Humming in ear: Nat Mur.
- Diminished hearing: Mag Phos.
- Glueear: Plantago.
- Middle Ear infection, known as Otitis Media, is very often tied into allergy to dairy products or to eggs, especially the whites. Doctors seldom suspect or advise about this as they suggest the all too often over prescribed antibiotics.

Pulsatilla drops are a universal Earache remedy.

Quite often simple Ear problems have been solved by holding nostrils (i.e. pinching), opening the mouth as if to take a deep breath or yawn, then vigorously blowing the nose, or by treating with Ear drops by piercing a Vitamin E capsule and putting into Ear. *Turn to Noise also Hearing captions*

EARS RINGING

See Tinnitus Caption.

EATING

'You are what you eat'. If all were to take this adage to heart, abiding by or conforming to it, partaking of only pure natural additive free foods and drinks also taking exercise, there would be much less call for medicine. Natural foods can be termed 'live foods'. When eating, relax, eat slowly, masticate and chew properly to enjoy food and the benefits. Eat in moderation, exercising self-control. Don't mix foods that fight because here is one of the chief reasons for indigestion and stomach problems. *See Hay Diet caption* if you have continuous digestive problems, combining the advice given with the partaking of natural additive free foods. Eat small meals regularly rather than one large meal in the evening. This is very important, as it helps to keep the blood sugar levels balanced and constant. Having a salad starter or a side salad lays a good foundation for the digestive system to work from. Fresh fruit and vegetables should be the consideration of all main meals. Practice the rule of fish, meat, eggs, and cheese to be eaten every fourth day. Food produced locally is best, especially organic. Much of that marketed has come from abroad, often being anything but fresh. Eat pure, live well. *See DIET, Food Pyramid also Fruit and Vegetables captions.*

ECHINACEA

Echinacea is one of our greatest natural remedies and preventatives. It's uses as a tonic, detoxer, antiseptic, blood purifier, natural and therefore non-toxic antibiotic, alterative and much more are renowned. A super remedy to help banish microbial infections, including boils, septicaemia, also for relief of respiratory tract problems such as laryngitis, catarrh and sinus. Can be used on cuts and sores as a lotion. It is a stimulant for the immune system. If small children dislike the drops give them Echinacea lozenges. As an anti cold and flu remedy it is a wonder herb. There are three types of Echinacea. Purpurea is regarded as best. *When asked, as I often am 'Should I have the flu injection'? My reply is, 'Echinaceaforce has never failed me for cold or flu'.* I have prescribed it many times, to be taken from early October to March. I have yet to see one who used it diligently have cold or flu. Echinacea should not be taken if with Asthma or Diabetes.

ECZEMA

There are many types of Eczema such as wet, dry, children's, teenagers, fungal, infants and those bordering on dermatitis. It is vital to search for the root cause of the Eczema. For instance infantile Eczema is almost always as a result of milk allergy. Breast fed children seldom have this problem. The need for pure, natural, additive free Diet, as promoted in this Guide, is emphasised. If an allergy is suspected suspend all dairy or gluten products for seven/ten days, then re-enter them one by one to the Diet to find out what the allergy is. *See Allergy caption.* Children who change to goat's milk often have the problem banished within days. Chickweed Ointment as an external application has proved to be good

Other natural remedies, which have helped remove Eczema, are Udo's Choice Oil or Evening Primrose Oil Extra Strength, Combination D New Era, with Kali Sulph Tissue Salts. Also in conjunction with additive free natural food take a slow release Multivitamin tablet. The wonder of nettles as an Eczema remedy is not appreciated. *Turn to Nettles caption.* Take four to six tablets of Effamol Evening Primrose Oil high strength daily. Low doses are ineffective.

Often with the use of natural remedies and change of eating habits there has been vast improvement, bringing freedom from skin problems in a very short time, even after a few days. In some instances it has taken weeks of perseverance and discipline to eliminate the Eczema, because it may take some time for the body to detox, when natural foods are introduced. *See DIET caption.*

EFA

See Essential Fatty Acids Caption.

EGGS

A good food, giving protein. Free range Eggs, twice every eight days, is the recommendation to add to a well-balanced Diet of natural foods and drinks.

ELBOW

Puffed or swollen elbow can be treated as Synovitis.

EMOTIONAL IMBALANCE

See Nervous Exhaustion Caption.

EMPHYSEMA

This bronchial progressive respiratory disease is indicated by shortness of breath, repeated chest infections, also tiredness. The chief factors acknowledged are smoking and chronic bronchitis. Why apparently sensible people smoke is beyond understanding? The use of tobacco products is taboo. Change to pure natural additive free Diet has helped, also avoiding dairy products. Supplement daily with Vitamins A, C and E also Kelp, Echinacea and Folic Acid, or take a good Multivitamin tablet. Regular exercise such as cycling or walking in fresh air is strongly advised. *See DIET and Exercise captions.*

Exercise caption advises the need to speak with your doctor about this discipline if on medication.

ENDOMETRITIS

Remedies are Helonias, Echinacea and Agnus Castus.

ENERGY DRINKS

Any intelligent person reading the ingredients labels on these chemical filled unnatural 'drinks' would avoid them. Water mixed with sugar would be equally as good, giving short time boost and eventually leading to ill health. There is nothing better than cool clear water to refresh the thirst. Properly balanced and energy giving supplements such as Spirulina would prove much more beneficial and healthy than the many so called 'energy drinks' which are on offer. Sports personalities are paid enormous sums to promote these over sweetened liquids. Fizzy Energy or Soft 'drinks' are not worthy of further comment except to emphasise their dangers to health of body and mind. *See Fizzy 'Drinks' caption.*

ENTERITIS

See Gastroenteritis Caption.

EPILEPSY

Complementary therapies can help one to deal with the problem. Three things, which I have recognised as being of immense help are Diet, Acupuncture and Aromatherapy. Include in the Diet, as suggested in this guide, plenty of raw fruit, also fruit and vegetable juices. Obtaining a good juicer and juice recipe book will never be regretted. Change of lifestyle often helps. Many do not obtain enough sleep. Yoga is a wonderful form of exercise for mind and body. Acupuncture therapy friends speak of successful treatment where patients were disciplined to take the full course. Avoid stress and emotional problems. *See Yoga, Sleep and DIET captions*

EPHEDRA

One of the few herbs to be avoided. It is not written about or recommended in this guide.

EPISTAXIS

See Nosebleed Caption.

ERECTION OR ERECTILE PROBLEMS

This is known medically as Erectile Dysfunction. *Most men are notorious for disregarding anything pertaining to illness or good health. This is a fiercely broad ranging statement, sadly all too true. They regard themselves as being tough, resilient, with the idea being it 'can't happen to me'. They are reluctant to either complain or seek medical advice. This is entirely wrong.* All-too-often I have seen the consequences of this Manish attitude.

There can be many reasons for Erectile Problems. With reasonably good health, man's sexual interest and activity should be life-long. When the problem arises it can be due to heart or circulatory problems, diabetes, aging process, smoking, often being psychological due to stress, depression or worry.

Synthetic medication is often the cause of the problem. *We are now told of the dangers of Viagra in relation to infertility. Within hours we are told that this is alarmist and to continue taking it. The latter comes from somebody in the Viagra camp. Here is an example of where mistrust is best. If in doubt leave out.* Erectile and sexual problems can be treated by some of the complementary therapies listed in this guide. The repeated theme of a natural balanced Diet, with supplement aid, can lead to better health and a zest for life, helping to eliminate stress, worry and psychological problems. *Turn to DIET caption.* Orthodox medicines, including Viagra and others, also injections into the penis, as prescribed by a doctor, may be at a cost other than monetary. None are aware of the health consequences, long or short-term.

For those who have not been able to reverse the problem there is a truly natural remedy or therapy. Rapport tm Premier, is a unique vacuum therapy system, specifically developed as a user friendly, effective treatment for Erectile Problems. It does not involve the use of drugs. With its unique and easy natural pumping, Rapport tm Premier creates a vacuum around the penis. This quickly produces a satisfactory erection by drawing blood into the penis. The pump is then removed, leaving the ring at the base of the penis. This will maintain a firm erection for up to thirty minutes. Unlike drugs, Rapport tm may be used over and over again, as often as required. Because Vacuum therapy means a man does not have to take any drugs, there is no risk of interaction with any existing medications he may be taking.

Rapport tm Premier is available on prescription for patients suffering from specified medical conditions. For people outside of this category, it can be purchased from Owen Mumford Ltd., Brook Hill, Woodstock, Oxfordshire OX20 1TU. Tel 01993 812021 Fax 01993 813466. There are other somewhat similar vacuum therapy aids available, but I have no hesitation in recommending the Rapport tm Premier. Before starting any treatment for Erectile Dysfunction ask your doctor if your heart is healthy enough to handle the extra strain or joy of having sex. *Very seldom will the medical profession, or those who write about Erectile Problems, bring to the attention of the public this type of natural aid. All-too-many suffer from tunnel vision as they prescribe drugs, many of them harmful to health.*

ERYSIPELAS

homeopathic doctors can treat successfully.

ESSENTIAL FATTY ACIDS. (EFAs)
See Fatty Acids Caption.

ESSENTIAL OILS
See Aromatherapy Caption.

EVENING PRIMROSE OIL (EPO)
Here is another of nature's aids to better health and well being. It comes from the seeds of the Evening Primrose plant, being so called because it's flowers open at dusk. The key ingredient is Gamma Linolenic Acid (GLA), which in the body is used in the production of important prostaglandins, which regulate the menstrual cycle, immune system, circulation and blood. The hormone type of substances which are prostaglandins regulate the power of sex hormones. It is a woman's friend, being a valuable aid for PMS, menstruation also the menopause. It is an aid to banish eczema and acne also to maintain healthy skin. Being anti-inflammatory it is good for arthritis, rheumatism and joint pains. Helps asthma. Like most natural remedies, supplements, vitamins and minerals, the real or true goodness of Evening Primrose Oil comes about in conjunction with partaking of natural Diet. Pure unprocessed additive free food and EPO work wonders health wise. 'Enfamol' is arguably the brand, which has pioneered the research into this priceless herbal remedy. Ask for high strength EPO. Those who suffer from epilepsy must not take Evening Primrose Oil.

EXAM NERVES (FEVER)
Pure natural, additive-free Diet of food and drink lays a foundation for the elimination of the problem. Supplements are Bach Flower Rescue Remedy, Ginkgo Biloba also the tonics Biostrath or Floradix. The tissue salt Kali Phos is also very good for mental faculties and exam nerves. *See DIET caption,* with the advice given, leading to better health of body and brain.

EXERCISE
When told we must Exercise regularly, the reaction of many is of a feeling of something difficult, evoking ideas of a gymnasium, weight lifting or training, repetitive workouts, squats, press ups or other exertion. This may all appear as being difficult and over-tiring to those who are unfit, being regarded as worse than hard work. Don't falter here. Read on, because my idea of Exercise is that it should be enjoyable. ***Many who have been active participants in sport as well as those who have never competed, become almost lazy, using the simplest excuses to put off any form of Exercise from day to day, or week to week. All too many who will not admit to it become couch potatoes.***

Before the advent of the motorcar people walked or cycled. They were Exercising in order to get about. Now TV, the computer and of course the motor cars are enemies of reasonable health, as all too many sit in their comfortable seats. The word couch potato, quite new to our vocabulary, is very apt. *Many, especially the young, are grossly at risk of injurious health, taking little or no Exercise. Children should be encouraged to do so. Perhaps their parents should be too.* Now few walk to or from school, having little if any chores to carry out at home, principally because of all the modern conveniences available, with the majority not interested in or involved in sport or team games. If the rigours of Exercise are not instilled into the youth, who can blame them for opting for an idle life, dare one say lazy. Added to this almost dilatory way of life, is the kind of food and drinks, which our youth and many adults are fed. Much of it is processed, sugary, also flavour enhanced, with a vast amount of it being of little nutrition, leading to obesity. This is for a later subject. Exercise or lack of it is the problem. *Before deciding to Exercise, strenuously or otherwise, those with heart or other serious health problem must speak with their doctor. One can take the matter of Exercise too seriously. It must be enjoyable and not undue or excessive.*

Three things, which lead to better health are Diet, Exercise and Sleep which are paramount to better health and can be found under relevant captions. Exercise we will concern ourselves with here. Yes – don't falter now. Read on, and when you combine the Diet and the Exercise together you arrive at something, which is an exhilarating feeling of goodness.

An energetic 84 year-old woman whom I know well and who was extremely ill over twenty- five years ago, now enjoys good health. She could be taken for a person of 60, as she gave her recipe for health, attitude and outlook on life. On rising each morning she stands in front of open door or window, doing some breathing Exercises or deep breathing, also some gentle stretching and loosening up Exercises for three or four minutes. Her Diet consists of natural meals, with breakfast of porridge and two slices of wholemeal bread being a priority. Added to this for one week were food supplements consisting of a Multivitamin tablet also Udo's Choice Balanced Omega 3 and 6 Oils. The following week she took that wonderful natural tonic Floravital, alternating each week as set out. Rain or shine she took a brisk walk of 35/45 minutes duration. She spoke of the need to be properly attired and of wearing comfortable walking shoes. She told of how she had trainers, which she discarded, maintaining they were no good for the health of her feet. Her dog is her constant companion.

Exercise can be as hard or as simple as you wish to make it. No matter how unfit one is it can be pleasant and satisfying provided it is not overdone. As pointed out 'Pace Yourself, Enjoy Yourself.' Not alone can you become physically fit, but in so doing you will feel a whole range of improvements in your daily pursuits, being stronger, with better circulation, clearer brain, with improved good feeling towards others, also being a better person in many ways. Exercise can be tailored to meet your needs, according to how mobile you are, or as to how energetic you feel. Just pick out whatever you like or might enjoy and get with it. Physical activity helps to keep the blood pumping or circulating, which in turn acts like anti-inflammatory drugs, helping to prevent narrowing of the veins and arteries. Inflammation is a major factor in heart disease, being linked to atheroma and heart problems.

Did you ever hear of a doctor giving a prescription for Exercise, with change to Diet of pure and natural food, for a health problem? It cannot be registered or patented as a medicine, so there is nothing in it monetary wise for either the drug companies or the medical profession. It is one of many free prescriptions, which could be issued. Many need to change their lifestyle, Diet or manner of living.

If you have the time and wish to play golf or squash, do so. The latter can be extra strenuous. Also for the energetic, there are organised sports; such as aerobics, running, jogging, tennis, cycling, the gymnasium or other physical activity. Age, health, weight, also mobility must be taken into consideration before deciding.

Writing about Exercise here is done with the idea of improving ones state of health. Therefore if you so desire there is no need to take up anything more difficult than will tone your body, will have your heart beating a bit faster, not too much so, that you are warmed up, but not overly so. *When Exercising you should at all times be able to converse without undue pressure.*

Many with injuries to legs, joints, or muscles, have come to me for treatment. Some who exercise, perhaps do so too severely. There are easy ways of keeping fit. Walking costs nothing except for outlay on comfortable, good-supporting sensible footwear, together with loose fitting protective clothing.

If walking after dark wear reflective clothing. Be highly visible, especially in the headlights of motor vehicles.

A walking stick to which easily obtained reflective adhesive tape has been affixed is as a companion. Few realise the need to keep all parts of the body warm when taking Exercise or the need to be well clothed to keep the muscles warm. This keeps them lubricated, so helping to attain fitness quicker, apart from the fact that there is less danger of muscle damage. It is most annoying to see a person out training or when jogging or running, have bared legs and arms exposed to what is often cold and inclement weather. They would be just as well off to sit at home and forget about Exercise. Fewer still are unaware of the need to keep the head warm, this being an area where much body heat is lost. This is probably one of the reasons for so many sniffling and sneezing throughout the winter months. Seldom does one see hat or cap worn. *Yoga is very much more than just an Exercise. It can control all*

...spects of health, both mentally and physically, even though it is gentle Exercise. There are various types of Yoga.

Read the Walking and Yoga captions in this guide to learn the benefits of these easy workouts.

One might pose the question: "What is there to learn about Walking". Reading the caption on walking you will be surprised to find that you have discovered something new. We are told, one could say warned, almost every day of the need for Exercise and proper Diet. *It can be condensed into a few words.* <u>*To improve and to attain reasonable good health we must take natural foods, exercise and have a regular sleep pattern.*</u>

EXERCISE BICYCLES AND TREADMILLS.

There are compact Exercise Bicycles and Treadmills available for use in the home. They can be adjusted to ones own pace and speed of walking or cycling. The tempo can be regulated with speedo, energy use and other gadgets attached to help the enjoyment. One can listen to the radio, music or watch TV while putting in the miles. Keeping a logbook of the fun run or cycle ride can be interesting when the workout pages are reviewed. Skipping is another form of indoor exercise. It can be extremely good for young people. One seldom sees a skipping rope in use now. Is this another sign of the couch potato era?.

EXHAUSTION

See under respective headings, Nervous Exhaustion, Fatigue, Jetlag, Lethargy and Tiredness.

EYES

Many just take their faculties, including the Eyes and vision, for granted. They must be looked after, being precious possessions. They must be fed, exercised, relaxed, palmed and appreciated. *See Bates Method caption.* Prevention of optical problems is the easy way to good Eye health. Excellent aids are the Multivitamin Visionace, specially formulated for eye health, also pure carrot juice taken daily. *See Juices caption.* Keeping the Eyes exercised is very necessary. From the Bates caption you will learn how to obtain information on Eye Health including the necessary exercise. **Bilberries or pure Bilberry Juice and Vitamin C are to the eyes as pure nutritious food is to the body.**

Remedies are;

- Baggy Eyes: Often caused by kidney problems. Drink Parsley Tea also plenty of liquids.
- Blepheritis: Evening Primrose Oil. Ferr Phos.
- Blood Shot: Ferr Phos and Silica alternated.
- Cataracts: I have witnessed many cases where Manuka honey warmed to

make it viscous, then placed as drops in the eyes removes the cataracts. This to be done for four or five nights before retiring to bed. An optician friend states that whatever substance is in the pure honey breaks the film covering the eye, this being the cataract. Other opticians have verified this. Manuka Honey is available at any good health food store.

- Conjunctivitis: (As if grit under the eyelids). Aloe Vera gel, white of egg or Ferr Phos.
- Hordelum: *See Stye caption.*
- Iritis and Macular Degeneration: Very often due to inferior Diet. *Turn to DIET caption.* This can be aided by taking a Multivitamin, also Nat Phos and Echinacea.
- Macular Degeneration: This occurs as grey or blurred spot in the field of vision, usually in the centre of it. There may be wavy lines, with printed word being blurred or with objects being proportionally out of size or shape. If with any of these symptoms, see optician immediately. People with blue or blue/green eyes are more prone than others to the disease. Antioxidants and nutritious food are preventatives and can also help if with Macular Degeneration. *Turn to Antioxidants also Diet captions.* Be guided by your optician or ophthalmologist, to whom you will probably be referred.
- Night blindness: Vitamin A.
- Tired Eyes: Bathe with tepid tea.
- Eyes watery: Nat Mur.
- Eyelid twitching: Codeinum 6c.
- Twitching in Eyelid and Eyeball: Agaricus 6c. Twitching is a sign of Magnesium deficiency, which can be taken in tablet form.
- Inflammation of Eyelids: Pulsatilla 6c.
- Glaucoma prevention: The serious Eye problem of Glaucoma can come on without warning and vision loss from the disease cannot be repaired. Some on being questioned admit to not having had Eye tests for up to three or four years. This is a serious mistake.
- Short-sightedness (Myopia) We are told that short-sightedness could soon reach epidemic proportions because children and young adults are spending too much time looking at television screens and playing computer games.

With all bodily health and this includes the Eyes, pure food DIET is all-important.

It is imperative to pay regular visits to the optician for check-up in order to help eliminate or treat eye problems. Look after your Eyes and be rewarded handsomely.

F VITAMIN

See Vitamins and Minerals Caption.

FAINTING

Medical term is Syncope. It occurs due to blood supply to the brain being insufficient. Experienced sometimes on rising suddenly from a sitting position. It often happens after standing for long periods, to those who are unfit, after illness or if with sedentary habits. It can occur through fright or after physical injury. Avoid prolonged hot baths. To treat, loosen clothing, including collar, also belt around waist. Do not force liquids down the throat as choking may occur. Fainting often happens in teenagers who are growing quickly. Recovery takes place quickly and without any apparent ill effects. It is associated with a shortage of vitamins and minerals, therefore proper natural Diet, aided by food supplements, can help correct the problem. A good tonic is suggested. *Turn to Tonic also DIET captions* and be guided.

FARMERS LUNG

Occurs when the lungs are exposed to the spores or dust of mouldy hay, straw or grain. Allergens must be avoided. See your doctor who will arrange X-ray. Fresh air, pure natural nutritious food, also the natural remedies, Echinacea, Garlic and Iceland Moss are all aids for the illness. Homeopathic doctors have much to offer by way of relief. Prevention is all-important by use of dust mask.

FAST 'FOODS'

Most Fast 'Foods' are junk food, so for convenience sake (no pun intended) both are treated as one. Almost all are of little or no nutritional value, containing additives, including bulking agents, fillers and chemicals. They should be shunned, not to be written about except to be publicised in order to expose the harm. Here is one of the chief causes of obesity, also of our present day ill health, including various niggling ailments, many of which lead to something more serious. *The remarkable chef Georgio Locatelli sums it up well: "I think that food is a very serious thing and people should pay a little more attention to what they eat." He said: "People who spend two hours choosing a pair of shoes would then spend 30*

seconds cooking their dinner in a microwave".
The majority have no idea what is in the fast 'foods', or of their dangers to health.

Examples of how big business places the monetary result first and the health of what they sell nowhere, is the research which has gone into designing bun and burger which needs little if any chewing as it slips down. As with the makeup of much of the stuff on offer, including coke and other fizzy or caffeine drinks, the partaker seeks more, not knowing when to stop. Obesity and very often ill health can be the result. ***Most Fast foods should be avoided.***
The attraction of the palate to chips and crisps can be dangerous. Even simple food like breakfast cereals do not escape the money-orientated processor. Some have up to 30 ingredients, many of them unnatural, being of little food value. Read the ingredients labels, leaving the additive-filled undesirables on the shelf, including those with added synthetic vitamins and minerals. If the 'foods' were wholesome these additives would not be needed. Almost daily we hear criticism of burgers, fast 'foods' and fizzy 'drinks' also of the dangers of junk 'foods' and sugarised products, including 'soft' drinks. People need educating about the risks involved in eating and drinking these types of so called 'food' and 'drinks'. If they refuse to be educated at least they can learn. *Turn to DIET caption* to read about nutritious foods and drinks which are health giving. There are other ideas included which should help to improve the lifestyle of many.

FAT

Fat is only a three-letter word, which has grown into bigger matter for contention than ever before, now being a political issue because of our obesity problem. We heard little about Fat in the past, except when some guru launched another faddist Diet, usually with short-lived propaganda as to its effectiveness with regard to losing surplus weight.
It has taken me some years to understand about the different Fats, with various research, analysis and study done, with many and varying answers. Fats are the most concentrated origin of our food energy, giving twice the amount of calories of protein or carbohydrates. *We need some Fat in our system but serious health problems arise when we have too much, as is the case in our modern lifestyle of fast foods, additives and quick preparation, with much unnatural.* Nutritionists now tell us we should avoid margarines, using butter instead. This is something those interested in natural health have always practised. Some margarines should carry a health warning because of 'excess' fatty acids, which with saturated Fats should be avoided.
Having studied, debated and argued about the Fat topic, friends and myself are convinced that proper additive-free natural Diet, *as set out in DIET caption*, goes far towards avoiding the dangers of excess Fat intake. The processed, fast foods,

hydrogenated cooking oils, confectionery, which are a wide-ranging collection, and much else, sold as 'food' should be avoided. Also to be missed out on are anything with sugar, which should be regarded as a Fat, also many Fat-free or low-Fat foods and spreads, highly- promoted, displayed and advertised. Replace with avocados, nuts, bananas, vegetables, fruit and everything natural as suggested in the *Diet caption*. Hydrogenated Fats, used as additives to give long shelf life, are to be avoided. They can cause LDL Cholesterol, the bad type, and excess triglyceride levels - heart evils. Most people are not aware of the dangers of transfats to health. The healthy, polyunsaturated oils when refined, processed and heated can be completely changed to what can only be termed inferior oils. This occurs too when using for frying purposes. Margarine is an example of where hydrogenation of oils can and does occur. Another reason why margarine is unnatural and best left on the shelf. *Turn to Margarine caption.*

A low-Fat Diet might make you look good on the outside but inside it may be completely the opposite. Low-Fat Diets deprive us of the Fats that are healthy, the Fats that heal. This can lead to dry skin, low energy, hair loss and proneness to inflammatory and auto immune conditions, increased glucose sensitivity and insulin resistance, mood and behaviour swings. One could safely add that Low-Fat Diets can lead to ill health.

Dr. Udo Erasmus has done much in the study of Fats in relation to our health. His book, *"Fats that Heal, Fats that Kill,"* which is available from bookshops or the health food store *(See Bibliography)* is extremely detailed about the role of what to avoid and what to use. The simple guide is to avoid saturated Fats as in pastry, cheese, animal Fats and confectionery. Polyunsaturated Fats, to be taken in moderation, can come from pure olive oil or fish such as mackerel, herring and trout. Eating too much of the wrong type of Fats can lead to heart problems including stroke, obesity and other circulatory diseases.

In order for our bodily system to function correctly it is imperative that we supplement our Diet where necessary with the correct type of Fat, the good Fat, the essential Fat! *See caption Fatty Acids (E.F.A.'s)*

FATIGUE

Lack of energy, exhausted, weary, lethargic. There is no quick answer on how to regain energy unless the root cause is known. It can be mental or physical. It may be as a result of illness or especially from poor Diet that is lacking in nutritives, including vitamins and minerals. I have found that the majority who had little energy and felt listless were Iron deficient. The food intake must be natural foods, well balanced for better health, energy and well being. Good nutritious food is often the best medicine for the wearying problem. *See DIET caption.* An Iron-based tonic such as Floradix or Biostrath, also food supplements, which include Vitamins C, E and B Complex can go far to solving the problem. 'B' at Eze, which is a little known complex multivitamin, is an excellent restorer of energy. Rhodolia has marvellous herbal constituents for fatigue aid. The lethargy can be due to boredom, which means taking up a mind-occupying hobby or pursuit. *If the Diet is adequate and the tonic or supplements do not help, with the trouble persisting, see your doctor. Ask for a blood test. A low blood count or anaemia could be the problem, or there may be other underlying factors. I know some who had felt lethargic and tired for many years and when blood tests were taken they showed up the problem. If diagnosed earlier in life the health of those affected could have been improved enormously. Also see Lethargy and Tiredness caption.*

FATTY ACIDS (E.F.A's)

These are a chain of countless beneficial aids to health and well being. Eating a well-balanced Diet of natural foods is the key to obtaining the necessary EFA's. The low and extremely low-fat Diets so frequently advocated by the slimming gurus ignore the health of the dieter. Supplements are available to ensure sufficient EFA's, including the excellent Udo's Choice blend of omega oils or Organic Choice Omega 3 + 6 + 9, which is a balanced blend of EFA's. Essential Fatty Acids are - as the name suggests -essential. They cannot be created by the body and must be consumed in the correct ratio, as too much of one will cause a deficiency of the other. There are two types of essential Fats – OMEGA 3 – Alpha Linolenic Acid and OMEGA 6 – Linoleic Acid. Many systems within the body rely on the correct ratio or amounts of essential Fats. Because of the gross interference with the food chain and the introduction of 'Foods' which are additive- filled, the chances of a balanced Diet, with EFA's included, has diminished considerably.

EFA's have positive effects in:

• Increasing energy production

• Reducing sugar cravings

• Boosting the immune system

• Helping to reduce cholesterol and for circulatory health

• Helping to maintain healthy cardiovascular function

• Skin, hair and nails health

• Helps brain and mind function

• Good for the digestive system

Those on a low-fat Diet, if overweight, with dry skin, brittle nails or dandruff, may need extra Essential Fatty Acids. Other signs of being low in E.F.A's are if with frequent colds or other infections, rundown, with dry eyes or suffering from cold hands or feet. If pregnant or breastfeeding consult your doctor before taking supplements. See book ***"Fats that Heal, Fats that Kill"*** as recommended in Fat caption and described in Bibliography. Visit the health food store and be advised further. *Turn to Diet also Udo's Choice Oils captions* if you wish to learn more about Essential Fatty Acids.

FEAR

I have seen the huge success of the complete shutout of both fear and anxiety, which are closely related, by change of Diet to natural additive-free food and drinks. Added to this was the use of some food supplements such as Vitamins and Minerals. ***When the health of mind and body improves, no matter at what age, the fears and cares of everyday life can be shrugged off.*** This has been proved many times. *See DIET also Anxiety captions.* Natural nutritious food is as medicine to body and mind, which may need building up, therefore enabling one to shrug off cares, worries and fears.

FEET

Seldom do we give sufficient attention to ensure healthy Feet. Often it is only when something goes seriously wrong that we seek a remedy. They are a sign of our general health. *Wash weekly in warm - not hot - soapy water, unless working in an environment which means washing more often. Don't rub between the toes, just dabbing to ensure they are COMPLETELY DRY.* Avoid talcum powder. Smear a little cream, such as non-steroidal Allergenics, between the toes to help ward off athlete's foot or inflammation. Cut nails regularly, straight across, not too short, with a proper nail clippers. Keep the Feet warm, wearing good clean wool or wool mixture socks. If with Foot problems visit a Chiropodist. Avoid wearing footwear which does not allow the Feet to breathe, such as rubber boots or plastic trainers. For Feet that perspire or smell excessively this signifies a change of Diet, with any of the following supplements being extremely helpful to eliminate the problem: Zinc, Silica or Sage. If with diabetes, do not self-treat the Feet. Burning Feet sensation is usually a sign of poor circulation. Taking Vitamins E and B Complex also Hawthorn and Zinc can help this. Exercise, even regular walking is necessary. If on medication see your doctor and tell him what you wish to do, such as walking regularly or taking other form of exercise.

FEMALE TONIC

When one feels the need for a pick-me-up the most important thing is to consider the Diet. Is it balanced with nutritious additive-free, pure and natural food? Bad Diet leads to ill health, fatigue and various ailments. Food supplements, which are an aid to better health, are a Multivitamin such a Wellwoman, or the iron tonics Floravital, Biostrath, or Floradix. Exercise and Sleep are equally important. *See both captions.* Ask the health food shop personnel for further advice. *Turn to DIET caption* and be guided about natures best medicine - unprocessed natural food. This also gives much information about supplements, vitamins or minerals, which may be necessary to attain better health.

FERR PHOS

See Tissue Salts Caption.

FERTILITY

See Infertility Caption.

FEVERFEW

This herb, which is of the Pyrethrum family, has many small chrysanthemum-like flowers, grows almost wild, being regarded by many as a weed. Few know of its excellence as a remedy. It is used to treat headaches, arthritis and is now looked upon as a migraine preventative. Take one or two large, or three or four small leaves daily, made up into a wholemeal sandwich or in mashed banana. Alternate week about, with capsules of Feverfew, obtainable from the health food shop. Not to be used if pregnant, breastfeeding or if taking contraceptive pill. Here is a glaring example of the medical or pharmaceutical industry ignoring something highly efficient, Feverfew being a wonderful remedy. This is simply because they cannot patent or register it. There is no monetary gain in it for them, as they continue to promote expensive and less reliable, synthetic medicines.

FIBRE

Dietary Fibre and roughage have only been headlined in recent times. Much of the need for Fibre, soluble and insoluble, has arisen because of the unnatural Diet which the Western world is offered and accepts without question. The highly processed, refined, additive-filled foods contain little roughage. On its own the essential Fibre contains a small amount of sustenance, but is invaluable to maintain good health. It is found in fruit, green vegetables, pulses, nuts, natural cereals, grains, brown rice, stewed prunes, dried apricots also pure, natural unprocessed wheat bran. White and most brown breads, other than whole meal or grain, contain little or no Fibre. Those who partake of natural Diet as promoted in this Encyclopedia, have very much less of the diseases many are plagued with. Pure natural wheat bran is a Fibre which when moist becomes softage, which is not so with the majority of the sugarised breakfast cereals available. Bran is invaluable as a Fibre and as a dietary aid, to be taken as required, not continuously, mixed with breakfast cereal such as porridge.

FIBROIDS

Linked to use of oral contraceptives, also to high oestrogen levels. Natural Diet and Yoga have proved very helpful. The Diet helps to reduce weight, eliminating unnecessary fat intake, with the Yoga assisting the pelvic area. *See DIET, also Yoga captions.* Supplement with Agnus Castus and a good natural Multivitamin. If anaemic take Floradix or other Iron tonic. Be guided by your doctor, especially if pregnant or with excessive bleeding during menstruation.

FIBROMYALGIA

This word covers more than just pains and aches. Very often it comes with fatigue, headache, insomnia, swollen joints, even digestive symptoms. Some doctors tell patients diagnosed with Fibromyalgia to rest. They seldom tell them that the main causes are poor Diet, bad eating habits, additive-filled food and drinks. The thought often occurs *'That it pays them to keep people ill'.* *If with this aching, tired and worn-out feeling, change your Diet by following the suggestions under DIET caption, or if you can discipline yourself to follow the Hay Diet, as under that caption, return to normal health will come even quicker.* Exercise is vital. *See Exercise caption.* To aid the problem, supplement with St. John's Wort to increase Serotonin. Calcium / Magnesium tablets, Devils Claw, Spirulina, Garlic and Udo's Choice Oil have helped immensely. The Calcium / Magnesium tablet is best taken before bedtime with warm milk or water, to which is added two teaspoons of pure natural honey, as sold by the health food store. This will help restore sleep pattern which is vital to better health.

FIBROSITIS

This is inflammation of back, other muscles, or of connective tissue, sometimes called muscular rheumatism. Usually due to wear and tear of the joints or when muscles react to abnormal immune system. Clears up quickly if muscles are not pulled or torn. Use Arnica external remedy or take Combination I New Era, Devils Claw or Cider Vinegar and Honey. A good remedy is to chop or liquidise some raw cabbage mixed with two teaspoons of Cider Vinegar, adding some apple and banana, eating with wholemeal bread daily.

FISH AND FISH OILS

Eat Fish regularly. They are a good source of nutrition, with valuable health giving oils, protein and mineral salts. Heart disease is a minor ailment where much Fish is eaten. Fish, frozen or fresh, is equally good as the freezing process is now well organised, with perfect hygiene in place. Avoid smoked or tinned Fish, unless the former is cured naturally like Manx Kippers. Fish is now seldom smoked with timber; being treated with artificial smoked flavour and colour. Most tinned foods including Fish have an analysis showing traces of chemical substances.

We are told that smoked flavourings are dangerous as the EU instructs that the amount used be reduced. At the same time we learn of the salmon colouring scandal. It is nothing less. In the past all salmon was natural. Not so now. *Farmed or battery caged and reared salmon has much been laid against it. For instance the European Commission has ordered that a colouring agent fed to farmed salmon and laying hens be reduced in administering, as it can affect the eyesight of humans. The product, Canthaxanthin, makes the grey flesh of farmed salmon turn pink, as we expect natural salmon to be. This product is also used to make egg yolks yellow. In the batching, weighing, and dispensing of these harmful chemicals we depend on the human element. Nobody can police this instruction. As well as the EU issuing what is a denunciation of the overuse of the chemical, a United States study has shown up to 10 times the level of cancer- causing chemicals are in farmed salmon as against wild salmon. Now we have the Salmon Growers Association telling us that the United States study set out to scare customers away from salmon unnecessarily. THERE IS DOUBT, BIG DOUBT. It is obvious that we are being dictated to by another breed of corporate food barons in that we must eat what they produce and put on the shelves. Farmed salmon is not natural. Apart from the toxic chemical being used to colour the flesh, we must ask ourselves: "Is salmon as produced now really fit for human consumption" They are incarcerated in their thousands in cages, infested by lice, infected by disease, for which they are often over-treated with chemicals. Many of these are dangerous, like the colour, which is now being trafficked by denial and counter-claim. As usual the unsuspecting public are expected to accept these harmful substances as food.*

There are many kinds of fresh Fish to choose from, all natural. Also available are Fish oils, bottled or as capsules. These are extra supplements to be used long-term even when Fish is on the menu. They are good for circulation, blood pressure, arthritis and skin. They aid brain memory also the heart, assisting in keeping one free from colds. *See Udo's Choice Oil caption* to find information about his unique blend of health giving oils. Visit your health food shop and be guided about natural Fish oil supplements. As advised in this Encyclopedia, *Eat Fish Regularly.*

FIZZY DRINKS

These also include the so called 'energy drinks' which are highly advertised. Four words could cover this subject as far as I am concerned: THEY SHOULD BE AVOIDED. Why? They are one of the main causes of obesity, also because there is much evidence of the dangers of saccharin, the toxic aspartame, excess sugar and other chemicals added. They can lead to ill health in the partaker. Cunningly the manufacturer tells us how some are sugar-free, although loaded with artificial sweeteners. Figures released show that Irish people consumed 384 million litres of effervescent drinks last year. The cost is estimated at €450 million. In the UK the figure is a little over eight times the amounts shown. These are staggering figures if one dwells on the fact that most of the liquid is additive- filled and most unhealthy. The quality of the water is unknown to the drinker. The question again arises: 'Who cares about what is put into the most intricate system in the world' – The Human Body? As mentioned in this Encyclopedia: 'Many look after their cars better than they do their bodies'.

Recently we hear of the 'fizzy drinks' makers having to remove their brand label from sales cabinets. Some schools and colleges in both Europe and America have banned their distribution or sale. The multi-national producers of these concoctions have agreed to this. Even though it is only a percentage of a percentage this is like an admission of guilt. Need one comment further?

It has now been found that the increase of cirrhosis of the liver is linked with huge increase in the consumption of fizzy 'Drinks'. Many of these high additive, often caffeinated 'drinks' contain up to the equivalent of 10 spoonfuls of sugar in a 500ml container, as well as the many other chemicals so detrimental to health. Now we learn of a study where scientists have issued a warning about the risk of cancer of the oesophagus (the gullet). Apparently there is a strong link between this type of cancer and the consumption of 'fizzy drinks'.

Schools promotions are highlighting the fact that these effervescent, highly sweetened drinks are not alone causing obesity but also how they are destroying teeth, with the drinking of water being encouraged. This will be extremely difficult to foster. **Do you or any persons who care about reasonable health read the ingredients labels on the aluminium cans or plastic Fizzy 'Drinks' bottles? Most of them are psychedelically presented in glaring garish colours in order to catch the eye. Here are the ingredients of one of the best-known brands: Water, Carbohydrate blend, Glucose syrup, Maltodextrin, Citric acid, Acidity regulator, Sodium Citrate, Preservatives, Potassium Sorbate, Sodium Benzoate, Antioxidant, Ascorbic Acid, Sweeteners, Aspartame, Acesulfame K, Flavouring, Stabiliser, Acacia gum, Vitamins, Niacin, Pantothenic acid, B6, B12, Colour, Beta Carotene, contains a source of Phenylalanine. Even the vitamins are synthetic, being nullified by certain of the other chemicals. Phenylalanine on its own, also the Aspartame, can be toxic.** *Turn to Aspartame caption.*

A valid and worrying aspect of the intake of these frothy effervescent, processed and unnatural waters is that the youth - both male and female - are not obtaining sufficient calcium because the drinking of milk is shunned. Milk is so very important, in order to allow dense bone formation. It is not realised that whether milk be skimmed, half or full fat, the calcium content is the same. It is extremely annoying to see some of our sporting heroes accept big money, exhibiting for advertising purposes and promoting these unhealthy, additive-filled and sweetened 'drinks'. They are paid enormous sums to do so. Again money is the all-important factor. ***Young people, to whom it seems the drinking of the carbonated, additive-filled water is the norm, must be taught the dangers. They should also learn that THEY SHOULD BE AVOIDED.*** *Turn to Energy Drinks caption.*

FLATULENCE

This makes one feel as if with bloated feeling. Caused mostly by inferior Diet. Remedies are Charcoal, Carbo Veg, Combination E New Era, Slippery Elm or Molkosan. Also recommended are fresh Parsley or Parsley tea. *Turn to DIET caption* and learn how to be without Flatulence long-term.

FLORADIX AND FLORAVITAL

These are excellent tonics. Floradix contains easily assimilated organic Iron, herbs, and fruit juices also Vitamins C, D & B Complex. Suitable for men and women, (including expectant, nursing mothers, those convalescent, or vegetarians). Kindervital, which is from the same laboratory, is equally suitable for growing children and teenagers. Floravital includes similar ingredients to Floradix, but is yeast and gluten free, with no added sugar, also suitable for vegetarians and vegans. I have known about and recommended these tonics for many years. Taken from September onwards, in combination with pure food Diet, one can be completely free from colds, flu and much illness, with a general feeling of well being throughout the winter. To me they are on a par with Echinaceaforce, taking the place of the flu jab, as they do for many who praise their efficiency and health giving goodness.

FLOWER ESSENCES

See Bach Flower Remedies Caption.

FLU

See Influenza Caption.

FLUID ON KNEE OR ELBOW

See Synovitis Caption.

FLUID RETENTION

See Water Retention Caption.

FLUORIDE

This is a toxic chemical. It is added to water in many areas. It is mandatory in Ireland where the water is the most Fluoridated in Europe. Fluoridated public water supplies have been banned by 98% of Europe. The majority are against its use. The principles of democracy have been thrown out the window as the Government and civil servants foist the harmful Fluoride substance on us. In some areas including small towns and villages, Fluoride that is a hazardous industrial waste and pollutant is not even metered into the drinking water, being poured in, if and when it is thought of. This comes from a water board operative that even went so far as to say: "We sometimes put in extra if it has been forgotten about".

A doctor cannot force a patient to follow his orders. Similarly there is nothing in any Government act that specifically permits a water system to be used for the dispensing of a toxic substance added to it, for the purpose of effecting bodily or mental function. *To find out how Fluoridation is an affront to human dignity, how it is forced on the unsuspecting user, See Bibliography for details of the best sellers,* ***Fluoride - Drinking Ourselves to Death?*** *by Barry Groves or* ***Fluoride Deception*** *by Christopher Bryan.* **Despite the dangers, Fluoride is included in the makeup of toothpaste. How many with young children know that those under the age of two should not use Fluoride toothpaste. Not only is Fluoridated toothpaste used too soon in life, but too much was used in 80% of cases. Dental decay has decreased not because of the use of Fluoride, which is of no help whatever, but simply because most people can now afford to visit the dentist regularly. Older dentists confirm this, having seen the massive growth in the numbers of patients attending the dental clinic over the past 40 years. Many dentists are against its inclusion in water or toothpaste. More chemicals mean more sickness. All too few are aware of this as they seek synthetic pills for all ills and continue to drink Fluoridated water.**

Hexafluorosilic acid - which is Fluoride, is supposed to help teeth. There is no evidence that it does so - in fact the opposite is the proven case. It is a toxic substance, a by-product of Agri chemicals which forms dangerous substances when it comes in contact with aluminium. It accumulates in parts of the body. Because of its overuse it has been recommended that there be a reduction from the current level of 0.8 to 1.0 part per million to 0.6 with a target level of 0.7 parts per million to be added to the water. It is a fact that the use of this amount leaves it of no value for what it was proposed for in the first instance. Common sense should therefore be used and the fluoridation ceased. **Because of the chemical content, mothers are now advised not to use tap water when making up baby foods, including bottle-feeding.** It is a sad state of health affairs when it comes to this kind of directive or advice. Not alone are there additives in much of the 'foods' being given the child but now the Fluoridated and Chlorinated water is harmful. We are told this now, despite it being foisted on us for years. *Turn to Chlorine caption.*

FLUSHES. HOT

See Menopause Caption.

FOLIC ACID

Part of Vitamin B Complex formula. Needed for healthy hair, skin, appetite, digestion, mind, mental and emotional health. Found in fresh green vegetables, especially spinach and broccoli, also in fruit, grain, liver, wheat germ, soya flour and brewer's yeast. Folic Acid can help to prevent birth defects, including Anencephaly and Spina Bifida *Research shows that few women give thought to the need for additional Folic Acid, which is extremely important before conception and during pregnancy.* It has been proven to reduce the risk of neural tube defects, such as Spina Bifida. Women are advised to take Folic Acid supplements daily. Like proper Diet this vitamin is one of life's essentials. Ask at your health food store for Folic Acid, also tell your doctor, who has only recently deigned to prescribe the vitamin, because it is wholly natural, even though those who promote natural remedies and way of living have for many years harped about the need for this essential member of Vitamin B Complex. Originally found in spinach, it does not remain stored in the body and must be replaced daily. **An excellent method to ensure required amount is to take Pregnacare, which is an invaluable pregnancy supplement.** If you visit your Health Food Store they will advise further.

FOLLICULITIS

This infection of the hair follicles, which can cause itchy, red, boil-like spots, is usually brought on by inferior Diet. Added to this can be allergy to wearing apparel, including sanitary towels, or it can be as a result of improper hygiene. Calc Sulph, Combination D New Era or a tonic such as Floravital will help clear the problem. *See DIET caption* which is one of the main remedies to correct impure blood and related problems.

FOOD

Because so much of our 'food' has been purified/processed, one feels like using the word putrefied, we are becoming a sicker nation due to malnutrition. Taste is now created in the laboratory, using fragrances and additives attractive to the taste buds, especially that of our children. I must repeat the need to leave the additive-filled, so called 'foods' on the shelf. Only a minority read the ingredients labels. In situations like this it is certainly true that *'There are none so blind as those who see and will not read and understand'.* Partaking of good food leads to good health. Much of what we eat today is foodless. There is no nutrition in most of the over 5,000 substances with which our 'foods' are filled. The only people who benefit are the 'food' stores, supermarkets and the 'food'-producing conglomerates. As with the drug companies they have little interest in anything natural. There is no money in it. To be healthy, think healthy and eat natural food. *Turn to DIET caption* to read about nutritious health giving FOODS, additive-free, unadulterated, non-processed, and purely natural.

FOOD ADDITIVES

See Additives in 'Foods' and 'Drinks' Caption.

FOOD ALLERGIES

See Allergies Caption.

FOOD CHEAP

Almost daily we are led to believe that there is a price war, that one supermarket or food store is cheaper than another. Their loss leaders, the promotions of the day or week, may be cheap but this does not necessarily mean good. Additive filled 'food' is like food diluted. Some of what we are offered is so nutrient-deficient that the processor has to add synthetic vitamins and minerals to warrant its being called 'food'. Do you look at the ingredients label? Often it can be frightening. Health wise cheap 'food' can be terribly expensive.

FOOD COMBINING

This is often the answer for relief and total freedom from stomach and digestive problems and much other illness. **It is the safest, surest, health-giving and best slimming Diet ever.** The Food Combining Concept, which was introduced by Dr William Hay, is to eat proteins such as milk and fish, with vegetables or salads but not with carbohydrates such as potatoes, pastas or bread. The carbohydrates are to be taken with the neutral foods to be eaten, some hours later at the next meal. The foods are divided into three categories: protein, carbohydrates and neutral. The latter to be taken with one or other, which must not be mixed. Following the diet has proved exceptionally health giving. Many with M.E. (Chronic Fatigue Syndrome) and other health problems have benefited enormously, as have those who have used this form of food combining Diet in order to lose weight. The results have been extremely good. *See HAY DIET caption.*

FOOD PYRAMID

Set out in the chart of daily health food choices is an example of what is needed to augment the pure natural Diet promoted and advised in this Encyclopedia. Study the *food pyramid* and note that it is very easy to abide by the rules of using required or suggested amounts of daily portions. The erroneous ideas can be put aside that large servings are needed and that there is much work involved in following the advice set out. Also *see Fruit and Vegetables caption* for a simple understandable explanation as to what can easily be provided.

The pyramid is simply a guide to what should be a balanced daily diet. Avoid food and drinks with additives which are not natural. *Guidance and advice is given under DIET caption.*

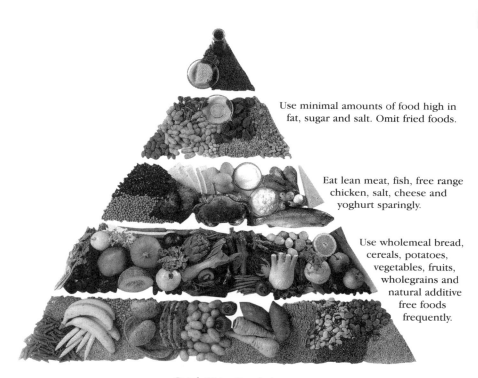

Use minimal amounts of food high in fat, sugar and salt. Omit fried foods.

Eat lean meat, fish, free range chicken, salt, cheese and yoghurt sparingly.

Use wholemeal bread, cereals, potatoes, vegetables, fruits, wholegrains and natural additive free foods frequently.

Drink Water Regularly

FOOD SUPPLEMENTS
See Vitamins and Minerals Caption.

'FORESIGHT' *How this Charity can help Infertility*
Known as the Foresight Association for the Promotion of Pre-conceptual Care, this organisation has proved extremely good in its treatment for infertility. It is run as a charitable concern, using dietary approach to maximise the producing and

conceiving of a healthy baby. Figures show an over 80% success rate. Here is a wonderful example of how natural is best. Foresight has been highly commended for the natural methods adopted. They can be contacted at FORESIGHT, 28 The Paddock, Godalming, Surrey, GU7 1XD UK. Tel: 01483 427839.

FREE RADICALS

These molecules produced by our metabolism can become uncontrollable if not attended to quickly. They occur mainly as a result of inferior Diet or lifestyle, also from environmental toxins. They are associated with ageing, coronary heart disease, also weak immune system, rheumatoid arthritis, Alzheimer's disease, cataracts and other ailments. The type of damage they cause plays a major part in the progression of these and other degenerative diseases. Properly balanced Diet of natural additive-free foods, aided by important antioxidants such as Vitamins A, E and C, also Coenzyme Q10, Selenium and Zinc are vital to help eliminate Free Radicals. These help slow the ageing process, giving zest and energy with better all round health. *Also turn to DIET caption* and be guided further.

FROZEN SHOULDER

If not as a result of stroke or injury treat as osteo arthritis also taking regular gentle exercise. *Turn to Arthritis Osteo caption* if relevant.

FRUIT JUICES AND SQUASHES

With many of the Fruit Juices on offer pure is not always pure. The majority are made from concentrated Fruit Juice. What is added is the problem, including the water! Here again it is advisable to read the ingredients label. Even this does not tell the full story of the manufacture or make up of these juices. Juice made up from concentrates is best avoided. Many pure Fruit Juices are available, such as Aspells, Biota and other brands, all free from additives, with no sugar or sweeteners. Often these must be searched for, noting the contents label, remembering that the word pure is often a lie. *To be sure of obtaining pure natural Juice it is advisable to make up your own with a juicer. There are simple juicers on which you place half an orange or fruit. There are more elaborate Juicers on offer, some of which will extract Juice from carrot or other vegetables, as well as fruit. Fruit and vegetable Juices mixed are extremely health giving, being full of vitamins, minerals and other goodness.* The health food stores carry a range of Fruit Juices, all pure and natural.

FRUIT AND VEGETABLES

When it comes to writing about good health, the need to extol the virtues of, to praise the goodness of, to emphasise the need for daily intake of fresh Fruit and Vegetables, would require a book on its own. Space does not permit all I wish you the reader to know about their wholesome, beneficial, health giving excellence.

Many, especially those who have to provide, including those who accept the advice that accompanies the food pyramid chart, are put off, believing the following:

- that 4 plus portions of Fruit and Veg is a large amount
- that they are to eat the Vegetables raw.
- that they are dull, boring, not needed.
- that something which fits in the microwave will replace their value or goodness. These are entirely wrong ideas.

For those with large families or on low income, budgeting is often necessary. Many become alarmed when told to serve four plus helpings of Fruit and Vegetables daily. Put your mind at ease, realising that a serving consists of :

- half glass of Fruit juice
- or one medium sized fresh Fruit
- or two tablespoons of cooked Vegetables or salad
- or one small bowl of home made Vegetable soup,
- or two tablespoons of cooked Fruit.

These can be permutated in any way in order to use up whatever is provided or available. There is no need to dash out to purchase some if ample of others are at hand.

Instead of sugary or additive filled snacks use apples, even half will suffice, bananas, grapes, nuts, raisins also raw Vegetables such as carrots, celery, cabbage or others, diced or chopped up.

Oranges are not an economical buy, with one 250 mg tablet providing ample daily requirement of Vitamin C.

All Vegetables are good, especially carrots, cabbage, French and runner beans, leeks, courgettes, garlic, celery, rhubarb and cauliflower, with broccoli and beetroot being regarded as superior vegetables. Beetroot and broccoli contain a multitude of essential vitamins, minerals and nutrients. *Vegetables are best when steamed, with much of the goodness being retained.* Boiling is not advisable. In Wintertime a stew including Vegetables is nutritious and warming. The use of a pressure cooker is highly recommended for quick and easy cooking with the vital nutrients kept within.

Avoid buying reduced priced Fruit and Vegetables offered close to sell-by-date, as the valuable nutrients of fresh produce have probably been depleted. Do not leave Vegetables soaking in water. If possible buy every couple of days rather than weekly. Store in the fridge where possible. All Vegetables and particularly Fruit should be washed thoroughly before cooking or eating. Vary Vegetables in presentation and cooking by adding to soups, omelettes, and casseroles or even mixed with mashed potato. Raw Vegetables can be puréed with Fruit to add to salads. *Turn to DIET caption* to be guided about the natural foods needed for better health.

FUNCTIONAL FOODS

Here is another idea recently introduced by the 'food' industry. Functional means useful or working. If ALL foods are functional why now offer something different to the trusting public who have relied on and continue to believe in the retailers and suppliers. The belief that what we purchase is edible and healthy food cannot be sustained. Many of the 'foods' processors and additive manufacturers are no longer reputable or principled as they pedal the stuff called *'food'*. They know that what they sell is lacking in goodness. Now they have the effrontery to promote what they refer to as Functional foods. We are officially informed that :*"They are 'foods' and 'drinks' that tend to make specific health claims of some kind on the packaging or in the advertising".* At the same time we are told: *"That Functional foods are not a replacement for eating a healthy, balanced Diet, but could be used to supplement such a Diet".* You, the reader are, I presume, as wise as I am after reading that explanation. Probiotic products are an example of what the 'food' and 'drinks' industry is once more trying to force on the unwitting public as they plug these so called Functional Foods. How did we manage without these things in the past? It does not make scientific sense to add them to the countless 'foods' we are offered. Part of the blurb tells us: 'Probiotics is an exciting area for the consumers and the food industry at present'. Here is another example of where the bottom line – MONEY – is the end product. The quality of the additive-filled 'food' will not improve. All too much of the manufactured stuff stacked on the shelves and colourfully advertised is far from being FUNCTIONAL.

FUNGAL INFECTIONS

To correct and improve the bloodstream, pure, natural Diet of additive-free food is necessary. *See DIET caption.* Consider what you eat as a first step to help eradicate the problem. Aids to the Diet for Fungal Infection eradication are the whey-based Molkoson, also the plant remedy Spilanthes. Acidophilus, obtainable from the health food store is another safe way to help eliminate Fungal Infection. Tea Tree Oil, such as in Thursday Plantation Anti Fungal Gel is a powerful, natural antiseptic which is used extensively for Fungal Infections. Combined with change of Diet they are extremely good to help remedy the problem. Ask at the health food store for these simple natural remedies, including the Non-Steroidal Allergenics cream or ointment, which helps control athletes foot and groin itch. Vitamin B Complex is usually lacking in the system and should be taken as a supplement.

GALL BLADDER INFLAMMATION & GALL STONES

Linked to inferior Diet, where sugar and fats are overeaten, also much more prevalent since the introduction of oral contraceptives. Being overweight, also ageing, increases the risk. The inflammation is due to bacterial infection, causing extreme pain or may be due to Gallstones being present. They may have lain dormant for years. Devils Claw, Milk Thistle, Dandelion, or Echinacea can help to remove the inflammation where stones are present or for protection from them. Vitamin C, up to 750mg daily, can reduce the cholesterol in the bile. Boldo has proved to be exceptionally good for both prevention of and if with Gallstones.

Over 30 years ago the following remedy was given by a lady who said it worked for her husband also a friend, both of whom had Gallstones, with operations pending. This remedy has been passed on to many for whom it has worked. In all cases where the advice was followed operations were no longer necessary. Drink about 2 litres of PURE apple juice (as Aspells) over six or seven days in order to soften the stones. Omit the evening meal on the last day of taking the apple juice. At 9 pm take two level tablespoons of Epsom salts dissolved in 2 or 3 tablespoons of water. One hour later add the juice of two large lemons to half a cup of pure cold pressed olive oil, into which is stirred two teaspoons of Manuka honey, to be well dissolved before taking. Go to bed immediately and lie on the right side with the right knee drawn up towards the chin. Stay in this position for 30 minutes to allow the liquid to drain into the body and to assist its restorative action. During the night a similar mixture of the Epsom salts, honey & lemon, may be needed, so prepare one and leave by the bedside. Next morning soft green jelly-like substances will pass without the partaker feeling anything. Some can be as big as a small marble. Only last week I had a letter from a lady to say: "Thank you" for the remedy. The operation, which had been arranged, was not necessary.

GARDENING THERAPY

In all my years of dealing with natural healthy way of life, with suggested relief or therapy, also being addicted to gardening, I have never heard anyone mention 'Gardening Therapy' except when I introduce the subject. Many who are attracted, dedicated or drawn to this wonderful hobby agree that when one enjoys the feeling of tilling the soil, cutting the grass, watching the birds, the trees, the flowers, the changing seasons, and much more which is natural and beyond comprehension, here is a Therapy where no pills, potions or tablets - chemical or otherwise - are needed. It is a good form of exercise. Those not interested in gardening or gardens miss much.

GARLIC

This is one of the oldest medicinal herbs or plants in the world. Garlic, with the lovely herbal title of Allium Sativum, is universally recognised as being one of the herbs that has curative properties for so many illnesses, that it should be in every home and on every table. Here is one of our greatest supports in times of ill health. Try telling that to the medical or pharmaceutical profession. They cannot patent and therefore have no interest in this marvellous root and herb. With no multi-million pound chemical company to advertise the health value of Garlic, its goodness remains untold except by lone voices like that of myself and those who have similar interest.

Therapeutically Garlic is far above most of the synthetic chemical, so called medicines, we have to contend with.

Long before the Christian era it was recognised for its healing powers. Only in recent years has the discovery been made that the goodness of Garlic is in its highly potent oil. It can help reduce instances of stroke and coronary heart disease, helps lower cholesterol and blood pressure, also assisting the immune system. It contains many trace elements, having anti-fungal and anti-bacterial properties. Helps alleviate symptoms of colds and flu's, being an aid to remove catarrh, no matter how stubborn. We are told of how it can dissolve the crystals deposited in muscles and joints, which cause rheumatism and arthritis. It is used to cleanse the system through kidneys, skin and liver, also for relief of colitis and laryngitis. It is recommended for fatigue and lack of energy. When travelling, especially when going abroad, take a garlic capsule daily to protect and guard against bacterial and stomach ailment. There are no known or recorded side effects, other than when too much is taken in its raw or vegetable state it can sometimes cause mild digestive problems, also there is the often unwelcome odour, including smell of breath.

The health food store and most chemists can supply it in odourless supplement form as either tablet or capsule. They are equally as good as fresh garlic, especially the capsules. Garlic is both a medicine and a food to be used by all. I would not be without my Garlic capsules.

GASTRIC ULCER

See Ulcers Caption.

GASTRITIS

Comes as inflammation of the stomach, brought on following illness or disease, usually by excess alcohol, stress, inferior Diet, smoking or taking aspirin or other chemical medicines. Needs careful treatment. Fasting for 24 hours, drinking only tepid water, is recommended. Then take onion soup with Slippery Elm stirred in, followed by pureed or crushed ripe banana. Avoid hot food or drinks, as these will aggravate the inflammation. It is caused by infection by Helicobacter pylori (H. pylori). Dietary change is most necessary but the body must be cleared of the bacteria. Mastika, which is a natural gum or resin-based formula, obtainable from the health food store, can actually eliminate the H. pylori, at the same time reducing the inflammation and helping restore to better health. When the appetite returns choose nutritious foods and soups also Slippery Elm drinks or milk puddings. Supplement with Calamus Tablets, Vitamin B Complex and Floradix iron tonic, later changing to a good Multivitamin tablet. *Turn to DIET caption*, which it is recommended to change to, in order to help avoid stomach ailments.

GASTROENTERITIS

Usually brought on by food poisoning, bacteria or virus, which may have come from impure water or meat, animals, dogs, pets or perhaps milk. Take extra liquids, including Slippery Elm drinks, until the attack eases or has passed. Then take small portions of banana, rice, apple and dry toast with Slippery Elm drinks. Follow on gradually with return to pure natural food Diet including milk puddings, gruel and liquidised fruit juices and vegetables. Calamus and Combination S New Era also Papaya tablets are a valuable aid to recovery. Gastroenteritis in children must be watched carefully. If it persists for over 24 hours or if alarmed seek medical attention. The extremely high instances of this stomach problem can very often be put down to the unnatural, processed, additive filled 'food' including junk and fast 'foods', which are served regularly. *Turn to DIET caption* to find out more about natural foods, so necessary for bowel and body health.

GENETICALLY MODIFIED FOODS (GMF)

Democratically elected representatives, but certainly not in a democratic fashion, are now having Genetically Engineered Foods foisted on us, without our say so. It appears as if the mighty industrial tycoons, who are certainly not interested in our better health, are dictating to us.

Modern technology now allows us to alter the genetics of the food we eat. No long-term tests have been done, let alone completed. Very short-term experiments, health-wise, are not acceptable. The issues are far too complex to fit in the allocated space in this Encyclopedia to all things natural. Suffice to remark that GMF's are no cheaper and certainly no better than what we buy. There is little if any control over the amount of herbicides or pesticides used. The crop will not be damaged. The environment will. Who cares? The central issue for all of us is what GMF's will do to our bodies.

As with cigarettes, thalidomide and many banned medicines, we are again being used as guinea pigs, often finding out too late about their dangers. It appears that much of the trials are supposition and guesswork. Again the unsuspecting public have to bow to the whims of the all-powerful chemical manufacturing multinationals and the almighty food producers as they pursue their policy where the end line is monetary gain. Our health is way down their agenda, if there is any.

Additive-filled food can be left on the shelf, therefore we have a choice of the unnatural or the natural. Despite this GMF's will infiltrate all, with our having to accept them whether healthy or otherwise. *This is a scandalous interference with our right to choose. So much for democracy! The voices of the nation must be roused and heeded before it is too late.* Like the thousands of substances in our 'foods', which the general public appear to have no interest in, the forcing of GM 'foods' on us is also casually accepted. Our Government representatives must certainly be regarded as foolish, or worse, if they allow Genetically Modified Foods be introduced, before all are totally satisfied as to their present and future significance, especially health-wise.

GERMAN MEASLES
Seek Medical Attention.

GERMS
Many do not realise how easy it is to spread germs through touch, having picked them up similarly. Wash hands frequently and scrub thoroughly.
If possible use the same drinking container so avoiding the spread of germs or bacteria.

GIDDINESS
See Dizziness Caption.

GINGER

Here is an example of the maxim repeated in this Encyclopedia: 'That pure food be your medicine with medicine being pure food'. The root of the Ginger plant contains several substances, which, like Garlic, contains Oil. The supplements or powdered root available in the health food store help control or prevent motion, travel or morning sickness. Ginger is an aid to digestion and digestive problems, also Raynauds Disease, cold hands, feet and circulation, osteo or rheumatoid arthritis. It also helps to lower cholesterol and aids in fat breakdown. Not to be taken if with kidney problems. Ginger is another of natures natural gifts to all, pure food.

GINGIVITIS

See Gums Captions.

GINKGO BILOBA

This wonderful herb is one of the oldest known. It has been through many clinically controlled tests, all resulting in high appraisal. Ginkgo improves blood and circulation, helping to strengthen blood vessels, assisting varicose veins. Has helped those with tinnitus, multiple sclerosis and rheumatoid arthritis. *It is a brain and memory aid, being used also to offset early stages of Alzheimer's Disease and dementia.* It is usually only after six to eight weeks of use that results are evident. Rare cases of sensitivity to Ginkgo Biloba have been reported, with stomach upset or skin allergy. Consult your doctor before taking, if on blood-thinning agents.

GINSENG

For many years we have read or listened to the promoting of this much over-hyped herb. It may have its devotees but I have not been convinced of it being a panacea or an elixir. There are several types, all giving varying results. A herbalist should prescribe it, as its makeup or attributes do not suit everyone. It has many contraindications. Certainly not one of my favourite remedies because I have found that after three or four weeks of use it no longer benefits the partaker.

GLANDS SWOLLEN

Often a sign of being run down or if with debility. Diet of pure natural additive-free food is important to help restore to better health. With care the swelling should only last two to four days. Allied to good food, valuable aids to restore to health are drinks of juiced carrot, onion and apple. Take two teaspoons of each Cider Vinegar and Manuka honey in a full glass of warm water three times daily. Poke Root and Echinacea are excellent restoratives. Include with the natural Diet a Multivitamin tablet. For children use Kindervital Tonic or Junior Multivitamin. *Turn to DIET caption.*

GLANDULAR FEVER

Seek Medical Attention. Aids to recovery include rest, balanced Diet of nutritious foods, warm drinks also raw vegetables pureed with fruit or fruit juices. Supplement with tonics such as Floradix, continuing when this is finished with a good Multivitamin tablet. Proper and natural food DIET is as medicine.

GLAUCOMA

See Eyes Caption.

GLOSSITIS

This is Inflammation of the tongue, which may be caused by anaemia, Vitamin B Complex deficiency or candidosis. There may be underlying conditions, which should be diagnosed before treating. Aids to help recovery include a change to natural nutritious Diet. *Be guided by what is set out under DIET caption.* Take Vitamin B Complex, Ferr Phos also a tonic such as Biostrath or Floradix. If with candida take Acidophilus.

GLUE EAR

See Ears Caption.

GLUCOSAMINE

This is now used successfully in conjunction with Calcium, Vitamin C and other minerals in helping maintain joints, muscles, ligaments and bones. It should be formed naturally in the body, but with the modern Diet not providing sufficient Glucosamine there is reason for supplementation. It has been shown to be as effective as synthetic steroidal anti-inflammatory drugs in the treatment of osteo arthritis. Ask at the health food store for further advice. There are several remedies, which include Glucosamine with Aloe Vera Joint Complex being extremely good.

GLUTEN FREE DIET

See Coeliac caption. Included is reference to recommended reading by Ann O'Dowd Fogarty, which gives much enlightening advice. *See Bibliography* for details of the book **'Eat With Joy On a Wheat Free, Gluten Free Diet'.** This also contains excellent and easy Gluten Free recipes.

GLYCAEMIC INDEX TESTED FOODS.

Many are confused with the advice and propaganda turned out by the supermarket, 'food' and slimming industries. We now hear of Glycaemic Index tested foods in relation to weight control. Nowhere will one read or be told of the additive-filled stuff offered as 'food'. The Groceries information machine will keep all ignorant of the true facts as it is meant to do. Forgetting this idea of G.I. things and using only pure natural, additive-free food will help control weight problems and lead to better health. G.I. is just another gimmick of the 'food' industry to hide the many shortcomings of what they concoct and sell, much of it foodless. Some doctors and others are recommending it but fail to dwell on the need for additive free *NATURAL FOODS*.

GOITRE

See Thyroid Caption.

GOLFERS ELBOW

Treat as Tennis Elbow Caption.

GOUT (PODAGRA)

This arthritic condition occurs in fingers and toes because of deposits of uric acid around the joints. Insufficient intakes of fresh fruit and vegetables also excess alcohol, meat and starchy foods all have a connection. Banish by taking fresh or tinned Cherries or Cherry juice. Devils Claw, Runo or Combination A New Era are further remedies. Kordel's Celery 6000 plus capsules are an extremely good aid to remove the aggravation. Diet must be changed to avoid recurrence. *Turn to DIET caption* to read about what is probably our greatest remedy for Gout and very much of the illness with which we are plagued. Drink plenty of pure water. Up to eight or 10 glasses daily act as a medicine. *See Water caption*. Morello cherries and cherry juice are excellent remedies. Morello cherry spreads, full fruit, sugar free, are available from the health food store. Many suffer from Gout, doing little about it. The remedies mentioned have all treated the problem successfully, especially the cherries and juice.

'GRACE' MAGAZINE

For over 40 years each Spring, Summer, Autumn and Winter the wonderful uplifting, nature's way, easily read **'Grace'** magazine has been published. It is devoted to positive thinking, spiritual refreshment, healing by natural methods, contributing to social and spiritual development. No adjective could compliment sufficiently this publication. Available by very reasonable subscription from Grace Publishers, Mulberry Court, Stour Road, Christchurch, Dorset. BH23 1PS.

GRAPEFRUIT

The Grapefruit Diet was so simple and natural, being health giving, as well as helping people lose weight, that it is amazing why any health-conscious person does not use it. The evidence is there that it works, but then one supposes that being eclipsed by the glib writings of the Dieting book industry, it is just forgotten about.

Studies show that it works extremely well where adults eat half a Grapefruit with each meal three times daily. *When the Grapefruit Diet was in vogue people were not aware of the dangers of sugar, as they spooned it on to Grapefruit, so nullifying its goodness. Even today many do not realise the health implications of excess sugar. Turn to Sugar caption.* As a natural food and sweetener, to take with Grapefruit, there is nothing better than pure Honey as supplied by a beekeeper or the health food shop.

Pure grapefruit juice, natural and unsweetened, is equally good. Grapefruit can also help reduce the risk of diabetes, as it helps break down the sugars, which are responsible for fat.

GRAPES

The goodness in Grapes is not recognised by most. There are many cases recorded where people, even some with cancers, have turned to a Diet of just Grapes and Grape juice, returning to good health. Books and articles have been written on the outcome, several of which I have passed on to those who were seriously ill. As with all fruit, Grapes should be thoroughly washed before use.

GRAVES DISEASE

See Thyroid Overactive Caption.

GREASY SKIN

See Skin Caption.

GREENS

Only recently, as the health gurus realise there is much wrong in our food chain, has the word Greens been highlighted. Apparently many thought they could live without them.

Although it is in relation to fruit and vegetables that there is a fresh arousal of interest, it should be remembered that Greens cover much else, which can be equally or perhaps more health giving. Included are invaluable herbs, fruits, grasses, cereals also the high protein Chlorella and Spirulina which have come from Greens, being a foundation for good health. The latter two are available made up as food supplements, obtainable from health food store. Few realize the good of sprouted seeds, pulses and grains, which can truly be said to be true Greens in their natural state.

All through the years those who were referred to as cranks or nut cases, those interested in natural food, have praised or promoted the value of these natural Green foods. Only problem was they did not and still do not have the financial backing to promote and highlight them in a big way, like the money-orientated food processors who cunningly and now in full colour, advertise and promote their over-processed, watered, additive- filled so called 'foods', much far removed from farm and earthy *GREENS*.

Greens are seldom if ever advertised. Because they are natural they have been in this world since day one, being so easy to come by we take them for granted. All too many do not realise or understand about their nutritious health-giving goodness. Dr Udo Erasmus, who pioneered the use of fresh oils, including omega 3 and 6 as in Udo's Choice Oil, has also formulated his 'Beyond Greens' and other oil and green vegetable-based aids to better health. ***Greens make the oxygen we breathe, provide us with water, trace elements and antioxidants. They are a rich source of chlorophyll, enhancing immunity, detoxifying the body, improving digestion, curbing the appetite, increasing energy and cleansing body systems. Most health problems will improve with use of Green foods. This typifies how the natural can be as medicine. One has yet to hear of side affects or the consequences of an overdose of Greens, or anything natural. I prescribe Greens as being excellent, superior medicine. Imagine a doctor doing so! The pharmacist would look at the prescription scornfully.***

We are constantly told how over-eating brings on obesity. It certainly is so, but not by over-indulging in and enjoying pure, unadulterated foods, including Greens. This includes the wide range of Greens referred to here. Intake of good foods including ample amounts of Greens and the drinking of plenty of water, leads to better health, also weight control. Greens should not be micro waved. The use of sprouted food as mentioned can be regarded as extremely good medicine. *Turn to Sprouting of Seeds and Pulses, Fruit and Vegetable also DIET captions* setting out the goodness of greens in our foods.

GRINDING TEETH

See Teeth Caption.

GROWING YOUR OWN FOOD

Few give thought to the fact that in the very near future there will be a world shortage of petroleum products. This will include the thousands of by products of the oil distillation column. Maybe they know something I don't or else they live in hope that something will turn up to keep the wheels turning.

We may yet be grateful to the farmer, now almost unwanted, as we search for a local source of fruit, vegetables, greens and other edible foods or we may have to revert to Growing Our Own Food.

GROWING PAINS

Children may have pains when growing up, but the term growing pains is a bit of a myth. This can very often be put down to rheumatism, or more often to inferior, processed, additive-filled 'foods' and 'drinks', usually lacking in Calcium/Magnesium / Vitamin D combination and other nutrients. Provide a balanced Diet of pure additive-free, nutritious foods. Supplement with combination P New Era, Calc/Mag/Vit D also a good tonic as Kindervital, all available from the health food store. When recovered don't forget that proper Diet is as medicine as well as being a food. If in doubt seek medical advice. *See DIET also Children and Teenagers Health captions* and be guided by what is advised, especially for young people.

GUMS

Gum disease, including gingivitis, gums soft, sore or receding, can almost always be diagnosed as being due to inferior Food, also bad dental hygiene. The modern Diet of processed, sugary, acidic, refined, additive-filled foods, mostly lacking in the necessary vitamins, minerals and nourishment, is the chief cause of gum troubles. There is little realisation of the relationship between bad dental hygiene and ill health. The gums and teeth are a pointer to state of well being. All who wish to take care of their health should take care of teeth, gums and sterility of the mouth. *A report shows that heart disease is linked to poor gums and teeth. There is an increased risk of stroke where there are long-term gum infections. The advice to dentists has been to send patients with bad teeth for heart checks.* Sage is an all-round gum tonic, available as Menosan.

Other natural remedies are
- Sore gums: Niacin taken as Vitamin B Complex.
- Gums painful on pressure or if with gumboils: Silica.
- Gums bleeding on brushing: Calc Sulph alternated with Silica also Rutin.
- Gingivitis: This is gum disease in its very early stages with perhaps bleeding gums, bad breath and sore red gums which when healthy should be pink. Proper DIET combined with a tonic such as Floradix or Bio-Strath will help correct gum problems, returning one to better health. The use of a good Multivitamin is recommended when Tonic has been taken for four to six weeks.

Coenzyme Q10 has also proved to be an extremely good gum health aid. As an antiseptic mouthwash, which is a huge aid to gum problems use Menosan or Tea Tree Oil, adding ten drops of the Tea Tree Oil to a glass of warm water. Also *see Teeth, Toothpaste and Periodontal Disease captions.*

THE DANGERS OF MIXING ALCOHOL WITH ANY MEDICINES, NATURAL OR SYNTHETIC,
CANNOT BE OVERSTATED. THE PARTAKERS SHOULD BE REMINDED OF THIS
REGULARLY. IT APPEARS ON SOME LABELS, BUT SHOULD BE ON ALL REMEDIES.

HAEMORRHOIDS

Commonly known as Piles.

They occur because of enlarged veins in the rectum, which tear easily. This may be due to poor circulation, lasting constipation, or maybe as a result of overstraining on visiting toilet or during pregnancy. Diet to be of high-fibre foods, taking plenty of fruit and vegetables, especially Brussels sprouts, cabbage, cauliflower and broccoli. Bilberries, pure Bilberry Juice, Bilberry tablets or capsules are excellent as a Haemorrhoid remedy. A liver tonic such as Milk Thistle or Dandelion is suggested. Drink plenty of pure water. Up to eight or 10 glasses daily is recommended. Take one dessertspoonful of Olive Oil on retiring to bed and supplement with Rutin, Aesculus (Horse Chestnut) or Combination G New Era. The health food store can also advise about their natural pile remedies, which are usually Psyllium Husks, Senna, Aloe Vera or Potters Lion Cleansing Herbs. By using certain of the remedies or aids mentioned, find out which suits best and use when necessary. Constant or long-term use of chemical or indeed any laxatives is not advisable. Sitting on the toilet and reading leads to over-stretching of the anus veins and is to be avoided. A change to natural foods, with extra fibre, including an amount of bran, can solve the problem or steep one dessertspoonful of linseed in water overnight. The bran or the linseed to be taken with porridge or muesli at breakfast time. Four or five dessertspoonfuls of bran every four or five days, combined with linseed, are usually the remedy to keep bowel movement good. Visit your doctor if bleeding persists.

HAIR

Shiny lustrous Hair is a sign of good health, also of good food intake. A well-balanced Diet of pure nutritious, additive-free foods brings better health, including that of skin, Hair and nails. Have you ever noticed the pale complexion, dull Hair or tired look of those who crash diet, slim, or try losing weight quickly? The essential nutrients to cover all aspects of health are drained away, not being replaced. Many shampoos contain chemicals, which may be harmful to Hair and scalp. Ask for the natural kind, as sold by the health food shop. Read the labels. Ask questions.
Dry Hair naturally. Hair dryers may dry the Hair quickly but sap out and destroy the natural oils emanating from the skin. Do not wash the Hair in water where chlorine

A to Z Guide to Good Food and Natural Over the Counter Remedies • 153

or fluoride is present. *Turn to Water caption.* Aids to Hair health are Vitamins C & B Complex, also Zinc, Iron or that excellent combination of Hair, skin and nail nourishment Perfectil. The latter, taken with recommended natural Food, makes a perfect combination for health of Hair and body. *Turn to DIET caption* **to read about the greatest medicine there is for Hair, skin and nail health, which is simply, proper nutrition.**

Other Hair problems can be treated naturally
- Hair falling out: Combination K New Era
- Hair oily – use Thursday Plantation Shampoo for oily hair
- Hair dry – use Thursday Plantation Shampoo for dry hair
- Lack lustre Hair: Silica.
- In-growing Hair: Take 1 or 2 tablets of Echinacea daily until condition improves.
- Dandruff: This Hair problem is also associated with inferior Diet and lifestyle. It is amazing the range of shampoos containing dandruff remedies. Most of them are of little use for the problem. The only permanent remedy is that taken internally as medicine, which will eliminate the scaling. Take Perfectil, as already recommended for Hair health, also Combination D New Era, to help banish the dandruff.

HALITOSIS (bad breath)
Stomach acid, teeth or gum problems, the drinking of coffee or breathing through the mouth almost always causes this. The latter is often caused by catarrh, or the simple act of not blowing the nose regularly, especially before retiring to bed. The other health problems, especially the acidity, mostly arise because of poor Diet. Most doctors will reach for the prescription pad. Pure, nutritious, additive-free food, which is as medicine, is unknown to many. In conjunction with pure food can be taken Acidophilus, Vitamin B6 or Kali Phos. The Iron tonics Floravital or Floradix are naturals for better health. *Turn to DIET caption* and be amazed at the difference the advice given can make, if followed.

HAMBURGERS
Like many processed fast foods, most are best consigned to the garbage bin unless homemade with good wholesome ingredients. The Health Food Store can supply burger and sausage mixes, which are delicious when cooked, being meat free.

HANDS
Hand care is necessary for all. Women are much more careful of them than men.

Many don't wash the Hands regularly, not realising that they are perhaps our greatest germ spreaders. Use soap, nail brush and hot water, scrubbing properly, drying the Hands carefully to avoid chapping or other problems.

Natural remedies are:

- Hands chapped: Combination P New Era
- Hands cracked including tops of fingers: Calc Fluor. Cracks are often due to lack of Vitamins B Complex and C.
- Palms sweating: Take Sage, which is obtainable from the health food shop as Menosan.

HANGOVER

To be avoided in the interests of better health. Nourishment is much better than punishment. Take two or three glasses of water after imbibing, or take Milk Thistle and eat a Banana. Another good help is to take Slippery Elm tablets or powder made up as a drink. An old remedy is to sip water into which pure lemon juice has been mixed. Avoid fizzy drinks when with a Hangover and at all times.

HAPPINESS

Health and Happiness go hand in hand. This cannot be denied, the proof being that when we feel good the tendency is to be Happy. To feel good we must be reasonably healthy. Here it is repeated, as is done many times in this Encyclopedia, *'Let food, sleep and exercise be your medicine and medicine be sleep, exercise and pure food.'* We cannot be Happy all of the time otherwise there would be no enjoyment. Happiness is a wonderful preventative medicine, easily swallowed, especially by children.

Happiness is chased, as if it were at the end of the road or the tunnel, when all the time it is round about us, in the friends we meet and greet, the things we do and the places we visit. A proper attitude leads to Happiness. Very often it only needs a change of lifestyle, especially DIET, to help find Happiness, because of the improved health, the spring in the step. *'HAPPINESS is not about having what you want, it is about wanting what you have'.*

HAWTHORN (Crataegus)

When as a boy I ate Hawthorn berries, little was the realisation that here was one of the best heart and circulation tonics available. It helps to keep the heart and heart-related problems normal, either stimulating or depressing its activity as required. Assists in control of high blood pressure also being a wonderful aid when with angina. Excellent for athletes and sports competitors to help maintain maximum performance. It is non-toxic, there being no reports of side effects. Again here is one of nature's greatest natural remedies. The drug companies have no interest. It cannot be patented or registered because there will be no monetary gain. An Irish man, Dr Greene, who practised in Ennis, Co. Clare at the beginning of the 20th. century, was internationally renowned for his successful heart treatment. When he died it was revealed that his remedy was Hawthorn-based. It is available in tablet or tincture form from your health food store or some chemists.

HAY DIET

Although referred to as a Diet, it does not mean cutting down on food. I have seen results of the completely natural HAY DIET in the elimination of several problems of ill health, some of them serious, also where used to reduce weight. Like many things natural and good for the body it has no scientific basis, having worked for many, requiring only discipline and self-control. When unwell these come easy if one is searching for better health. It is the best and healthiest SLIMMING DIET ever devised. It is safe, strength and energy giving, being a sure and good way to attain normal weight. We hear little about it, because being purely natural, there is no commercial, money-orientated interest.

The word HAY does not mean eating hay! The name is taken from the prognosis or teachings of Dr William Howard Hay (1866-1940). He was an American surgeon who had serious ill health at the age of 40. Grossly overweight, he had extremely high blood pressure, heart trouble and acute kidney ailment known as Bright's Disease. Little hope was held out for his survival. Being desperate he turned to naturopathy. The theme of this Encyclopedia includes very much the practice of this therapy, which includes the incorporation of a purely natural Diet, nothing processed. Everything partaken has to be free from additives, sugar, and other processed so-called food 'baddies', referred to over and over in this Guide. Dr. Hay turned to the basics of the therapy, which means the use of pure whole foods, including cutting down on salt and sugar as set out in *The HAY DIET* and as harped about in this book. Salt especially was his health enemy.

The big difference in his approach to the various foods is very briefly explained here. He ate fish, and fresh meat in moderation, mostly liver dishes. Natural cereals, grains, pulses, also dried fruits, fresh fruit and vegetables, including raw foods and salads were the chief foods used. He recovered extremely quickly. In three months he was quite well and in less than 12 months fully recovered. *His weight was reduced by over 25 kilos, over four stones, which was phenomenal.* He then led an extremely active and strenuous life until aged 74, when he died after an accident. *The whole ideas, view, call it a doctrine, is that food comes in three categories: protein, carbohydrates and neutral. When all three are mixed they are very often the cause of digestive and other health problems. Dr Hay aimed to prove that proteins and starches did not combine; setting out that either category should be taken with foods that are neutral. Protein and the neutral foods should be at one meal and three or four hours later carbohydrate and neutral fare to be partaken of.* He believed that proteins made the stomach produce acid, whereas carbohydrates need an alkaline base to be digested in. *The HAY DIET, which he developed, put Dr Hay on the road to recovery. It has also helped many to regain better health. The writer has seen the results of observance and discipline of the guidelines set out.* Sufferers of M.E. (Chronic Fatigue Syndrome) have recovered completely, as have those with allergy, food intolerance such as to gluten or dairy products, candida, digestive problems, hormonal imbalance and PMS. These are just some of the health complications which lead to a host of other ailments like irritable bowel syndrome, diarrhoea, headaches, depression and many other niggling disorders. The proper combining of the foods listed and the partaking of, have resulted in detoxing of the body, where one did not set out to do this.

Those who abide by the HAY DIET method of eating, unwittingly lose weight. Many have been amazed at their return to normal weight and trim-like figure, arrived at without having to resort to calorie counting or cutting down on sustaining food, with resultant under nourishment. **The HAY DIET could safely be said to be the paradigm, the truly real Diet, for those wishing to lose weight, remain trim and have better health. It has no celebrities to advertise, publicise or launch it further. It is too natural. Nobody writes about or promotes it. There is no money to be made by doing so, as has been done by many of the Diet gurus of the past. Most of their Dietary advice has been left aside, because often it is unworkable, unsatisfactory, even unhealthy.** Many use the HAY DIET. It means becoming organised, disciplined and determined to adhere to good natural foods, which are divided into their respective three categories, being eaten as set out.

In this Encyclopedia I can only gloss on a subject, which I firmly believe in. Perhaps this is because of my experience when asked to help where M.E., also Meniere's Disease, have been diagnosed early. Having already seen and heard about the return to good health of those who had adhered to the Hay form of food combining, it was wonderful to see the return to fitness of the M.E. and Meniere's Disease sufferers. *Two books are on my shelf, both good guides about this excellent form of Diet. They are referred to in the Bibliography section. There are other publications and guides about the Hay Diet and its excellent health-giving results. Here is a Diet, which has much to be said in its favour, being both healthy and health giving, at the same time acting as a weight- reducing or slimming aid. If I were trying to lose weight, I would most certainly be using the health giving and weight-reducing HAY DIET.*

HAYFEVER

In Spring and early Summer for many years, I have listened to the appeal: *"What can you suggest for hay fever?"* Thoughts about treatment must begin at the start of the year. Hay Fever sufferers should make a New Year resolution to discipline themselves to be free from the nasal congestion, taking early steps to do so. Refer to the Diet caption in this Guide, follow it, and you are well on the way to part or very often, full relief. If with allergy you must also avoid dairy products, including milk, cheese and yoghurt. Set out also in this Encyclopedia is how much of our 'foods' are now lacking in the nutrients required for good health. *How can it be good when in some instances up to 75% of certain 'foods' contain bulking aids, fillers and much more, which do not add to the nutritive, calorific or energy value? We are then glibly told by some of the medical profession and others that we do not need extra Vitamins and Minerals. Proper Diet is not in their sphere, certainly not as medicine.*

Hay Fever is very often brought on by a weak immune system, which may need building up. Nettles taken daily are an excellent preventative of Hay Fever. *Turn to Nettle caption.*

Visit your health food shop and seek advice about natural substitutes such as the various types of Soya Milk, also asking about the natural remedies suggested here. They will have pure Honey such as Manuka, which when taken with Cider Vinegar is an excellent aid to banish Hay Fever. Other remedies which have protected many from or cured Hay Fever are: Nelson's Homeopathic Hay Fever Remedy, Luffa Complex, Butterbur (Petasites), Kordel's Perilla 6000, Combination H New Era, Vitamin B Complex, with Devils Claw helping the immune system, which when healthy will help guard against Hay Fever. I have listed these in the order of their good, as found for the relief of the problem. What suits one may not suit another. A change from unprocessed, additive- filled foods to natural DIET is very often the only remedy required. Reflexology therapy has proved to be an outstanding remedy for Hay Fever.

HEADACHES

This ailment is amongst the top five everyday health problems. Headaches are a symptom, not a disease, a warning that something is wrong. Take proper steps to correct. On visiting the pharmacy, many shops, even D.I.Y stores and filling stations, one sees the many Headache remedies. Almost all are just stoppers of pain, repressors, not being remedies. Here is an example of where the root cause should be found, before attempting medication by the intake of chemicals, with no idea of the consequences.

Tension is often the main reason for the attack. Headaches are often brought on through lack of exercise or by anxiety, stress, allergy and low blood sugar, especially on becoming hungry, with eyestrain, lack of sleep or over-consuming of alcohol or coffee. They can be from side effects of medical drugs or painkillers. High blood pressure almost always leads to Headaches or dull throbbing head, with the most common cause being constipation. To diagnose the cause calls for more than just human pronouncement. Incorrect Diet, constipation and excess alcohol are the predominant reasons for being with Headache. *Turn to Diet caption,* following the advice given, where resultant better health helps relieve tension and many niggling things, which lead to Headaches, including the troublesome constipation. *Up to four or five dessertspoonfuls of unprocessed bran every four or five days can be the remedy for constipation and resultant Headaches as can a heaped dessertspoonful of linseed steeped overnight in water and taken with porridge or muesli at breakfast time.* If you are sure that the Headache does not require a visit to your doctor, such as with blood pressure, or if severe and persistent, look up the natural remedies in this Encyclopedia for whatever the condition may be and treat accordingly (i.e., migraine, constipation, tension etc). The Dietary change to natural foods is almost always the answer. Common Headaches usually respond to natural remedies such as Petasites, Devil's Claw, Combination F New Era, Petaforce or Garlic, all of which can be obtained in tablet or capsule form from the health food shop, being entirely natural.

HEAD LICE

We were led to believe they came because of poor hygiene. They were like a stigma, with a family reproached. They are not a sign of bad hygiene or dirty hair. As a matter of fact Lice like cleanliness. Young children who are in close contact with one another are usually affected, often being the cause of spreading them through the family, including the parents. They are not easy to banish, requiring a little thought and energy for some days. People now realise the dangers of synthetic chemical treatment, as some may be carcinogenic. Excellent natural remedies are available in the health food shop.

Killing the Lice is the easy part, with the eggs being the problem, as it is almost impossible to slay them. It is important that the carrier be found and also that they or their parents be informed, as they may not know about the infestation. Diluted Tea Tree Oil, Riddance or Neem have all been used successfully. What must be remembered is the need to fine comb, after leaving the treatment on for the required time. Work through each section of hair thoroughly to remove dead nits and eggs. Next day wash and shampoo, adding the diluted Tea Tree Oil or whichever natural remedy you have selected. Dry naturally and thoroughly. Fine comb thoroughly, again catching the eggs, also live Lice, if any left. Next day, which will be the third day of treatment and every second or third day after, or as per instructions on container, apply the lotion. Fine comb, examine and destroy the eggs found in the hair. Continue this until all is clear. Tea Tree or Neem Oil natural shampoos are recommended. Comb over white paper to make detection easier. Thiamin (Vitamin B 1) taken for three to four weeks is both the cure and a preventive, just as it is for protection from insect bites, especially if travelling abroad. Be guided by children's dosage guideline.

HEARING

Many do not realise that they have excessive wax in the ears, just waiting to be removed, going through life, not realising that a visit to the doctor can improve the Hearing. Temporary Hearing loss can be helped by taking Pulsatilla and Hawthorn together. *Turn to Noise also Ears captions.*

HEART

Scourge of the health of the Western world, the most widespread disease in so-called developed countries, is cardiovascular. In short the word means circulatory, heart and heart-related problems. The ratio of incidence of heart affliction or disorder in this country is more than double that of cancer.

Why do we hear so much more about cancer than we do about heart disease? As a voluntary worker and organiser for the Heart Foundation, having had a heart attack, I have met and talked with others with heart problems, to their relatives, also to doctors, nurses and heart specialists. They will tell you of the trauma, of how so many only care about their health after a heart attack, stroke or other serious illness. These are the lucky ones - they got a second chance.

Unfortunately we have the highest rate of death for heart disease in Europe before the age of 64. Last year the combined total heart death rate for the UK and Ireland was over 160,000. The ratio of heart attack only a few years ago was four to one in favour of women. *This has changed dramatically in recent years with a huge increase in female arteriosclerosis. As mentioned, the incidence of heart disease, including the most common condition, which is CHD or Coronary Heart Disease, is more than double that of cancer. This is emphasised in order to highlight the fact that in general the public worry about cancer, whereas they appear to trust to luck that they will not have a heart attack or heart problem. Could this be because cancer is usually a lingering illness, whereas heart attacks, if not fatal, are short or sharp? The word sharp here means horrendous pain. The attitude of many appears to be: 'OH NO IT WON'T HAPPEN TO ME!'*

See the multitude of voluntary cancer workers, including the younger generation, as they collect for their organisations. Compare this to the equally excellent but very much less number of volunteers for the Heart Foundation. Except for the many students who collect for the heart organisation, the rest of the volunteers are made up mostly of elderly relatives or those recovered enough from heart problems.

Men do not look after their health like women, who are much more particular. The female gender should realise that heart disease is up to 10 times more prevalent in women than breast cancer.

Heart problems are caused by a build-up of fatty 'plaque' on the artery walls, this being known as Atheroma. It comes about mostly because of our lifestyle and the adulterated, processed, all-too-rich, sugarised, additive, preservatives, fat and colour filled 'foods' we eat. *A Diet of fast food, couch potato attitude, with lack of exercise, added to stress, pace of life, also a bottling up of emotions and the terrible evils of smoking, all combine to make us susceptible to heart attacks. Granted a small minority are born with the problem, often only becoming apparent in later years, possibly hereditary.*

Consider your lifestyle because this is what leads to coronary heart disease, angina, stroke, poor circulation, blood pressure and high cholesterol, also hardening of the arteries. Diabetics are increasingly susceptible. As should all of us, those with diabetes must be extremely particular in endeavouring to reduce the risk of heart attack and strokes. Prevention is better than cure, more especially as many do not get a second chance. I write on the subject of heart disease from experience, having brought it on by lifestyle and mode of living.

We are told that DIET causes between one third and a half of some cancers. I am convinced that here lies the main cause of heart disease and very much of the other sicknesses with which we are afflicted.

Government Cardiovascular Strategy advises those with cardiac disease:

- Stop Smoking.
- Make Healthier food choices: reduce fat, salt intake and increase fruit & veg.
- Become physically active – walk for at least 30 minutes or longer four or five times a week or daily if possible.
- Achieve an ideal weight for sex and height.
- Consume moderate or little amounts of alcohol or better still none.
- Have a blood pressure of less than 140/90mmHg.
- Use appropriate medication.
- Have total cholesterol of less than 5.0mmol/litre

We hear all too little about the prevention of the disease, where the advice given above would certainly help. The combined total spend in the UK and Ireland on prevention of illness and education of the public, on how to achieve better health, is a paltry 0.08% of the billions poured into the health service. The Government advice set out here about food intake or choice is in one sentence - *'Make healthier food choices'* with just a few more words. What they mean by healthier food choices is to avoid the 'stuff' we are expected to use which is over-processed and mostly unnatural. *Do you think for one moment that the bureaucrats or anybody in authority with regard to our health would elaborate on something like that? As usual the softly, softly tongue-in-cheek approach to the all powerful 'food' industry is apparent.* Much more must be done to warn the unsuspecting.

Despite being told that a significant amount of cancers and heart disease are caused by the food we eat there is no condemnation of the additive-filled 'tack' we are expected to consume as 'food', much of it without any nutrition, with much lost in the processing.

Always be extremely choosy about what is being eaten, partaking only of pure natural additive-free food. *To learn about this see DIET caption, also reading the Sleep and Exercise captions which are equally important.*

It is extremely meaningful that some kind of workout is used daily, that some form of exercise be taken if at all possible.

The Diet caption sets out the need, where relevant for use of Vitamins, Minerals and Supplements. To help the heart Vitamins A, C & E are excellent antioxidants, one working in conjunction with the other to help prevent plaque, keeping the arteries flexible. Folic Acid is also required. One of the best ways to obtain these is to take daily a good slow release Multivitamin tablet such as Wellman or Wellwoman. At bedtime take a Calcium/Magnesium/Vitamin D supplement. Take Fish Oil or other Oil such as Udo's Choice to obtain the necessary Omegas required to protect the heart. Garlic tablets or capsules, Lecithin granules, Hawthorn or either Horse chestnut or Rutin also help to keep the heart healthy. The Lecithin helps in breaking down the fats in the food we eat. *We must return to a natural way of living, dare one use the word primitive.* All the natural remedies mentioned are available from the health food shop, with some chemists or pharmacists now stocking them. When there, ask questions and seek answers about the natural health-giving remedies they offer. *If on medication tell your doctor what you are doing. Discuss what you intend to do.* Anything mentioned is compatible with synthetic medicines.

In this 'Encyclopedia about Good Food, Natural Remedies and Better Health', my intention at all times is to convey my experience and that of the many who have used natural remedies, in a return to improved well-being and vitality. Everything written about is natural. Included is advice about the need for Exercise, Sleep and much more, all of which should lead to better health and which are described under the various captions. At no time has illness been diagnosed or medical advice been given. Do not self-treat without proper diagnosis. Before starting any form of exercise if on medication seek medical advice. There are many like myself who have turned successfully from chemical or synthetic medicines. The use of anything suggested in this Guide is entirely discretionary.

When I went for annual check-up and told the specialist what natural supplements or remedies were being used side by side with the synthetic prescribed, his reply was: "I know nothing about them but whatever you are taking keep doing so. They appear to be doing you good". It is a pity he and his associates wouldn't learn something about them. We would certainly have much less illness if people like him prescribed natural foods and remedies alongside the synthetic.

HEART ATTACK, HOW I FOUGHT IT AND NOW ENJOY LIVING.

What I write here is from experience after a heart attack. Some years ago, having ridden my bicycle, on a warm day, some 60 miles in the Welsh mountains, not feeling well, being uncomfortable in the saddle, not enjoying myself as was usual on a trip like this, I returned home in the evening to shower and then dinner. It must be added that for many years tours of up to 120 plus miles daily were normal at least once a week.

Later I felt unwell, becoming cold and clammy, gasping for air, my chest being as if in a clamp. My wife with her nursing experience, including that of heart problems, on noticing my greyish colour- her words- telephoned the hospital. Whisked there, the diagnosis was heart attack. My thoughts were: 'If only I'd looked after myself in days past this would not have happened'. I have never admitted it but I was frightened. I was diagnosed with Angina.

Being warned to take it easy, rest, not to garden, lift, or do anything strenuous, including riding my bicycle and much more restrictions to life advised, also prescribed aspirin and other tablets, I returned home. Over the following months I had days when I felt without a health problem. Other days I was ill, tired, and lethargic, often with chest pain. In between times I sometimes did not take the medication as I felt that bit better. The result was another attack, after helping to install a heavy cooker.

On returning home the second time the determination was there to fight the disease. The book entitled **'Your Arteries Can Clear Themselves'** *(See Bibliography)* proved to be the first step towards rehabilitation and recovery. Later I learned much more to add to my knowledge of heart disease. This strengthened my resolve to fight the affliction. Just as previously, there were bad and good days, doubts, chest pains if I did too much, often having to take afternoon sleep or rest. Cycling or exercise was the least of my thoughts. Even walking had to be curtailed. *Here must be added a word of warning to those who have had a heart attack or any form of cardiovascular or serious circulatory problem. What is described here is my experience, also that of others who have done or are doing similarly. No claims are made that what I write about will work for any.* Seek advice from your doctor, being totally honest. It is your prerogative what you do. Tell of what you are doing or what you intend to do. You may already be taking natural remedies, or intend to do so. None of us are alike, including those with heart or circulatory problems.

The question of exercise, how to become fitter or more active must be

discussed with the GP. This is very important. *See Exercise caption* to discover that it does not entail serious workout, visiting the gym, or what appears to be strenuous hard workout. No, I found an entirely enjoyable way of exercising, of keeping the blood circulating freely, simply by walking. This can be done at one's own chosen pace or speed, with the walker gaining better health simply by the amount of energy put into the walk. One can get to the stage of walking briskly and fast, often for many miles, which should be the eventual aim. *Turn to Walking also Exercise and Sleep captions.*

After reading about how the arteries could be cleared, I spoke with herbalists and doctor friends, also read much, discovering that others had followed and practised the use of natural remedies and supplements to assist the circulation, thereby regaining better health and well being. ***Having given up smoking many years ago there was no problem with what is one of our biggest health enemies. The cigarette packet tells us 'Smoking Kills'. This is naked truth.***

In previous years, although I did try to adhere to a reasonable Diet, I could have done very much better, especially in the avoidance of sugar, alcohol, confectionary, fizzy 'drinks' and the hundreds of processed products with which we are now faced. ***Sugar is an enemy of good health. I don't say it kills, it certainly helps to.*** Therefore I had to become almost fastidious, to be extremely particular of what was taken by way of food and drink. ***I did not tell my doctor or consultant what I was doing or intended to do. That was my decision.***

To regulate the cholesterol, blood pressure, circulation and to help clear the arteries, alternative or natural remedies were selected. Many with high blood pressure (hypertension), often referred to as the 'silent killer', have brought it to normal by using the remedies listed. Cholesterol has been brought under control similarly.

This is my food and remedy pattern. A glass of tepid water, one slice of wholemeal bread with pure honey and a banana first thing before walking for 30 to 90 minutes. At the outset I could walk at most for 15 minutes, having to stop frequently because of chest pains and breathlessness. I then return to breakfast of porridge, one dessertspoon of each Lecithin Granules and Wheat germ, also two slices of wholemeal brown bread with Morello Cherry Spread, which is sugar free. Every four or five days I take four or five dessertspoons of natural bran. Taken either immediately before or with the breakfast are a 400iu Vitamin E capsule, two each Rutin, Kelp, Hawthorn and Vitamin C tablets, also one each Oil of Peppermint and Garlic capsules, together with a 75mg Aspirin, as prescribed by heart consultant. This is the only synthetic or orthodox medicine taken. I stopped taking the others. Two hours later one slice of wholemeal bread with pure honey and a cup of tepid water are taken. Midday lunch, I call it dinner, consists of additive-free, natural foods selected from what is set out in DIET caption in this Encyclopedia. With this, the main meal of the day, one slow-release Multivitamin is taken daily. Sometimes this is replaced by taking the tonic Floradix, which is taken once daily. They must not be taken on the same day, being alternated. Two hours later a cup of tepid water and a slice of wholemeal bread are taken. The last meal of the day comes before 6pm, which again can consist of anything mentioned in the Diet caption, all of which is wholly natural. Daily up to 10 or 12 glasses of pure water are consumed. *Turn to Water caption.*

When a heart attack occurs it is a dreadful, alarming experience. For some weeks perhaps three to four months afterwards, the need for care including rest, must be emphasised to allow for healing. The tendency is to adopt a defeatist attitude, especially if the person has been active in the past. As my doctor friend, a cardiac specialist told me:

"You did the right thing, you fought it, you did not lie down under it".

Doing everything recommended, taking all the advice given, I am also convinced that four things have helped my return to better health. These were natural Diet as set out, Exercise, proper regular Sleep pattern and the natural Remedies combined with the prescribed aspirin. Aspirin, which can be dangerous, comes from a natural ingredient, originating from Willow. It must be added that being disciplined is vital in order to follow this course. I can now walk for hours, garden, do manual work, all without feeling overtired, which must not be allowed to happen. *Advice passed on is: "Pace yourself and keep brain and body active even if only pottering about".* Now I have found a book which sets out much of what I learned by trial and error. Any person who desires to help prevent a Heart attack or who has Heart problems would do well to read what to me is admirable advice. It is set out in '**The Healthy Heart Programme, How to Prevent, Treat and Reverse Heart Disease in Three Easy Steps**', an excellent guide by Dr. Richard Fleming. *(See Bibliography.)*

I recommend that you also turn to chapter at beginning of this Encyclopedia, headed '**Are You Prepared To Volunteer To Help Make Yourself And Others Healthier?**' *See DIET, Exercise, Sleep, Heart, also Blood Pressure High captions.*

HEART ATTACK SYMPTOMS IN WOMEN

Studies show that the symptoms may be very much different from those of men or of what a woman expects to experience. The typical chest pains may not occur, leading to unrecognised Heart Attack, mistaken diagnosis, or too hasty discharge from hospital. Research finds that some experienced extreme fatigue, others had sleep disturbance, with different percentages with indigestion, anxiety, or shortness of breath. Less than one third experienced chest pain. Females need to be vigilant, more especially because what was a man's disease is now almost equally that of women. Another disturbing factor which has come to attention is that grandmothers who care for grandchildren are at increased risk of Heart Attack. *Turn to Heart, DIET, Exercise, Sleep and Blood Pressure High captions.*

HEARTBURN

Just as for headaches we see many remedies on display for Heartburn, acidic dyspepsia, gastric problems, including gastritis. The long-term use of these acid-suppressing chemicals can cause serious health problems. Smoking, alcohol, caffeine and more especially inferior Diet of additive-filled foods, also fried, fatty and spicy intake are all linked to Heartburn. Natural remedies are Charcoal tablets, Combination C New Era or Centaurium, the latter to be taken 15 minutes before food. Charcoal tablets seldom fail to ease the problem. Taking as little as half a peeled apple after food has been a favourite remedy. *Turn to DIET caption* and if with Heartburn frequently this is usually the answer to the problem. *Also see Indigestion caption.*

HEART BYPASS OR STENT

Many do not know about how the use of the Stent can perhaps lead to the avoidance of a Heart Bypass. It is used when the arteries are being re-opened or widened when under angioplasty and is highly successful. Whether one opts for Bypass or Stent it should be remembered that during convalescence and at all times later there is a need for healthy lifestyle. There must be a change from the kind of foods and drinks and the manner of living, which created the problem.

HERBS OR HERBAL FORMULAS

There are many recommended in this Guide, either as Herbs or Herbal remedies, all available from Herbalists, Health food store, or some Pharmacies. There are many books on the subject. The author recommends '**Bioforce Publications**', '**The Complete Herbal**' by David Hoffman or '**Encyclopedia of Herbal Medicine**' by Thomas Bartram.. *See Bibliography section.*

HERBAL TEAS

See Teas Caption.

HERPES SIMPLEX

See Cold Sores Caption.

HERPES ZOSTER

See Shingles Caption.

HIATUS HERNIA

This is where part of the stomach enters through a rupture or hole into the cavity of the chest. May have been present from birth or can be caused by partaking of extremely hot foods or drinks. These and very cold items are to be avoided so as not to aggravate the ailment. Inferior additive-filled or processed foods, low in nutrition, are enemies of the problem. Hiatus Hernia can be controlled by proper eating habits, also by use of natural remedies, all of which have no side or other harmful effects as found with drug treatment. Triggers of the Hernia can be pork, cheese, peppers, salt, spicy foods, salad dressings, anything containing raw eggs, white bread, also white flour as in pastry, confectionery, etc.   Avoid alcohol, anything acidic, citrus foods, fatty or rich foods. No solids to be taken for three hours before bedtime. Two bananas daily, mashed and mixed with pure honey, act as a lubricant, also being health-giving. If overweight it means taking steps to correct, because the extra pressure placed on the flabby diaphragm aggravates the condition. Hypnotherapy treatment has given excellent relief, even for long periods of time. Exercise is extremely important. *See Exercise caption.*

Shedding excess pounds and toning the muscles, with regular moderate exercise such as walking, can help relieve Hiatus Hernia. The individual concerned will learn by trial and error as to what triggers the ailment. *See HAY DIET,* because pure natural food, plus everything advised under that caption can be the answer to Hiatus Hernia complaint as well as being a weight reducer.

HICCUPS

Remedies are: Papaya Tablets with a teaspoon of Pure Manuka Honey or a Lemon Wedge Saturated In Angosdura Bitters.

HIGH BLOODPRESSURE

See Blood Pressure (High) Caption.

HIVES (Nettle Rash)

Usually due to a particular food, fruit or food additive which should be avoided. Associated with warm weather.   Rhus Tox, Echinacea or boiled nettle water, taken as a drink, have eliminated the itch and the Hives. *See Nettles caption.*

HOARSENESS

Usually occurs with colds or from excessive use of the voice. It often comes on for no apparent reason, sometimes lasting for several days. Two teaspoons of each Cider Vinegar and pure Honey three or four times daily usually brings relief, as does the tonic and remedy Comvita Herbal Elixir. If it persists seek advice from a doctor. *See Laryngitis caption.*

HOLIDAY AILMENTS

See Travel and Holiday Health Caption.

HOLISTIC MEDICINE

Much of alternative therapy treatment and line of thought is based on the Holistic approach. Thomas Bartram in his excellent **'Encyclopedia of Herbal Medicine'** *(See Bibliography)* tells us: "Holistic medicine relates disease to a patients personality, posture, diet, emotional life, and lifestyle. Treatment will be related to body, mind and spirit. It encourages positive psychological response to the disease from which a patient suffers. For instance, its gentle approach to cancer embraces stress control, meditation, forms of visualisation and other life enhancing skills".

The foundation or basis to the Holistic or natural approach to much of our illnesses is pure additive-free, unprocessed food, *as set out in Diet caption* and repeated many times in this Encyclopedia. If all were to rigorously adhere to this principle there would be little need for chemical treatment for the all too many niggling, simple ailments, which plague us daily.

HOMESICKNESS

Take Bach Remedy Honeysuckle.

Homeopathy

This is a method for treating illness, which uses very small doses of carefully chosen and prepared homeopathic medicines. Put in simple terms homeopathic medicine is likened to the poison that causes the illness, being treated by a similar poison. This may seem a rather brusque or abrupt explanation. When consideration is given to the fact that the medicines are diluted many times in order to make stronger, with sufficient likeness to treat and arouse the self healing aptitude of the patients body, the definition or interpretation of Homeopathy appears complex. *'The medicines promote the body's own power to heal itself'.* They are based on the hypothesis or view that *'Like Can Cure Like'.*

Hippocrates, the father of medicine, formulated the idea in the 5th Century BC, laying the foundation for this natural way of treatment. Over the centuries the belief was kept alive, with treatment given by various doctors, many of whom believed that plants and natural substances, such as vegetables, herbs and pure food were the key to better health, encompassing the *'Like Can Cure Like'* theory. Homeopathy like many words in the English language, is derived from Greek words, in this instance, 'Homoeios' and 'Pathos'. Translated this means 'Like Suffering'.

The present day use of Homeopathy stems from the work of Dr Samuel Hahnemann, a German physician in the late 18th century. His methods were to spread to different countries, with many other eminent medical practitioners expanding his theories in the 1800's. *In the period 1930-1970, Homeopathy, like most alternative or complementary medicines, including the natural things akin to this way of thinking, was swept aside, as the influx of the modern synthetic pills and potions was unleashed on the then healthier people than are to be seen now. Only in the past 20/30 years has it been realised that many are not well, despite the thousands of drugs being prescribed. A huge turning has now been made to the many homeopathic and other natural alternative remedies, as people realise that these are in many instances a less harsh antidote or medication.*

This is one of the main reasons why homeopathic and many other doctors have resurrected and worked on improvement of homeopathic knowledge. They are essentially natural healing and assist regaining of health by stimulating natures vital forces of recovery. The majority of the medical profession grudgingly realise their efficiency, with no side effects.

All-too-many, particularly those with serious illness, turn to Homeopathy, as a last resort, often too late, when orthodox synthetic medicines have failed. Had they visited a qualified homeopath in the first instance the results might have been very much different. How often, even today, have I been told: "Oh, Homeopathy was tried. It was of no use". The full story was not told. It was too late. When the subject of Homeopathy was brought up on one occasion I was told: "I don't like it, I have never tried it". Sounds like the wording of the advert of old.

Homeopathy is now included as part of the National Health Service in Britain. When using Homeopathy remedies always remember to stop the treatment when relief is obtained. If the illness or ailment returns, recommence the natural medication. 'Like is been treated with like', hence the need for this advice.

Here is a brief guide to selected and often-used homeopathic medicines all of which are available through health food stores, some chemists and specialist homeopathic medicine suppliers. Further remedies are in the captions of this guide under the various illnesses listed. homeopathic doctors use and prescribe many other remedies, which they fully understand, prescribe and direct the use of. Like prescribed synthetic medicines they are not available off-the-shelf.

The following are obtainable, over the counter; -

Aconite 6 — Beginnings of influenza and colds; fear; shock.

Actaea rac 6 — Headaches; neuralgia; painful muscles and/or shooting pains; depression; menopause.

Allium cepa 6 — Common cold, with much sneezing and watering of eyes; hay fever; hacking cough in cold air.

Apis mel 6 — Burning, stinging pains; chilblains; cystitis; boils; swelling of lower eyelids; insect stings; hives.

Argent nit 6 — Anticipatory fear; dyspepsia; headache; mental strain; conjunctivitis.

Arnica 6	After injury; mental and physical shock; before operations, visits to dentist, etc; bruises and sprains; rheumatism.
Arsen. alb 6	Restlessness; vomiting; diarrhoea; stomach upsets from food poisoning.
Belladonna 6	Hot flushed face; shiny eyes; sore throat; facial neuralgia; severe throbbing earache; throbbing boils; throbbing headache.
Bellis perennis 6	Lumbago; bruises
Bryonia 6	Chesty colds; coughs; arthritis
Calc carb 6	Profuse periods; cold extremities; cramp; depression; craving for salt.
Calc fluor 6	Piles which bleed and itch; for the prevention of tooth decay and the stimulation of the formulation of tooth enamel.
Calc phos 6	General debility associated with arthritic conditions particularly if indigestion also suffered; general debility; mental debility.
Calc sulph	Blood purifier, healer; body cleanser; prevents cold and sore throats if caught in early stages.
Cantharis 6	Burns and scalds before blisters form; cystitis; burning pain in bladder both before and after passing water; sunburn.
Carbo veg 6	Indigestion with excessive flatulence; varicose veins.
Causticum 6	Raw, burning, sore pain with chesty cough and sore throat; hoarseness; stiff neck; rheumatism; contractures of tendons; incontinence.
Chamomilla 30	Teething; irritability and restlessness; colic; green slimy diarrhoea; total intolerance to pain.
Cina 6	Worms; itchiness of nose and anus; nausea with white diarrhoea.
Cocculus 6	Travel sickness; nausea with hollow sensation in stomach; nausea during pregnancy.
Coffea 6	Sleeplessness due to mental activity; tension, agitation
Colocynthis 6	Colic; stomach pains; flatulence; cramp; stitching pains.
Cuprum met 6	Cramp in extremities; poor circulation; whooping cough; vomiting.
Drosera 6	Coughs; whooping cough, persistent, irritating cough with retching and vomiting.
Euphrasia 6	Conjunctivitis; inflamed, burning eyes; hay fever; catarrh.
Ferr phos 6	Colds; inflammation of the respiratory tract; a tonic for general debility resulting from influenza.
Gelsemium 6	Colds; influenza; sore throat; runny nose; tight headaches; nervous anxiety.
Graphites 6	Dry skin eruptions on scalp and body; eczema; dry, cracked fingertips; dandruff; catarrh.
Hamamelis 6	Varicose veins; piles; chilblains; bruises.

Hepar sulph 6	Purulent discharges; body odour; choking sensation; general hypersensitivity.
Hypericum 6	Very painful cuts and wounds; blows to fingers or toes; horsefly bites.
Hypericum/Calendula Ointment.	Topical application for painful cuts and wounds, particularly where nerves are involved, as in crushed, punctured wounds, animal bites.
Ignatia 6	Weepiness; bereavement; hysteria; loss of appetite
Ipecac 6	Any illness where there is constant nausea and sickness; morning sickness in pregnancy; bronchitis; asthma.
Kali bich 6	Sinus troubles; catarrh with stringy discharge; coughs; sore throat; nausea and vomiting, particularly after alcohol.
Kali mur	Eliminates catarrh and mucous; aids digestion by helping to provide hydrochlorine.
Kali phos 6	Nervous exhaustion; nervous indigestion; bad breath; giddiness with exhaustion and weakness.
Kali sulph	For respiratory problems. Good for scaly skin or scalp and for hair health.
Lachesis 6	Hot flushes and depression in menopause; menstrual pain when relieved by flow.
Ledum 6	Puncture wounds produced by sharp pointed objects; muscle pains after stings; puncture wounds and injections; insect bites.
Lycopodium 6	Excessive flatulence; constipation; excessive hunger; anxiety; headache
Mag phos	Relieves pain and cramps including spasmodic pain; indicated for neuralgia; neuritis; sciatica; headaches; take with a sip of warm water for more efficiency.
Merc sol 6	Bad breath; body odour; sore throat; mouth abscess.
Mixed pollen 30	Hay fever where triggered by pollen.
Nat mur 6	Sinus troubles; sneezy cold; runny nose; cold sores; migraine; craving for salt.
Nat phos	Good for joint pains; stiffness and rheumatism. An aid to digestive problems.
Nat sulph	A liver tonic, promotes healthy bile; aid for biliousness and where feeling is weak or languid as in humid, oppressive weather.
Nux vom 6	Nervous indigestion; early morning liverishness; indigestion 2-3 hrs after eating; travel sickness; irritability; stuffy nose; hay fever.
Phosphorus 6	Bronchitis; dry cough; hypersensitivity; night sweat.
Phytolacca 6	Mastitis; ulceration of mouth and throat; sore throat; stiff neck with inability to swallow; shooting pains likened to electric shocks.
Pulsatilla 6	Weepiness, particularly in children and pre menstrual women; menopause; catarrh; styes;, prostate.

H

Rhus tox 6	Rheumatism; lumbago; sciatica; strains of joints or tendon; herpes; shingles; chicken pox.
Rhus tox ointment	Topical application of rheumatic pain and stiffness of joints, tendons, ligaments and strains from over lifting.
Ruta grav 6	Bruised bones; fractures; dislocations; sprains.
Ruta ointment	Topical application for bruised bones, dislocations, sprains and sciatic pains.
Sepia 6	Menopausal symptoms; often combined with depression; hot flushes; pre menstrual tension and depression; morning sickness in pregnancy; debility.
Silicea 6	Boils; abscesses; general improvement of skin; hair, fingernails; sinus troubles; headaches.
Sulphur 6	Itching skin; dry skin problems; eczema; boils; inflamed red orifices; burning sensations - eg feet hot in bed.
Symphytum 6	Bone fractures; bone injuries; rheumatic and arthritic conditions resulting from broken bones.
Thuja 6	warts; styes; chronic skin conditions; dandruff; body odour.
Urtica urens 6	urticaria; stinging burns and scalds; itchy blotches on skin.

The excellent book *'The Family Guide To Homeopathy'* gives invaluable and detailed information on the subject. *See Bibliography section.*

HONEY

Much can be written about the goodness of pure natural Honey. As with Honey, the old adage of Hippocrates and our predecessors was never truer, 'Pure natural food should be our medicine, and our medicine should be pure natural food'. *Honey is probably the oldest natural food known to humanity.* Medieval physicians and healers knew about its properties, medicinal and food-wise. Many have written about its goodness. The Bible in the Old Testament mentions Honey several times, including how Jonathan, who was beloved by all, to restore his strength in battle, took it. *Listing the remedies, call them folk, natural, modern, old or whatever, all including Honey, many still used throughout the world, there would be hundreds.* Lelord Kordel in his brilliant book *'Natural Folk Remedies'*, *See Bibliography section,* wrote much about Honey and its health- giving properties. He tells us that: "With 1,600 calories to the pound it is the second highest natural energy builder, surpassed only by dates". Before those who are weight-conscious take this information to heart, they must realise that there is a vast difference in the calories which pure Honey contains and the 'empty' calories in fat, sugar, refined flours and other processed foods. Honey can be classed as medicine because the amount consumed is limited. Used for sweetening purposes it would certainly not be fattening, giving energy, with much else good for the body, as set out here. As a sweetener there is a vast difference between pure Honey, artificial sweeteners and the commercial refined sugars we purchase, just as there is between much of the Honeys we are offered from our supermarket or other suppliers and that from the health food store or direct from the beekeeper. The purest of Honey in that in the comb, as it is when removed from the beehive. Comb Honey is Honey in its raw form, still sealed in the tiny, airtight compartments of bee's wax, something at which to marvel.

Much of the Honey on supermarket shelves has been heated, mixed, often being the product of more than one country. It is sometimes with additives, even though we may not realise this. A purveyor of Honey told me that it is well nigh impossible to analyse sugar syrup when mixed with Honey. The best source of supply of pure natural Honey, other than direct from the beekeeper, is from the health food shop.

Manuka honey, a product of New Zealand, is the purest of pure. This comes in a sealed jar, being offered to us as the champagne or elixir of Honeys. Like champagne it is expensive, the difference being that its health-giving properties are much more so than the alcoholic drink. This Honey is sourced from New Zealand's remote, pollution-free forests, having unique properties. Honey is not recommended for diabetics. There is no food, which will keep as long as Honey, without losing its taste, texture or other properties.

Pure Honey, which is the greatest natural sweetener, contains vitamins and minerals, with much desirable nutritional ingredients, all assimilated easily. It is a gentle laxative, not oxidising in the stomach like sugar, neither does it affect the kidneys. The hydroscopic ability is inestimable with the ability to draw every particle of moisture out of germs, being a powerful antiseptic. It contains an amount of natural glucose and fructose also Vitamins C & B Complex, Amino Acids, Calcium, Magnesium, Iron, Copper and other supplements. The nutritional properties cannot be acclaimed or praised sufficiently. Many who purchase Honey insist it must be clear, regarding the crystallization as sugar. This is a wrong idea. Much of this is the equally edible, health- giving wax. Bear in mind that what appears as sugar in pure natural Honey is vastly different from commercial sugar. Because it is solidified, the intending purchaser often refuses to accept the good product. Seldom does one see crystallized Honey on the supermarket shelf. Is there not a pointer here, perhaps an omen, about its pureness or otherwise. Extreme heat destroys the goodness of Honey but if placed in tepid water it will become more viscous. There is no need for a sell-by date on Honey; it will keep forever, if stored in proper conditions.

There are many remedies associated with Honey. Research now shows that some kinds of Honey, the pure and natural, have out-performed even the strongest antibiotics. Two teaspoons of pure natural Cider Vinegar such as Aspells, as sold by the health food shop, mixed with two teaspoons of pure Honey, is an excellent natural remedy for many ailments including laryngitis, as a slimming aid, sore throat, as a general tonic and much more. There are books written about it. *Turn to Cider Vinegar and Honey caption.* Honey is excellent for treating bed sores, burns, wounds including those septic, scalds, skin irritation, also arthritis, when taken internally. It is an aid where there is gastro enteritis, stomach problems, including peptic ulcers, also bowel problems. Those who suffer from hay fever can benefit from eating pure Honey. It is a good heart stimulant. Manuka Honey is excellent for treatment of open leg ulcers. Many who have had the problem for years have been healed, with the odd exception. The broken skin can often be healed in less than three weeks. *See Ulcers caption.* It has also been warmed, in order to liquidise, with drops placed in the eye to clear cataracts. *Turn to Eyes caption.* As a sleep inducer, Honey in warm milk or water, plus a Calcium/Magnesium tablet, is excellent before retiring to bed. Sir Edmund Hillary when preparing to conquer Everest used Honey in quantity for Diet. Honey in its pure natural form is one of the great gifts to humanity. It is recommended under many of the captions in this Encyclopedia.

HORDEOLUM

See Stye Caption.

HORMONE REGULATOR

Take Agnus Castus which is known as a 'woman's friend' when Oestrogen levels are high or to help regulate excess Progesterone take Dong Quai. *Be guided by advice in Menopause caption.*

HORMONE REPLACEMENT THERAPY (HRT)

This was once seen as the wonder treatment for women undergoing the menopause. As with many other enthusiastically prescribed drugs, which either failed or had lasting side effects, some fatal, HRT now carries an extremely big question mark. Some 40 years ago, as the medical profession - especially the drug manufacturers - were taking off on their unholy quest of prescribing, manufacturing and off-loading what seems an endless flood of so called medicines, including tablets and pills, they told us of the wonderful virtues of Oestrogen. It was promoted as a youth enhancer and the cure-all for the menopause, good for skin, also to increase sexual desire, amongst other things. Here it can be added that there are many natural remedies with no dangers attached, which have helped enormously, certain of them far better than HRT, during this time of life.

Some 10 to15 years ago women were urged to accept the oestrogen and progesterone treatment. **At time of writing the American National Heart Lung & Blood Institute (NHLBI) tells us that all clinical trials have been halted because** of the alarming results, with increase in breast cancer, blood clots, stroke and heart disease. A review by Oxford University six years before this told us of the dangers. Why were these facts not discovered and made known before HRT was allowed on the market? Why were they not made public? Similarly with Thalidomide and many other drugs withdrawn because of their unmistakable dangers. These have nothing to do with HRT, just being mentioned to help correct the mistaken impression giving by the medicines and food regulatory boards or bodies, that before they merchandise all is safe. Here again is a blatant illustration of the unsuspecting public being made the guinea pigs. Like so many synthetic or chemical medicines, HRT has unfortunate side effects. I have seen bloating, stomach and bowel problems, weight gain, depression and certain allergies, which can be put down to the effects of the treatment. It is another therapy, which has certainly lost its appeal. The informative magazine 'The Ecologist' *(See Bibliography)* tells us ironically that one alternative to HRT has been available, being well hidden over the years. *'Progesterone the other major human female hormone is made cheaply from soya, being used to manufacture the hormones in HRT. In fact progesterone is safer and more effective than any of the patented products made from it. It has been available as medicine since the 1960's. It is a remedy for osteoporosis and the reason it has not been used to treat this disease is because it isn't patentable, therefore being unprofitable. Again we see money as the winner. It only serves to show where the interests of the mighty drug companies lie, certainly not in the health of those to whom they offer their chemical concoctions'.*

A well-known medical Professor tells us that he sounded the alarm about the dangers of HRT in 1997. He was ridiculed, even threatened. This is just one of a long list of harmful and injurious drugs removed from the synthetic medicine chain. The Professor referred to has now called on the almighty and seemingly untouchable drug giants to make public their information on adverse effects, which no doubt they are and have been aware of. In all probability we will never be told, it will not be in their interests to do so. The dismaying fact is that they can get away with this as they promote their toxic substances.

This Encyclopedia is about natural health, nutritious, additive-free Diet of pure food, exercise and lifestyle. Here lie the answers, as to how to sail through the menopause. The Japanese are evidence, or an example of this mode of living, as the majority of them enjoy proper Diet, with Exercise, especially Yoga, giving them extreme benefits to mind, body and general well being. They tell of the need for sufficient and proper sleep pattern. The majority of them find the menopause natural. On being questioned many of them self-assuredly told of how they did not remember having it. When told of the many menstrual problems, which women have to contend with, without being prompted, they were not too complimentary about the kind of food on offer here, asking if this was the normal Diet served in the country. They even went so far as to say that 'Many are too lazy to take

H

exercise'. Their words. Allied to, and in conjunction with the all-important Diet, there are natural aids, which can be taken before peri menopause and during the menopause. These include Menosan, Blue/Green Algae such as Spirulina, Black Cohosh, Vitamin's C & E, also Menopace, which is excellent. There are other remedies, which the health food shop can advise on. Those named have proved to be very good where the well-balanced Diet of natural additive-free foods has been followed and used. I believe that much of the remedy is in the pure food. Think very earnestly if contemplating HRT. *Consider the evidence. Remember the advice: 'When in doubt leave out'. At the same time it must be stressed or highlighted that you consult your GP before coming off anything prescribed, such as HRT, even if it is doubtful or dangerous. This is like contradictory advice but it must be said or written. Turn to DIET caption* to learn about what is a great aid to forego HRT, *also See Menopause, Exercise and Sleep captions.*

HORSE CHESTNUT (AESCULUS)

To strengthen the veins, those with varicose and circulatory problems will gain much benefit from Hawthorn (Aesculus) tablets or tincture. It helps in avoidance of phlebitis and where there are haemorrhoids. Its properties in this respect are similar to Rutin. It is an invaluable aid to help eliminate the problem of water retention. As an aid to the heart it is extremely good. *Turn to Heart also Blood Pressure captions.*

HOT DRINKS & FOODS

Few realise the dire effects of hot beverages on the alimentary canal, the long passage in the body which food passes through, including the oesophagus (the gullet). Extremely hot foods and drinks are very often the simple avoidable reasons for hiatus hernia, air swallowing (aerophagy), bowel and other intestinal problems.

HOT FLUSHES

See Menopause Caption.

HRT

See Hormone Replacement Therapy Caption.

HYPER ACTIVITY

See ADHD Caption.

HYPERTENSION

See Blood Pressure High Caption.

HYPNOTHERAPY

Despite the success of the use of Hypnosis in different ways it is still looked upon with some scepticism. It was at one time regarded as quackery, used in the music halls or on the stage, as an additional act for entertainment. Now it has moved to respectability and much more than that. Franz Mesmer founded modern Hypnosis in the 18th. century. From his name originated the word mesmerised. Hypnosis has moved to a position where it is much respected, being highly recognised by the medical profession as another worthy complementary therapy, although not yet fully accepted by some. How it works is still a mystery.

Patients must co-operate fully with and be guided by the Hypnotherapy practitioner in order to benefit. Usually the first session or visit entails being asked about your general state of health, mental problems, addictions or other worries, being just a consultation. You may be questioned about past annoyances or frustrations, according to what you seek treatment for. For addictions, questions will be asked and then at further sessions ideas may be put forward to the subconscious mind, in order to try to solve the problems. Scientists now realise and are favourably disposed to the fact that Hypnotherapy enables the patients to take control of their own health. The practitioner is there but only in the sense of helping the client back to better well being. For instance addiction often renders a person helpless, leaving one incapable of control of oneself. Here the use of Hypnosis can allow one become free of fear, worry or mental problems.

Many claims have been made, the evidence being there, that Hypnotherapy brings relief and aid for pain, skin problems, asthma, allergies, depression and much else. It has proved wonderful for addictions, insomnia, stress and hiatus hernia. Many with the latter have been free from the problem for from five to seven years after treatment.

There is more than one facet of the therapy, including self-Hypnosis. This is where one can learn to impel their own Hypnotism. This may be used to self-treat several health problems. There are now one-day seminars or teachings available to train in self-help. The treatments and teachings are provided and run by fully qualified Hypnotherapists. **It must be mentioned again that there is little, if any, point in seeking treatment if not prepared to co-operate to the fullest degree with the Hypnotherapist.** Find a fully qualified person before seeking Hypnotherapy.

HYPOGLYCAEMIA (low blood sugar)

Occurs to diabetics as a result of insulin over dosage. In others it can happen because of low blood sugar levels. Here is further evidence of the harm of over intake of sugar or sugary products, a problem almost epidemic since the over commercialisation of it's production in modern times. *Turn to Sugar caption.*

Nearly everyone has Hypoglycaemia, some serious, with others being unaware of their problem.

How does one recognise the symptoms? There are so many that it is extremely difficult to explain. The majority of doctors cannot diagnose it. Some even go so far as to say it is a psychological factor. Imagine riding a bicycle for a considerable distance, or taking extreme exercise, fasting and then feeling as if coming up against a brick wall. One feels weak, lethargic, fatigued, irritable, shaking, even with blackouts. Sugary products such as a bar of chocolate will give temporary relief. *If threatened with or having Diabetes be extremely careful, being guided by your GP.* This Encyclopedia repeatedly tells of the dangers of consuming sugar, confectionery and other sugarised products, including adulterated, processed, unnatural fare, much of it fast or easy to put on the table, with little if any nutritives. For example, a study to determine the effects of caffeine and response where Hypoglycaemia was diagnosed, showed alarming results, especially as it could put diabetic patients at high risk. An aid to help control blood sugar is to take a half-teaspoon of ground Cinnamon twice daily. It is doubtful if any remedy will work properly if not partaking of pure natural, additive-free food, *as suggested in DIET caption.*

HYPOTENSION

See Low Blood Pressure Caption.

HYSTERIA

Closely allied to stress, which leads to the problem. Sensible, stable, apparently easy-going, placid individuals can become hysterical when under acute stress. There is no over-the-counter remedy to cure the problem. *There is at hand one of nature's greatest remedies, namely proper food, as written about under caption in this guide. This will lead to better health including calm nerves, warding off of stress and everyday problems. Let pure food be your medicine to help eliminate Hysteria. Turn to Stress and DIET captions* which give much advice in relation to this ailment.

WASH HANDS REGULARLY, ESPECIALLY BEFORE EATING OR AFTER USING THE TOILET. USE WARM WATER, NATURAL SOAP AND A NAIL BRUSH.

IMMUNE SYSTEM

Of the various systems in the complex wonder which is the human body, the Immune needs care to work effectively. If in a healthy state it protects the body from harmful bacteria and germs, keeps one free from allergies, helping to heal from within the body. For instance if a cold is hanging on, slow to leave, or we have one after another, the Immune System is ineffective. Antibiotics are a big enemy, often doing harm. Harming our Immune System can lead to long lasting bad health, often irrecoverable. *Good health, and that includes the Immune System, can best be attained by eating pure natural unprocessed additive-free foods as suggested under DIET caption, also by exercise, which need not be rigorous, only as set out under that caption. The food suggested will include onions, garlic, leafy vegetables and all that is necessary to boost and maintain the Immune System, everything being natural.* Add to this some of the Vitamins and minerals mentioned, including Zinc also Vitamins E, C & A. Immunace, Pure Propolis, Molkosan and Coenzyme Q10 are recommended as Immune System strengtheners.

IMPETIGO

An infection of the skin which is contagious, usually in children. Good hygiene is vital in treating. Proper Diet is of extreme importance aided by Vitamins B Complex and C, Garlic and a tonic such as Kindervital or a junior Multivitamin. Children's supplements are available at the health food store. *Turn to DIET caption* to read about natural additive- free food, which is a very important skin aid.

IMPOTENCE

Inferior Diet, which leads to lack of vitamins and minerals such as Zinc, Vitamin A and others, can lead to impotence. It has been found that wearing extremely tight clothing such as jeans has not helped. *See Diet caption,* which explains about natural foods, also food supplements which may be necessary, what to eat, what to be avoided, all leading to better health and get up and go. Smoking kills. It also helps cause impotence. Avoid alcohol and coffee. Aids are Udo's Choice Oil, Ginkgo Biloba and Damiana. Horny Goat *Weed is known as the king of male sexual enhancement and is often used as a remedy for impotence.*

Take regular exercise, which will also help the circulation, boosting energy, being a stress fighter. Regular sleep is very important. Your doctor may diagnose an underlying health problem, which may be the cause of the Impotence. This should be treated accordingly. *See DIET, Exercise and Sleep captions.* Where relevant, *see Erectile Dysfunction also Aphrodisiacs captions.*

INCONTINENCE

Not to be confused with bedwetting. There are several kinds of Incontinence, which can occur on coughing or straining, from a full bladder, or they may be physical or psychological. Many are too embarrassed to ask the doctor for advice. Ask to be referred to a specialist. ***Tell the doctor you require drugless treatment. This is available and known as behavioural therapy, where both sexes learn the basics of how the urinary process works. It results in controlling the problem, if the person takes the initiative and asks for help.*** St Johns Wort has acted on some problems, as has the partaking of Cherries including Pure Cherry Juice, aided by Morello Cherry spread or tinned Cherries. Pure juice and spread are available from the health food store or they will obtain them.

INDIGESTION

This is the most common complaint in the western world, covering a wide range of symptoms. These include heartburn, dyspepsia, acid stomach, flatulence and belching. Heartburn can make a person feel miserable. There are several reasons for Indigestion, such as eating too quickly, not masticating or chewing properly, irregular meals, eating wrong types of food such as those with spices or fats, including fries. Anxiety, stress or fear can also bring on Indigestion or heartburn. Do you chew your food to a state where it is almost like liquid, where it almost swallows itself? Many who have taken the advice to chew thoroughly, not gulping, have told me of how it solves the Indigestion problem. It leads to losing weight when food has been chewed slowly and deliberately. You are the cause of the problem, knowing what you have eaten. You alone can eliminate it.

Inferior Diet is almost always the reason for the ailment. Today we are expected to eat additive-filled, processed, quickly cooked meals, with some eating as they go, on the trot. MANY ARE NOT AWARE OF WHAT THEY ARE EATING. Think, ask, examine and if prone to indigestion be much more careful about your FOOD intake. The many antacid remedies widely advertised and promoted are to be avoided. The average person has too little acid, this being the cause of Indigestion, therefore the antacid tablets merely makes one worse. Drinking too much liquid with meals often triggers Indigestion because it dilutes the necessary stomach acid. For some it is better to drink either before or between meals. As stated, the natural remedy lies in the hands of the sufferer. The remedy is simply what you eat, what you put into the body. Smoking, alcohol and caffeine are health enemies to be avoided. *Persistent Indigestion can lead to gastric or peptic ulcers. If the problem is repeatedly with you and it should not be if eating sensibly, seek medical advice, especially if over the age of 45.* Natural remedies to bring relief are: Charcoal, Slippery Elm, Papaya or Calamus Tablets, Combination C New Era, Carbo Veg or Liquorice tablets. Charcoal or Slippery Elm tablets are a marvellous remedy for Indigestion, seldom failing to relieve the problem. Eating half an apple is a good aid for the problem. Partaking of pure natural foods and drinks, *as set out in DIET caption,* is the sure way to avoid indigestion. *Also see Heartburn caption.*

INFERTILITY

We are now informed that: 'Many companies are beating a path to the doors of alternative practitioners, in search of a less drastic and intrusive solution than IVF (In Vitro Fertilisation) or 'test tube baby'. Fertility treatment like this is traumatic. Proper lifestyle is vital to improve fertility. Being overweight, poor circulation, bad sleep patterns with lack of vital rest, caffeine, alcohol and fizzy 'drinks' all limit the chances of conceiving. Lifestyle and Food change can work wonders for health and fertility. Be guided also by the advice given in the *DIET* caption regarding intake of Vitamins and Minerals which are often required to enable one battle the stresses and rigours of everyday living. Complementary therapies such as Reflexology, Homeopathy or Aromatherapy can also help. Acupuncture has proved to be highly successful for infertility. ***The charitable organisation Foresight, which is drug-free in its approach to infertility, advocating health improvement by dietary approach, to maximise the producing and conceiving of a healthy baby, has up to an 80% success rate. They can be contacted at 28 The Paddock, Godalming, Surrey, GU71XD UK. Foresight has received much praise and recommendation for their methods, which have proved highly successful, as the figures show.***
Turn to Foresight caption.

INFLAMMATION OF GALL BLADDER
See Gall Bladder Caption.

INFLUENZA

Many confuse colds with flu symptoms. A cold is usually a head cold and will not develop further or become more serious unless neglected. There is an old adage that a cold is three days coming, three days there and three days going. The many cures we see on the shelves do little or nothing to help. Keeping well wrapped up, wearing warm clothing and stockings are often the best remedies as the cold runs its course. Influenza is much more serious. It is an infection, which comes on suddenly, affecting the respiratory tract. Some of the symptoms are pains and aches, lethargy, loss of appetite, a feverish feeling, headache, dry cough or sore throat. It can be a serious illness, especially among the elderly if there is underlying ailment or other health problem. Prevention is easier than trying to cure. *The Winter months of October to March are when Flu is usually caught, therefore the word INFLUENZA should be placed on the calendar for the end of August. Why? Because it is then that plans should be made to be free from the problem. Proper natural Diet is as medicine and is repeatedly advised in this Encyclopedia. The slogan 'You Are What You Eat' is never more relevant than when coupled with better health and prevention of sickness. I always recommend Echinaceaforce, to be taken regularly from September to March, as prescribed on the bottle. It is equal to or better than the Flu jab with an extremely high success rate. It is entirely natural. Added to this is the need for a natural tonic such as Floradix or Biostrath, alternated each week or two with a good Multivitamin tablet also a Garlic capsule and extra Vitamin C. Kindervital also Echinaceaforce are recommended for teenagers and children too. As a pick-me-up after influenza this advice is equally good.* Turn to DIET caption in this Guide to be advised about natural additive-free non-processed food. This and Echinaceaforce I have used and prescribed for many years. I know many who follow this advice and do not have flu or need for a flu injection. *Also see Body Warmth caption*, with the advice given being so necessary in our climate.

INNER EAR DISEASE
See Ears Caption.

INSECT, BEE AND WASP STINGS
See Stings Caption.

INSECT REPELLENT
Citronella mixed with Neem Oil also Bioforce Neem Care have both proved good. An excellent remedy, which is highly effective against insects including mosquitoes, is Thiamin (Vitamin B1) taken in daily doses of 75/100mg for about 21 days before travelling, if going on holiday. The odour of the Vitamin in the skin acts as a repellent. It never fails to detract the insects. It is equally good for both prevention and cure of head lice but with children's dosage to be abided by. *Turn to Head Lice caption* where relevant.

INSOMNIA
See Sleep and Sleepiness Caption.

INTERTRIGO
Occurs where two moist skin surfaces keep touching, not allowing moisture or

sweat to evaporate or dry, sometimes inflamed (i.e. between thighs or under breasts). It is often with Candida and where this is present Acidophilus is the remedy. Taking Devils Claw and Echinacea has also cleared Intertrigo.

IODINE

This mineral, found in seaweed, fish, kelp and mushrooms is necessary for brain and thyroid health, hormones, also to prevent fatigue and sleepiness. It is particularly good for skin, hair and nails. Nullified by fluoridated water, which is forced on us by the relevant authority, which has been too weak-kneed to reject its use. Iodine should come from pure food Diet but can be supplemented by taking Kelp and Garlic where there is a shortage. The following is a simple Iodine check, easily carried out. Paint a small (two inch) patch of tincture of Iodine on the inside of the thigh before going to bed. When dry it should be yellowish orange. Next morning check results:

1. Colour completely gone: significant shortage of Iodine.
2. Colour barely detectable: shortage of Iodine.
3. Colour slightly faded or almost as strong: adequate Iodine.
4. Colour stays for several days: indicates Iodine excess.

If with thyroid problem it is advisable to consult your doctor before taking Kelp or Garlic tablets.

IRIDOLOGY

The colour part of the eye, which surrounds the pupil, the Iris, is unique to each individual, just as fingerprints are. The Iris can tell more about your health than doctors can. Iridology, the study of the Iris or eyes, provides information about every part of the body and can actually warn of potential health problems, even before developing symptoms. Iridology is very often an additional aid to those who practise Homeopathy and naturopathy. Some doctors spoken with claim that Iridologists can cause alarm, even mistaken diagnosis. So also can the medical profession.

I have witnessed several cases of diagnosis of illness and the advice on treatment by some Iridologists. No pun intended they were an eye opener, as they gave sound advice in the treatment suggested. Although it involves examination of the eyes Iridology is quite different to the work of an optician. The latter is concerned with the health of the eye itself, whereas *Iridology provides a means to determining the strengths and weaknesses of all organs and systems of the body. Nerve fibres from all parts of the body are located in the eyes, their structure and condition indicating the degree of health of individual organs.* If you have a disorder that has not responded well to other forms of treatment, it may be because the real cause has not been identified. For example, skin complaints may stem from a number of causes, such as poor digestive chemistry, stress, glandular irregularities, disorders of detoxifying organs, e.g. liver or kidneys. Although they may seem apparently unconnected, many disorders can be due to spinal misalignment. From observation of the condition of the nerve fibres an Iridologist may be able to identify in which organ, system or structure of the body the problem originates. ***Besides being an analytical tool that can identify the root cause of existing disorders Iridology can also reveal problems that have not yet become apparent, enabling the patient to take remedial action to correct the situation before disease sets in.*** Although Iridology is not a remedial therapy, members of The Guild of Naturopathic Iridologists are qualified not only as Iridologists, but also in another form of complementary medicine e.g. Herbal Medicine, Homeopathy or Nutrition. Having determined the body's weaknesses from the Iris analysis, the therapist will then be able to advise an appropriate form of treatment. As with all therapy it is imperative that one is privy to fully qualified Iridologist. ***It must be repeated here of the need to have eyes tested regularly by an optician, to guard against eye disease, particularly glaucoma.*** *Also see Eyes caption.*

IRITIS

See Eyes Caption.

IRON

See Vitamins & Minerals Caption.

IRON DEFICIENCY

Iron Deficiency was almost unheard of until the latter half of the 1900's, except where it was brought on through excessive loss of blood, or with certain medical conditions, which lead to anaemia. It is much more evident now because of our over-reliance on processed 'foods', many of which are of doubtful sustenance. Young people, especially those on slimming Diets also vegetarians, are at risk and often have to resort to Iron supplements or tonics. It must be pointed out that too much can be dangerous. Seek advice; asking for blood test should you feel anaemic, lethargic, constant tiredness or rundown. Iron supplements should not be taken with Vitamin E or Calcium. They should be taken at least four hours apart. Iron only supplements or medicines should not be taken unless prescribed by a doctor. Best source of Iron from the Diet is liver, beef, lamb, green vegetables and dried fruits, including apricots and raisins. Floradix is an excellent tonic which gives safe balanced requirements of Iron, with Brewer's Yeast and Kelp also containing an amount of the mineral. Nettles are one of the best sources of natural Iron known. *Turn to Nettles caption.*

IRRITABLE

Being irritable can be attributed to many reasons, including a deficiency of Vitamin B Complex, Calcium, or if with low blood sugar. It can be corrected, as can many of our everyday niggling ailments, by change to natural unprocessed nutritious food. *See DIET caption,* which also includes advice about the supplements, mentioned, which may be necessary. Here you'll find much that is required to calm the mind, banish the irritableness, also advice which can only lead to better health. *Also see Loss of One's Affection for Family caption,* where Sepia is a remedy. This too can be extremely helpful where one is irritable.

IRRITABLE BOWEL SYNDROME

This disorder of the digestive system is not a disease, being as a syndrome, a collection of symptoms, which tend to occur together. It is a common problem. Symptoms include constipation, diarrhoea, stomach cramps, bloated feeling and frequent change of bowel habits, passing mucus or rumbling stomach noises. Often it is a follow-on of food poisoning. Most in the medical profession fail to recognise Candida Albicans as very often being the cause of IBS. I have spoken with men and women sufferers, all of whom had been attending the doctor. They were reluctant to carry on with or accept conventional medication. All have been able to live normal healthy lives, where they disciplined themselves to follow the advice given in this Encyclopedia about Diet, Exercise and Hypnotherapy. Some have opted for the *Hay Diet,* with excellent results. Others follow the *DIET* set out in this Guide, using the elimination programme of omitting an amount of foods for 10 to 14 days and then returning them to the Diet to find the disagreeable ones. *This is described under Allergy caption.* These are noted down and not partaken of at any time. Left out were fizzy 'drinks', citrus fruits, coffee, scrambled or soft-cooked eggs, spicy foods, certain dairy products including full cream milk, sauces, strawberries, pork, beef, sausages, processed foods including additive-filled meats and fried foods. Alcohol is taboo.

Including the foods listed there may be the need to eliminate white flour, wheat products or pastry. One may be lactose intolerant where a dairy free Diet is needed. ***This food exemption list looks quite long. Examine it and you will find that much mentioned is not nutritious anyway, being easily omitted.*** The Diet recommended, with perhaps the dairy and yeast products or some of them left out is often the answer. Highly successful as treatment for Irritable Bowel Syndrome is the taking of Silica, which is available as Silicea. One dessertspoonful taken daily in water absorbs the toxins and irritants from food and waste matter. As well as natural Diet of pure food, other aids for the gut problem are Acidiophilus if with Candida, Slippery Elm, extra Wheat bran with porridge, Psyllium Husks, Calamus or Lactate supplements also pure Manuka honey. *Proven results* *ιeen seen in the use of Hypnotherapy. Statistics show that it has given lerful relief, with the problem not returning for some five to seven years.* ss is to be avoided. The need for exercise is vital for better health. The one person who can nearly always solve the IBS problem is the sufferer, who must do so by trial and error, finding out what can be or cannot be eaten, then keeping rigidly to the chosen Diet. *See Diet, Hay Diet, Exercise, Sleep, Dairy Free and Gluten Free Diet captions.*

ITCHING

This may not be looked on as a serious health complaint. To those who suffer from skin itch or pruritis it can be exasperating. It is more prevalent in the aged, often referred to by the medical profession as senile pruritis. It may be neither age or skin related, often being a symptom of some underlying disease. Can occur as result of dry skin, too many hot baths or showers which remove oils from the body, synthetic fibres in clothing, or over use of antibiotic treatment. Candida Albicans, also known as thrush, which leads to itchiness can be treated with Acidophilus.

My diary shows that it is a big Winter problem and with good body warmth it can often be avoided. Very often no other treatment is needed. Wearing of silk or cotton next to the skin is advised. Change of Diet has very often solved the problem. With the present-day additive-filled food there is often little nutrition, with the person lacking in Vitamin B Complex. Lack of this Vitamin is often the answer to this itching problem. *Combined with Aloe Vera and natural food, the homeopathic remedies Sulphur 6 or Calc Phos and Vitamin B Complex seldom fail as a remedy.* Allergenics Emollient Cream is suggested where there is dry skin with itch. Evening Primrose Oil capsules with three or four cups of Dandelion Root tea taken daily have helped to banish itchiness. I have found that Combination P New Era taken with Acidophilus is sometimes a good remedy. If there is persistent aggravating itch proper diagnosis must be made to find the health problem, to be treated accordingly. *One has sometimes to try several of these remedies, keeping to what works best to avoid or banish the itch, but as set out, the remedy which has most success is the Aloe Vera, Vitamin B Complex, Sulphur 6 or Calc Phos taken with natural food combination. Turn to DIET caption* and read about natural foods which lead to healthy skin and freedom from Itching.

JAMS, MARMALADES AND SPREADS

I visit the supermarkets regularly to read the ingredients labels, to see does anybody look at them, also to view the trolleys laden with inferior 'foods'. Recently I noticed a man select one pot of each, Jam and Marmalade. It was observed that they were the cheapest displayed. The list of ingredients was appalling, containing preservatives, additives, colours, sweeteners and chemicals. The Jams sold under 'Weight Watchers' brand contained much additives. Also noted were some diabetic jams, which have been condemned as being unsuitable for those who use them. *A varied selection of sugar free spreads is available in the health food store and some supermarkets. They are full fruit, being sweetened with pure fruit juice. They cannot be called Jams because of an anomalous or bizarre ruling by the EU where sugar must be used to ensure it is Jam, despite the all-pure fruit product being much healthier. They contain no additives, all being purely natural.* 'Whole Earth' and 'Meridian' brands are purely natural and highly recommended. At no stage on any of my visits to the multi-food stores have I noticed one person scan or run their eye over the ingredients lists. Few are aware of what they are putting into their bodies. This is one of the main reasons why we are a sick nation.

JAUNDICE

This is observed as yellow discolouration of the skin and eyes, caused by excess bile in the system. The liver, which may have become diseased, should deal with it or there may be a blockage in the bile duct. It often leads to anaemia because of the breakdown of nutrients, which aid the red blood cells. There are several types of Jaundice, with medical diagnosis necessary before attempting any treatment. Consult your doctor and be advised. What is mentioned here are aids to recovery, with proper Diet being the all-important factor. *See DIET caption.* This must be adhered to for some considerable time, or at all times if possible also being supplemented by a Multivitamin tablet and extra Vitamins E and C. Carrot juice, Dandelion Root and Milk Thistle are all aids to a healthy liver and relief from Jaundice. *Turn to Liver caption.*

JET LAG

See Travel & Holiday Health Caption.

JOGGING

This is not a form of training that appeals to me, even though much attracted by exercise and physical fitness. Unless preparing for athletics or other sports, for which extreme fitness is required, there are easier forms of exercise such as walking or cycling. Jogging jars the joints, especially the knees. As an ex-international athlete, who enjoyed the rigours of tough work out and training, it is most annoying to see athletes and those who train, running or Jogging on the road instead of on grass or a proper track, with the hard surface being of no aid to the joints referred to. Many do not understand the need to wear tracksuit or warm clothing in order to keep the joints and muscles warm. This is one of the golden rules of how to attain fitness, when exercising or if training seriously. *Turn to Exercise caption.*

JOINTS AND JOINT HEALTH

Unless as a result of sport or accident injury, Joint problems are usually as arthritis, rheumatism or if with osteoporosis. Here is another example of how almost always the type of Diet partaken of is the cause. Our whole body, including the health of the Joints, is dependant in the first instance on an intake of pure, natural, nutritious foods and drinks, which include the necessary vitamins and minerals. Inferior and fast 'foods' and 'drinks' which are highly processed, with little nutrition, only aggravate health problems including that of arthritis, rheumatism or other Joint ailments. *Turn to Arthritis, Rheumatism, Osteoporosis also DIET captions*, being guided by the advice given in order to restore vitality, which includes supple and flexible pain-free Joints. Many find the supplement Joint Ace a relief and healer. It contains several natural ingredients in one easily taken capsule. Aktiv Juice is another supplement to be recommended. Devils Claw, Runo or Aloe Vera Joint Complex, which contains Glucosamine, are probably three of the greatest natural remedies for Joint aches and pains. All are available from the health food store or some chemists. Some choose one as being the most satisfactory, while others make a different choice. To ensure better Joint health take Calcium/Magnesium/Vitamin D tablet daily long-term. The natural combination is available at the health food store. For other recommended supplements find the ones most suitable and continue using them.

JUICES

I have seen much evidence of and have witnessed recovery and return to better health by the consuming of pure and nutritious fruit and vegetable Juices or purees. This has happened where illness and sickness was present, some of it serious. I've always said that if with illness, whether simple, acute or even life threatening, this would be the most important method of treatment for me. ***Don't rush out to buy from the legion of cartoned or plastic bottles of Juice so nicely presented and psychedelically packaged. Many have the word pure or pure fruit Juice printed on, with most to be avoided. Pure all-too-often does not mean pure. The sentence 'Made from concentrated fruit Juice' appears frequently, showing that the Juice has been diluted. Many have added sweeteners. When the words free from artificial additives, colour or preservatives are written on, be even more vigilant.*** Even if these things are natural, who needs them in food or drink? Most of the colours or preservatives, artificial and otherwise are factory prepared. Much is not edible. *If you are serious about Juicing, the advice is to buy a good Juicer, which will process fruit and vegetables. You will be repaid many times, especially health-wise. There are many on the market. Select a strong rugged pulper and Juicer, which will crush and grind both vegetables and fruits into a pure Juice. You should also be able to produce purees and fruit sorbets.* Pure juices are health giving, detoxing, as they help cleanse the systems, making one look and feel better, strengthening the immune system, increasing your energy, vitality and mental alertness. *As this Encyclopedia keeps repeating, better nutrition, with pure Juices high up on the list, can help prevent or relieve many of our health problems.* A wide range of fruit and vegetables can be juiced. There are Juicing books available which will assist greatly. The health food store carries a range of Juices, all pure and natural. They may be more expensive, but as is usual, one pays more for the pure quality product.

JUNK 'FOOD'

Much of the additive-filled, so- called 'foods' and 'drinks' consumed are just that, JUNK. Here is one of the main reasons for the ailments and illnesses with which we are scourged. Refuse to eat them. Much of the 'food' on offer is unnatural, being filled with a combination of some of the hundreds of substances used to provide the JUNK, which means rubbish. People will not be educated, but at least they can learn. The additives, all too many of them not edible, are used to make the 'food' cheap, with little if any thought given to the health of those who eat it. *Junk 'food' can prove to be terribly expensive. Also turn to Fast Foods Caption.*

K VITAMIN

See Vitamins Caption.

KALI MUR, KALI PHOS, KALI SULPH

See Tissue Salts caption to learn about these excellent remedies. Few know about their goodness for the treatment of much of our present day niggling ailments.

KELP

This source of iodine, which is an anti-ageing protection amongst other things, contains Vitamins B Complex, D, E and K also Magnesium, Iodine and Calcium. It is recommended for many ailments throughout this Encyclopedia. It must not be taken if with thyroid problems before discussing with a doctor. *Also see Iodine caption.*

KIDNEYS

Kidney disease, Kidney stones, and the several individual Kidney-related disorders are potentially serious and need medical attention before treating. Much can be done naturally to prevent or impede the problem. One of the prime reasons for our ill health including that of the Kidneys is inferior Diet of 'foods' and 'drinks'. All should be purely natural. Change to the foods and drinks mentioned in Diet caption to feel and see the resultant change in well being, to help cleanse the Kidneys or as a tonic for them, also acting as a preventative of Kidney troubles.

If with minor Kidney problems take pure unsweetened Cranberry Juice, Pulsatilla tablets and Pumpkin Seeds, obtainable from the health food store. They sell only pure juices. Kordel's Cranberry 10,000, which also contains Uva Ursi and Buchu has proven to be excellent. Parsley liquidised, chopped, or pureed, mixed with plain natural yoghurt, is a Kidney tonic as is Solidago Complex, which also helps to remove puffy or baggy eyes. Strawberries can cause Kidney stones. *See Barley Water caption,* because this is a real Kidney tonic, when made up naturally. Drink copious amounts of pure water, up to eight glasses daily. If you keep on diluting the urine the stinging effect will be neutralised, thus allowing you to have a full bladder with no discomfort. The Diet as already mentioned is number one remedy, prevention and aid. *In the DIET caption* you will learn of the need to avoid caffeine, alcohol, sugar, fizzy drinks, salt and other things, which do not help the Kidneys. If with Kidney stones avoid tomatoes. *Turn to Cranberry Juice caption.*

LACTOSE INTOLERANCE

The assumption is that the sugar which milk contains is the main cause of milk allergy. I believe it is the fat content. Many who switch to goats milk or skimmed milk find the problem vastly improved, or even banished, therefore it cannot be the lactose which triggers off the allergy. Seek further advice from your health food shop. They can supply natural or alternative remedies such as Lactaid or Lactase.

K

LARYNGITIS

Where this ailment arises due to over exercise of voice, as when singing or when shouting, take two teaspoons of pure Cider Vinegar added to half glass of tepid water into which is mixed two teaspoons of pure Honey. This should be taken every hour for eight hours. Other remedies are Combination J New Era, Poke Root, or Iceland moss. If the loss of voice persists for more than four to five days see your doctor as there may be some related problem.

LAUGHTER

Aristotle said more than 2,000 years ago, that "it is a bodily exercise precious to health". There is nothing like a good hearty Laugh. Doctors used tell of its goodness to get the circulation going, to expand the lungs, to aid the heart. Now many are too serious, too rushed, to enjoy the value of talk, banter and laughter or to suggest having a good Laugh frequently..

LAXATIVES

The use of chemical drugs as Laxatives should be discouraged. There are many natural Laxatives, including mild or stronger as required. Visit your health food shop and be advised. *Also see Constipation caption,* remembering that with good natural food there is little reason to be constipated or in need of Laxatives. Pure bran or linseed seldom fails as a remedy. Take one dessertspoon of linseed daily or up to four or five dessertspoons of bran every four or five days or as required, to help keep bowel motion regular. Steeped overnight, taken with porridge at breakfast-time, it is an excellent remedy. Taking the mixture daily is inadvisable. *See DIET, Linseed also Fibre captions.*

LEARNING DIFFICULTIES

See Dyslexia Caption.

LECITHIN

This is referred to as Vitamin F. Forty years ago little was known about the wonderful health giving substance, which is Lecithin. Then it was used as an emulsifier in a small way, with little or no information available. Much analysis and research has been done by the natural food industry. Because it is pure and natural, coming from the earth, the mighty drug conglomerates are not interested in its goodness. It is another natural product, which cannot be patented or registered, with no money in it for them. Again the health of the partaker is secondary to their line of thought. The public will be told little about the many natural aids available. They will learn only by asking those, such as health food personnel or the minority, who understand about what is natural.

Everybody can do with Lecithin. It contains Phosphatidyl Choline and Phosphatidyl Inositol, both of which are phospholipids, which improve and complement the mind, ensuring better mental performance. It is a brain food and memory enhancer, helping to prevent Alzheimer's disease and Dementia. It is also good for the heart, helping to control cholesterol. It is an extremely good emulsifier, breaking down fats, being an aid to slimmers. Essential for regulation of liver and gall bladder including the elimination of toxins and drug residue, regarded as a liver protector. It helps to alleviate psoriasis also helping to restore strength during convalescence. An amount of research and documentation has been carried out. It is best taken as Lecithin Granules obtainable from the health food store or some chemists. Chemists will offer it in tablet form which is a most uneconomical way to obtain the goodness of Lecithin. Ask for the Granules. One teaspoonful of Lecithin Granules, to be taken with liquid, on porridge or other natural breakfast cereal, is equivalent to eighteen 270mg of Lecithin tablets. Eventually all pharmacists will stock it, because of customer demands. It is natural, something medical people know little about. They are in the chemical business where the end product and money go hand in hand. *For years I have recommended this all round health giving remedy, which is derived from soya. Almost always when it is specified the question asked is "What is that?" People are learning slowly, about the natural and the good. Lecithin is both.* **When purchasing look for the Genetically Modified Free Symbol which should be displayed on the container.**

LEGS

- Aching: Hawthorn, Combination P New Era, Pantothenic Acid.
- Burning sensation: Aesculus (Horse Chestnut), Vitamin E.

- Cramps: Take a Multivitamin tablet plus Calcium / Magnesium/Vitamin D supplement long-term. Calcium is best taken at night and the Multivitamin in the morning. Drink Raspberry Leaf tea three or four times daily or take Raspberry Leaf tablets.
- Giving Way feeling: Cramp Bark, Elasto.
- Heavy lead like: Aesculus (Horse Chestnut), Multivitamin tablet to obtain Vitamins A, C and E also Zinc.
- Pins & Needles: Pantothenic Acid, Cramp Bark, Combination P New Era
- Restless, Known as Restless Leg Syndrome: Multivitamin tablet, also take extra Vitamin E, Calcium / Magnesium / Vitamin D combination and Zinc/Copper supplement. It has been found that faulty Diet has been the cause of Restless Leg syndrome. *See DIET caption.* The supplements recommended here will help, provided one takes the advice to consume natural unprocessed foods and drinks. The need to drink plenty of water cannot be over emphasised. Drink eight to ten glasses daily.
- Swollen: Can be due to heart or kidney complaint. Often brought on by excess heat. See doctor for diagnosis, because the circulatory system may be effected. It is recommended not to cross the legs when sitting.
- Leg Ulcers: *See Ulcers Varicose Caption.*

L

LEISURE

In 1970 I wrote an article headed 'Leisure' setting out how necessary it was to take time out to relax, to enjoy oneself. It was pointed out that a healthy life consisted not alone of reasonable health but also of peace of mind, including freedom from everyday worries. Stress, depression and many other ailments were not much in vogue then. We were told of a new device which would give us ample time for Leisure in the future. Our hours worked would be shorter, our wages and salaries would not decrease, with the workload easier. This new, at the time mind-boggling gismo, was the microchip. We now appear to toil harder also longer than ever, with endless problems at work, also with our health and minds. **The theme must be repeated, only stronger than ever, of the need to take time to relax and enjoy so much that is good in this life.** Those who think that visiting the pub, partaking of alcohol or smoking, is leisure, are wrong. You are what you put into your body and how you treat it.

Peter Bermingham who was the Works Manager and key person responsible for construction of one of the largest contracts in the world, the building of the Channel Tunnel, used tell his employees **"Pace yourself, enjoy your work, you will obtain better results".** *Learn to unwind, take time for breaks, to refresh, relax and recharge the batteries. Turn to Relaxation caption.*

LETHARGY & TIREDNESS

These two words can also mean fatigue, sleepiness, listlessness, exhaustion and a host of other tired related words. Constant Tiredness must be looked into, because it is most serious, often being a symptom of ill health, such as heart disease. If persistently Tired see your doctor, possibly finding the root cause. Often all of these ailments, if they can be called a sickness, are due to the modern working environment. Included are stress, life's pressures and the difficulty of sustaining a proper balance between work and home life. The need for sufficient sleep and regular bedtime hours must be pointed out. All too many do not realize the goodness of proper and regular sleep. It is as good food.

Fatigue is one of the most common symptoms of sluggish or stressed liver. Few seem to realise that pure natural Diet of additive free, unprocessed food, is like medicine, very often the answer to the problems of fatigue, lethargy and other similar problems. See DIET caption, which is a wide-ranging subject, with suggestions regarding the use of food supplements, including Vitamins, Minerals and Herbal Aids. Milk Thistle, Boldo and Dandelion are good liver medicines which when taken can do much to reduce Tiredness. A tonic such as Floradix or Biostrath, which contain Iron, are good pick me ups, leading to better energy and well-being. Pay a visit to and confide in your doctor, tell him exactly how you feel. Some are not honest with the GP. Many times a simple blood check has quickly found the cause of being Lethargic or constantly Tired. *Turn to Fatigue caption.*

LETTER WRITING

See Writing Caption.

LIBIDO

See Sex Drive (lack of) Caption.

LICE

See Head lice Caption.

LINSEED (FLAXSEED)

Old time remedies very often included Linseed, even for animals. Its goodness is no less today. It is extremely health giving, being a bowel lubricant, a healer, cough remover and is good for heart and circulation. It is a remedy to ease constipation, for relief of bronchitis and catarrh. The seeds can be ground in a liquidiser, stored for daily use, sprinkling a dessertspoonful or more on porridge or muesli, every four or five days or when necessary, at breakfast time. May also be infused as tea by adding boiling water to two or three teaspoons of the ground seeds, drinking three or four cupfuls daily.

LIPS

homeopathic tissue salts almost always prove to be the simple remedy for lips and many skin problems.

- Chapped: Combination P New Era or Calc Fluor.
- Cold Sores or Herpes Simplex: L-lysine or Combination N New Era. A remedy which seldom fails is to take Lemon Balm Leaves which are also available as Melissa tablets.
- Cracked: Calc Fluor or rub on pure Manuka Honey.
- Dry with skin peeling: Combination P New Era or Kali Phos.

Folic Acid is often deficient where there are lip or mouth problems. *Also see Mouth caption.*

LIQUIDISER

No home should be without one of our greatest kitchen gadgets, which is comparatively cheap to purchase. In this Encyclopedia and elsewhere we are repeatedly told of the need for intake of extra fruit and vegetables. Liquidising them is a labour saving and extremely beneficial way of making up this nutrition. It is an easy way to make up natural dips, smoothies, mayonnaise, fruit juices and purees. Other goodies, which can be made, are olive oil salad dressings, milkshakes, ground- nuts, nutritious soups, and other things found in a natural food recipe book. Make sure the ingredients are thoroughly washed before using also take time to read the safety instructions. A child's first solids can easily be made up as purée, then frozen in whatever size cubes chosen, all to be used later. Just imagine the good in this compared to the additives in most of the off the shelf baby 'foods'. A Liquidiser is indispensable for those interested in using pure natural foods, all of which lead to better health of mind and body. If interested *turn to Baby Foods caption.*

LIVER

A healthy Liver means health and energy. It is one of the most important organs of the body, all too often being abused. Thankfully it can to a limited extent regenerate itself, the only organ within the body able to do so. This does not mean we should neglect the Liver. Apart from all it does through our intake of sugar, starch, protein, fats, edibles or alcohol, the Liver stores needed vitamins and minerals. One of its most important functions is as a detoxifier, destroying much that is alien to our bodies. *'Modern Nutrition'* volume 17, No. 4 tells us that fizzy 'drinks', which it seems are anything but soft, are causing cirrhosis of the Liver, just as alcohol does. Even young people are being effected. Milk Thistle, Boldo and Dandelion are all Liver medicines to aid its health. Lecithin, which contains the required Choline is extremely good as a Liver tonic. It should be taken regularly to help the Liver break down fat by emulsifying it. Nat Sulph is a good Liver detoxer, which like the body, needs help to perform properly.

LOBELIA

As a herbal remedy Lobelia is obtainable in tablet form. For those with breathing, respiratory, catarrhal or bronchial ailments, it has very often proved invaluable. Coughs, colds and sinusitis have all been banished by the use of Lobelia. A friend who has respiratory trouble caused by his work in a dusty environment in the past, to whom I recommended the remedy some twenty years ago, now retired, recently produced a box from his pocket saying, "I would not be without Lobelia".

LOSS OF ONES AFFECTION FOR FAMILY

The symptoms are of being irritable and snappy, difficult to live with, warm-hearted with friends. Sepia, a homeopathic remedy, which comes from cuttlefish, can alleviate this aversion. *Also see Irritable caption.*

LOSS OF SENSE OF SMELL

See Smell Caption.

LOSS OF SENSE OF TASTE

See Taste Caption.

LOWER BACK PAIN

One of the biggest reasons for time off work. Lower Back pain can be physical or emotional, making it extremely difficult to diagnose exactly what the problem is, or why the pain. It can come from lazy lifestyle or from how one sits or walks. Lack of exercise can lead to Lower Back pain or it can be as lumbago. In women it is often found to be a menopausal problem. Sometimes due to stress or overwork. Often pain in the Lower Back is actually a prostate or kidney problem. It can also be brought on by lifting a heavy object or may be due to arthritis in the Lower Back. Recently a farmer with the problem told of how he jumped off a fence some years ago, feeling sore for a few days. The same pain had only recently returned. Doctors, Osteopaths, Acupuncturists or other Manipulative Practitioners must diagnose what is wrong and treat accordingly. Chiropractic or Reflexology therapy, have given excellent relief. *Turn to the relevant problems in this Encyclopedia* in order to treat naturally. *Read the Alexander Technique caption,* which I have no hesitation in recommending for different kinds of back pain. Qualified therapists are listed in the yellow pages.

LOW BLOOD PRESSURE

See Blood Pressure (low) Caption.

LOW BLOOD SUGAR

See Hypoglycaemia Caption.

LUMBAGO

This is another form of lower back pain, which must be diagnosed correctly, in order to find the proper remedy. For instance, a young lady with what appeared to be Lumbago, found that it was gynaecological, where treatment with Agnus Castus and Dolomite brought relief. Lumbago has been successfully treated by taking Rhus Tox 6C or Aesculus, Devil's Claw or Black Cohosh. Sometimes the problem is not Lumbago, being disc or lumbar related. Treatment should then be by osteopath or chiropractic. *The Alexander Technique therapy has helped many with back pain. Turn to this caption.*

LUNGS

Vitamin A can help prevent Lung disease. If with any Lung problem do not self-treat. *See Respiratory Health caption* for advice and care of the Lungs with prevention of Lung problems being emphasised.

LUPUS

This chronic and debilitating disorder is the result of the immune system going awry as it protects itself. Sometimes misdiagnosed as ME. There are two types of the disease or a third if you take that brought on by reaction to certain prescribed drugs. Changing to a purely natural unprocessed food Diet, after coming off what were inferior foods, has helped treatment of effected patients by a doctor. Proper nutrition is the key to successful treatment, which sometimes gives dramatic improvement. Sometimes it can be a slow and tedious climb back to full health. Speak with G.P. and discuss the matter of proper natural Diet. Some may not be even interested, only prescribing immunosuppressive or cortosteroid drugs. Pure fruit and vegetable juices, especially carrot, are essential, as this gives the necessary Vitamin A. *Be guided by the natural DIET caption* which also includes the need to supplement with natural Vitamins and Minerals in order to return to better health. *Turn to Immune System caption.*

LYCOPENE

Found in tomatoes, being an antioxidant carotenoid, which gives the red colour. It is a very good disease fighter. Helps reduce the risk of prostrate gland trouble also good for heart health. Easy way to obtain is in supplement form.

LYMPH GLANDS

Sufficient emphasis cannot be placed on the need for a healthy lymphatic system. The vessels, which work parallel to and in conjunction with the circulatory system, drain and cleanse waste products from the blood also being a protector of the immune system. At the same time they convey to the blood the end product, the life and health giving properties from the digestive system. If toxins or blockages occur it spells trouble in the form of disease such as glandular disorders, joint pains, with ears, throat, nose and eyes being affected. Therefore the lymphatic system is vitally important in the body's immune responses. This caption explains only a little about the wonder of the lymph, which in itself is only a watery fluid, devoid of colour. In order to have a healthy lymphatic and immune system the greatest single aid is pure natural unprocessed food. *See DIET caption and be guided as to how to be with better health including that of the Lymph Glands.* Many of the illnesses we are constantly experiencing today are caused by an overburdened lymphatic system. Food, pure food, additive free is the best medicine.

The advice under Diet sets out the food supplements necessary to attain better health, when used in conjunction with natural food, also the need for Exercise and proper Sleep pattern. *Also turn to Immune System caption,* with the suggestions there being an aid to Lymph Glands health.

THE DEPARTMENT OF HEALTH - OR IS IT SICKNESS? SHOULD BE BLUNTLY TOLD:
"THAT A SIGN, PRINTED IN BIG LETTERS, SHOULD BE PROMIENTLY DISPLAYED
WHERE HEALTH PROFESSIONALS GIVE ADVICE AND WHERE THOSE WHO SEEK IT, CAN
READ THE MESSAGE".
MORE EDUCATION ABOUT HEALTH THROUGH USE OF NATURAL FOOD, DIET, EXERCISE
AND REGULAR SLEEP PATTERN, MEANS VERY MUCH LESS MEDICATION.

MACULAR DEGENERATION

See Eyes Caption.

MAGNESIUM

See Vitamins & Minerals Caption.

M

MAG PHOS

See Tissue Salts Caption.

MAGNETIC THERAPY

I have spoken with many who wear Magnetic bracelets and bangles. It is only fair to write about their apparent goodness to muscular pains, including arthritis and rheumatism, also helping to increase energy. They are natural, with no side effects, the only contraindication is that they must not be worn where one is with pacemaker.

MALNUTRITION

In the world, over 500 million people suffer from malnutrition and it is estimated that over 15 million children die from this cause each year. Over 70% of the world's grain is consumed by a little over 20% of the world's population. Here is much Food for thought. In the Western world many die young through the intake of factory-made, processed, additive-filled 'foods' and 'drinks'. In poor countries there are millions who would be delighted to grow their own food if tools and knowledge of how to do so were provided. We live in a badly orientated and divided world *'WHERE MUCH WANTS MORE'.*

MANGANESE

See Vitamins & Minerals Caption.

MANUKA HONEY

This pure food, produced in New Zealand, is probably the elixir of honey. It has excellent curative properties, especially to help dissolve cataracts of the eyes, for varicose ulcers, stomach ulcers, burns, skin and many other diseases. *Turn to Honey, Eyes or Ulcer captions.* It is available from health food stores.

MARGARINE

This is artificial, man-made, a modern concoction of the giant food industries. Most contain water, with fats of animal and vegetable materials, also other additives. The oils can be cheap, over-refined, denatured, hydrogenated and far from being pure oils. *See both captions Cooking Oils also Cooking Oils, How They Are Produced.* Many Margarines or 'foods', which contain them, should be left on the shelf, shunned. Have you ever purchased or eaten Margarine-filled products? Have you read the ingredients label? Are you aware of what is in much of the over-hyped, highly-advertised, unnatural 'food' which is sold as Margarine? Do you believe the jargon about it being good for the heart and cholesterol levels? Read the advertising jargon describing the product. It is done in such a manner that it would be impossible to prove that the facts given are either correct or otherwise.

A link between adult onset asthma and intake of Margarine has been found in a highly organised study. This is apparently due to the synthetic oils used in Margarine becoming hydrogenated. This is another of the reasons that 'WHEN IN DOUBT, LEAVE OUT'. *I will probably be told by the Margarine producers that I am wrong. The European Prospective Investigation into Cancer and Nutrition (E.P.I.C.) who studied the Dietary and Lifestyle habits of 25,000 adults will tell them otherwise.* **Study the chart set out under Cooking Oils caption and form your own conclusions as to what type of oils are used to manufacture Margarine.** Recently we learn of how Unilevers, one of the leading Margarine-processors, have awarded their retired co-chairman £1.22million (€1.76million) as 'compensation' upon the termination of his employment. His pension is also valued at £852,000 (€1.2million) per annum. Pure butter as a spread, used sparingly, is additive-free, natural, pure. Margarine is processed, unnatural. *Also turn to Fat caption.*

M.E.

See Chronic Fatigue Syndrome Caption.

MEASLES

Seek medical attention. Here is a health problem that can be serious if not properly treated. Despite the many medicines available we are no nearer a cure for this disease. In the past mothers of young children did not send for the doctor in order to treat Measles. There were few if any after effects or fatalities. The child's system was free from antibiotics and chemicals medicines. Little, if any, of these were used at childbirth. Everything was natural. Now there is mounting evidence of a link between the use of vaccination and autoimmune disorder. Perhaps this is why Measles were easily treated in the past, with the immune system being healthy. **Many complementary therapists are of the opinion that childhood illnesses serve a purpose by strengthening the system.** After illness, such as Measles, a tonic or pick-me-up is necessary. For children there are natural tonics, also junior Multivitamins, which contain Vitamin A, so vital after Measles. They are available from the health food shop. A well-balanced Diet of pure foods is very important to help regain good health. *See DIET caption.* Good natural food is as medicine to help prevent Measles and attain better health afterwards.

MEAT

Over 25 years ago, yes, over 25 years ago - well before the first cases of B.S.E. were discovered - the natural foods and health magazine **'Here's Health'** *wrote about and highlighted the abject stupidity of feeding bovine offal to farm animals. Because they were like so many of us who promoted the natural, being looked upon as 'weirdos' or bizarre, the dangers were ignored, as the provender millers went their merry moneymaking ways. What will never be understood is that those self-same animal food industrialists, who made significant profits from their vast and monstrous errors which have affected so many throughout the world, have not been penalised one iota. Here again, just as within the human food and drinks chain, the corporate barons can apparently dictate as they wish.*

Many eat too much Meat. Some eat none, practising vegetarianism. All are entitled to their own views. Of red Meats liver is especially good, containing an amount of Vitamins A with some D and E, being a source of B Vitamins especially B12 and Folic Acid. Pig's liver is exceptionally nutritious. To remove the bitter or strong taste so that it is to one's liking, soak in milk for at least 30 minutes, before cooking. It is excellent for casseroles with most of the goodness being kept in during cooking. Supplement other main meals with fish or chicken, if you can be sure of their origin. **Purchase the free-range bird if at all possible.**

I have viewed battery-caged birds reared in what must be described as artificial, barbaric, spurious conditions. This to many does not appear cruel. Observing the methods used to provide us with poultry put me off this kind of Meat altogether. It is unnatural for any fowl to be reared in these all-too-closely confined man made conditions. The difference between both types of chicken when cooked is incredible, especially the taste. What is highly noticeable to the watchful - to those who deplore the unnatural - is the difference in the joints. The free-range birds have no signs of horrible discolouration, as have most of the, one could say, factory-produced chickens. This is where the salmonella, of which we hear so much, stems from. *Turn to Poultry Meat caption.*

M

There is a huge difference between fresh Meat and the watered, additive-filled, pre- packed, polythene shrink-wrapped or tinned meat. Reading the ingredients labels on some of these 'foods' is frightening and begs the question and answer, 'why all this just for food'. Eat them at your peril!

The family butcher, with his display of fresh Meat as we knew it, is almost extinct, as are all too many of our corner shops. They should be supported before it is too late. *To those who are interested in the 'foods' on offer, there is much going on of which we are not aware and this includes Meat. I'll set out one of the many tricks of the trade. There is a packaging technique which confirms longer shelf life to packaged Meat. Oxygen scavengers are sealed in the pack with the Meat, to help keep oxygen levels very low, this preventing the Meat becoming brown during storage. When the pack is put on display, a tape covering the perforated cling film is peeled back. This allows the Meat to 'bloom' and therefore look highly attractive on the shelf, usually under lights, which makes it look even better. This is sold as fresh Meat. Fresh is very often not fresh, just as pure is not pure.* One day we will miss the butchers who used provide nutritious cuts of fresh Meat. Convenience is the word. Convenience; often dangerous to our health at an enormous cost. The twice-weekly rule is to eat

1. Meat or poultry   2. Fish   3. Eggs   4. Cheese

This ensures moderation, as it should be. Be vigilant, choose your foods carefully, think and eat natural, especially where Meats are concerned. Vacuum-packed, shrink-wrapped, packaged and tinned Meats are best avoided. *Support your butcher when you purchase Meat.*

MEDICINES

See Drug Therapy Caption.

MEDITATION

How many take time to slow down, relax, rest or Meditate? Meditation is a form of therapy which costs nothing. It is often associated with religion but is in fact just as the dictionary gives its meaning, 'deep thought'. Note the word deep, which makes Meditation different from just casual thought. There is much good to be found in Meditation, with wonderful benefits accruing by way of inner peace and knowledge, which with calmness and concentration bring an indescribable self-realisation, or one could say a detoxing of the mind. As well as keeping the mind and brain active it is a beneficial method to prevent aging. *'Cygnus Books'* have excellent reading available regarding Meditation. *See Bibliography for their address.*

MEMORY WEAK

See Brain Health Caption.

MENIERE'S SYNDROME

The combination of varying degrees of tinnitus, deafness, giddiness, vertigo, sometimes leading to fainting and vomiting, often leaves the person exhausted and worn out. Grommets insertion and conventional medicines, which may have helped some, sadly are all-too-often not a cure. Doctors do not realise that inferior Diet is perhaps the main cause of the syndrome and that salt is hostile to the illness. *Where the nutritious, well- balanced, whole-food Diet, as set out under caption in this Encyclopedia, has been used in conjunction with the Hay Diet, under separate caption, there has been wonderful improvement. It must be emphasised that it should be both gluten and dairy free. It is a slow programme, taking six to eight months before signs of recovery, with accelerated improvement over the next three or four months. If disciplined enough to follow the food-combining advice of Doctor Hay, using pure natural unprocessed food as set out in the main Diet, leaving out the dairy and gluten products, freedom from the syndrome may be attained.* The combined Diet nurtures and heals, the food being like medicine. *See DIET also Hay Diet captions.*

M

MENOPAUSE

Over many years I have built up several files on the subject of Menopause, the time when a woman reaches the stage where when it is passed she will no longer be able to conceive. These clippings, writings, snippets, advice and more have never been gone through down the years until commencing this Encyclopedia about 'Good Food, Over the Counter Natural Remedies and Better Health'. A full book could be written giving the advice contained in the files, some of it contradictory, some of it old folk and herbal remedies, with an amount of it giving current or up-to-date suggestions. Much of the modern-day advice is just the same as that promoted 40 years ago.

We have more and more chemical, synthetic or what is called conventional medicines, being advertised and prescribed for the various related Menopausal problems. Most of them do little to ease the complications, just as some of the herbal remedies do not give relief. At least with the natural remedy there are no horrible side effects. What suits one may not work for another.

Before setting out the natural remedies, aids, or treatment, which have worked and are top of the list of remedies for the Menopause, there are factors, which must be mentioned. With the old slogan 'Prevention is better than cure' very much in mind before the peri Menopause, leading to the Menopause proper, the important thing to remember is to take steps well before-hand in order to be well prepared to make it easier to deal with the problem, if there is one. Very often there need not be any difficulty. One of the reasons for Menopause problems is smoking. It leaks out much of the necessary nutrients, which aid the body systems. Why try to treat or help the body when going through the Menopause if still smoking. It is time wasted; only leading to further distress.

All women over the age of 35 should take long-term a tablet of Calcium / Magnesium / Vitamin D, all of which work in conjunction with one another. This is for the prevention of Osteoporosis or brittle bones, which is brought on by the depletion of Calcium before, during and after Menopause. Only in very recent years have the medical profession accepted what the natural remedies people have always known and recommended - that Calcium is a must.

Being overweight demands the need to lose some excess. What is suggested here will help enormously with this, including the recommended Diet.

A disciplined pattern of sleep is required of up to eight or more hours nightly. Being overtired makes life much more a burden at this time of life. As well as eight hours nightly have an early night every seven or eight days in order to catch up. Sleep and pure food are like medicine, certainly at the time which used to be called 'Change of Life'. All who lead a healthy life-style; keeping to a whole food natural Diet and those who maintain a good standard of physical fitness, find it much easier to cope with the problem.

I have spoken with many from the Eastern world who have sailed through the Menopause because of their extreme fitness, also the get-up-and-go attitude. Those who felt good were fastidious about the food they ate, decrying the rubbish additives used in much of the Western world. They spoke of the wonderful discipline or workout, which is Yoga. Female athletes, cyclists, and those who do manual work, also others who realise the benefits of exercise and proper Diet, have told of how the Menopause has hardly affected them. Some said they did not realise they had it. All that is written here comes from the mouths of hundreds of women who have had Menopausal problems, also those who have had little, if any, complications. Many on being questioned at first were reluctant to talk about it, especially to a man. Later they laughed at their timidity, realising that if with a problem, it is good to talk with or confide in somebody. *It is more than coincidence that those who had nutritious dietary intake and took exercise were the least affected.* Much advice and tips were passed on by those who came back to say *"Thank You"*.

Relax before you go to bed. Switch off. Keeping a diary is a form of unwinding, including writing down the chores for the next day, which is a help to de-stress. It is good on the following morning to know that all is listed and you do not fag the brain, thinking about what is pressing. Don't look at the list until you have had that all-important and enjoyable meal, the breakfast, which must not be skipped. You will find that things which were worries less than twelve hours before are often found to be irrelevant. So it is in our daily lives as we agonise needlessly.

Hot flushes can be controlled by the use of the homeopathic remedy Sepia, also Damiana or Goldenseal, which like everything natural mentioned in this

Encyclopedia are available at the health food store. Natural aids to help influence the levels of hormones within the body are to drink Sage Tea or take Blue/Green Algae such as Spirulina, or Black Cohosh, Wild Yam, or Evening primrose Oil. Agnus Castus, also the highly effective Menopace can be a woman's best friends at the time. Menopace is a combination of 22 nutrients specially formulated, which can be used before, during and after the Menopause. Another highly commendable aid is Lecithin granules taken with porridge or breakfast cereals. Where there is a big imbalance of hormones, with progesterone levels high, the Chinese herbal 'women's supplement' Dong quai has been extremely good as a balancer. Take this for 28 days and then use Equyfiam, which is also extremely good for the same purpose. Alternate both these remedies month about. Agnus Castus to be taken when oestrogen levels are high. *Three extremely important factors, as mentioned, are nutritious Diet, Exercise and Sleep. If these are watched and the other advice accepted, the Menopause can literally be taken in one's stride. Almost all are in agreement that once suitable natural remedies are found, it is best not to change, just as one must keep to the Diet.* Although Black Cohosh is recommended here it is not one of my favourite remedies. It must not be used when pregnant or breast-feeding, if using contraceptive or hormonal pill or if with blood pressure. It must not be taken long-term. The safe way to take it is: seven days on and four days off for three months and recommence after 28 days. *Turn to DIET caption, also Hormone Replacement Therapy (HRT), Sleep and Exercise captions.*

MEN'S HEALTH

I write on this subject with abysmal or profound experience - 'Big strong man, nothing can happen to me'. It did and it is happening all the time to men. ***They are notorious for their ignorance about health problems, showing no interest until they have to. At the age of 40 or 50 they realise that just like the parts of the car, too often not properly serviced and looked after, the human body begins to give trouble too. Mention the dictum 'You are what you eat, or put into your body' or other rules to abide by for good or reasonable health and they will not show interest. One must be dogmatic. Men need educating about their health.*** I cannot speak with them personally, only asking that they read this Encyclopedia, if only to *turn to the captions* that are relative to their health, including what they eat and drink. *This means reading the DIET caption and much more.*

MENSTRUATION

See Pre Menstrual Syndrome and Menstruation Caption.

METABOLISM

The Metabolism, which is maintained and therefore kept in a healthy state by intake into our bodies of well-balanced and nutritious foods, is vital for our well being. It involves a breakdown of constituents, liberating energy and other complex substances, including enzymes, so necessary to maintain good health. Healthy Metabolism filters and distributes those so necessary food nutrients, as well as what is stored in the body. It is not realised that being overweight is linked to Metabolic inefficiency or disturbance. Bad Dietary habits also lead to a breakdown in the Metabolic process, leading to ill health. *Turn to DIET caption,* which is the cornerstone of a healthy Metabolism. It is the foundation for good health. The food must be additive-free and pure, with supplements to be taken where necessary, as explained

MICROWAVES

Avoid Microwaved foods. We had to wait for a very long time to be told of the dangerous and fatal effects of smoking. No doubt some day we will be informed of the dangers of Microwaved foods. *Two Swiss scientists have carried out research into the effects of Microwaved foods on human organisms, in comparison to that conventionally prepared. They found that foods cooked in microwave ovens cause significant changes in the blood after having been partaken of. They noticed that these changes, some of which could be termed highly significant, indicated the beginning of a pathological process, e.g. the beginning of cancer.* They were forced to stop their investigations, one being dismissed. Microwaves at eye level have been proven to damage the eyes, reports the Journal of Natural Science. The tests referred to had gone on for some years, being carried out by the two eminent Professors.

Some within the electrical industry continue to inform the public, those whose health seems only to get worse; that the food does not continue to get hotter after the machine has been switched off. This is how it should be. *Those with monetary interests also inform us that far from destroying the nutrients, Microwave radiation is less damaging to vitamins and minerals than most forms of cooking. At the same time we are told that research carried out shows that up to 97% of antioxidants in broccoli were wiped out when cooked in a Microwave. This latter report comes from a reputable food laboratory.* Vitamin C for instance is destroyed by heat.

The use of Microwave ovens was banned in Russia in 1976 after they proved that they were harmful. We are told that if evidence of the dangers of Microwave ovens were made know that the electrical industry would be in turmoil. We must be guided by those who do not have vested interests. *In the circumstances it would be prudent not to use a Microwave or eat the foods from them until such time as it is found that they are a safe method of cooking.* Cook and heat naturally to retain the goodness of pure food. Again I repeat: IF IN DOUBT LEAVE OUT, and there is BIG DOUBT about Microwave Cookers.

MIDGE BITES

See Stings Caption.

MIGRAINE

This is the worst kind of headache imaginable. It is thought that enlargement or stricture of blood vessels in the brain leads to the violent headaches. Treating with conventional painkillers is not the answer. Often this leads to further headaches and who knows what the long- term consequences may be. *'Prevention Is Better Than Cure'.*

The advice given here has helped many seeking relief to be rid of migraine, but much more importantly it has prevented attacks. Several had suffered from anything up to 20 years, now being free by doing as set out. Avoid going too long between meals. Smaller, more frequent meals which keep blood sugars stable, are best. The theory of stress, anxiety, worry and psychological factors being the cause, has not being proven. The main reason for Migraine is to be found in Diet and lifestyle, including lack of exercise and neglect of proper sleep pattern. Change of Diet may mean the elimination of several things partaken of regularly. Included are cheese and dairy products, or perhaps glutinous foods such as wheat products. Also to be avoided are citrus fruits, alcohol, coffee and synthetic food additives, including Monosodium Glutamate. There will be a need to eliminate, one by one, whatever you think might be the cause of the Migraine, replacing them similarly, until the culprits have been found or eliminated. Before doing this, if you so desire, there are natural remedies worth trying which have proved excellent to either relieve or banish Migraine. Feverfew Essence, or in the form of tablets, or two or three leaves from the plant, is a well-known preventative. The leaves to be taken daily in the form of a sandwich. Combination F New Era, Rhodolia, Lobelia and Acidophilus have all helped relieve Migraine pain. The uses of any of these remedies plus attention to Diet of pure natural food have all led to a pain-free life. *See DIET caption,* and be guided about what is a leading remedy for Migraine as well as helping one attain better health.

Purposely left until last is mention of the HAY DIET. Those with excruciating pain of Migraine have banished the headaches completely, also saying how much better they felt when using the food combination programme. *See Hay Diet caption* to learn more about its goodness. *Also see Feverfew caption.*

MILK

See Dairy Products Caption.

MILK THISTLE

This is excellent as a liver stimulant or tonic. Helps detox, control cholesterol and is taken to relieve hangover. It is despised as a weed, being a good table vegetable when cultivated. The medical profession has realised that it has many qualities. More will be heard about Milk Thistle in the future as a medicine, when the realisation comes that herbal remedies have much to offer which is good. Like all remedies mentioned in this Encyclopedia, Milk Thistle is available in liquid or tablet form from the health food store.

MINERALS

See Vitamins and Minerals Caption.

MINER'S ELBOW

Treat as tendonitis. If swollen or puffed on point of elbow it may be Synovitis and should be treated as such.

MOBILE PHONE SAFETY

In this Encyclopedia I set out truthful facts, which have all been published, printed or written, with the sources logged and available for examination. It is up to the reader to accept the advice given if they so wish, or to form their own opinions. We have had many recurring warnings about the dangers of using Mobile Phones, especially if regularly held to the ear, which means the side of the head. Various researches have shown that the use of Mobiles, including digital and cordless, has been linked to brain tumours. Do we stop using them? Try telling that to the millions of users. The Mobile Phone conglomerates have resisted any insinuation of cancer links, even though they accept that their radiation does effect the electrical activity of the brain. Who are they to speak against the medical profession? *Dr Richard Sullivan, Head of Clinical Programmes at Cancer Research UK, where studies are carried out says: "It suggests a strong link between mobile phones and brain tumours. We now need a full scale study".* Here again we must practice the advice 'IF IN DOUBT LEAVE OUT'. Mobiles are here to stay, with the advice being to never use without a hands free headset or use risk reducing protective covers, which are available.

MOLASSES: BLACK STRAP

This is obtainable from the health food store. Used sparingly as medicine, pure Black Strap Molasses contains Iron, Calcium, Potassium, Vitamins B Complex and E, Magnesium and Copper. An aid to losing weight and for general health is to mix two teaspoons of pure molasses in a glass of warm water adding the juice of half a lemon. Diabetics must not take Molasses.

MONEY Worries and Problems

Much of our Money worries could be avoided by practising the old proverb:

'Buy Not What You Want, Buy Only What You Have Need Of'.

MORNING STIFFNESS

See Joints and Joint Health Caption.

MOTION SICKNESS

See Travel and Holiday Health Caption.

MOUTH

Menosan, which is Sage-based, makes an excellent Mouthwash, being good for gums and when used as a gargle for laryngitis and sore throat. Pure Aloe Vera can be used similarly.
- Acid or Sour Taste: Nat Phos.
- Bad Breath: Kali Phos
- Tongue coated white: Kali Mur
- Tongue coated yellow: Kali Sulph
- Cold Sores: *See Lips caption*
- Corners Cracked: Silica
- Dry: Kali Phos. It is often the result of medication which needs to be changed. If necessary speak with your doctor. May also be due to improper Diet or lack of Vitamins.
- Inflamed: *See Stomatitis caption*
- Cracked Lips: Calc Flour. Also rub on pure Manuka honey.
- Thrush in Children: *See Thrush caption*
- Ulcers, Ashy Grey: Kali Phos. White: Kali Mur. At corner of mouth: Kali Phos,
Vitamin A 700iu daily is recommended for all mouth ulcers. *Where relevant see Lips, Tongue or Gums captions.*

MUESLI

Muesli is a breakfast cereal, which can be made up with pure natural ingredients, chosen from the shelves of the health food stores or the supermarket. Examine to see that apricots and other dried fruits are natural, with no mineral oils, preservatives or other additives. The health food store can provide all natural ingredients. They may be more expensive but they do not use additives to cheapen the food. Pure Muesli is full of goodness as a breakfast cereal. To make your own delicious sugar free Muesli from natural ingredients, mix together:

56g/2oz dried apricots, cut small.	114g/4oz raisins
56g/2oz hazelnuts	454g/1lb natural porridge oats
56g/2oz walnuts	114g/4oz large oat-flakes
114g/4oz sultanas	170g/6oz wheat bran.

Store in an airtight container. Freshly chopped apple, also a spoon of pure Honey added, means a healthy start to the day. Some prefer to soak overnight. Add extra milk or Soya milk before eating.

MULTIPLE SCLEROSIS

Natural therapies have helped those with MS. Aromatherapy in the home can relieve anxiety and stress related problems. Yoga has proved beneficial especially where the simple breathing exercises help to motivate. The theme of this Encyclopedia is pure, natural, additive-free food, and a natural Diet, with nothing processed. This has helped many with MS and I give you some evidence. First there is the story of Roger McDougall who was in a wheelchair and became completely free from the symptoms. This did not happen overnight. He disciplined himself to use a process of elimination, whereby over a number of months he left out certain foods, then returning them to the Diet to find out which were alien to the system. Many have since followed the Diet with success as did Roger. His Diet was based on gluten free food, also the non-use of anything processed or with additives. Cream and all saturated fats were out. Butter to be used very sparingly. Bacon, pork, duck or goose was forbidden, with lean meats allowed. Another example is of the Diet recommended and used in the treatment of MS by Doctor Joseph Evers whose clinic is in Haachen, West Fallen, KR Arrensburg, Germany. Many have followed this with success. The foods must be completely natural and non-processed. Those which may be eaten are milk and milk products if not allergic to them, a raw egg daily, all root vegetables, organic if possible, including beetroot which is particularly good, with potatoes forbidden. Allowed were pure Honey, all fruits, with bread to be made from gluten free flour. We should be indebted to these men for their work in aiding to halt or prevent the onset of MS. *The Diet is somewhat similar to that set out under DIET caption in this Encyclopedia, with gluten advice given under the caption Coeliac or see Allergies-Food caption.* Here the MS sufferer has to decide which food to accept and to pick and choose what is best. There is no doubt that food as set out here, which has helped so many, is as medicine. There is a need for essential fatty acids. With the advent of Udo's Choice balance of Omega three and six oils, this can be met. To supplement the Diet it may also be necessary to take minerals, including Magnesium, Potassium and Calcium, also Vitamins B Complex, E and C, some of which can be covered by use of a good Multivitamin supplement. The Multivitamin should be taken in the morning, and the Calcium / Magnesium / Vitamin D combination at night, because this is also an aid to better sleep. Your health food shop will advise about everything natural written about here. **Using only pure natural foods and following the Hay Diet has proved highly beneficial for many with MULTIPLE SCLEROSIS.** One must be very disciplined to follow the Diet recommended by Doctor Hay, but if prepared to do so the results can be extraordinary. *Turn to DIET and also HAY DIET captions.*

MULTIVITAMINS

See Vitamins & Minerals Caption.

MUMPS

This infectious inflammation of the salivary glands, which usually occurs in school children, needs care and attention to ensure that there are no after effects. Where the immune system is not strong or healthy it is easy to catch this illness. Treatment usually means a few days in bed, keeping warm and staying indoors, until after the swelling of the glands has gone down. A Diet of pure natural food, aided by a tonic such as Kindervital, with a junior Multivitamin later, will help the patient back to normal health.

MUSCLE SPASMS

See Legs Restless Caption.

MUSCULAR RHEUMATISM

See Fibrositis Caption.

MYALGIC ENCEPHALOMYELITIS (M.E.)

See Chronic Fatigue Syndrome Caption.

MYASTHENIA GRAVIS

Sometimes wrongly diagnosed as Neurosis. This neuromuscular disease is often linked to unhealthy Thymus gland. Change of Diet to pure foods, additive-free and the partaking of 50mg of Manganese three times daily, one tablet at each meal, also Vitamin B6, Udo's Choice Oil and Lecithin have almost always ensured complete recovery within weeks unless there is an underlying or more serious health problem. *See DIET caption and be guided,* with all foods to be natural and Gluten Free.

MYOXEDEMA

See Thyroid Under active Caption.

NAGGING

See SADS Caption.

NAILS

Healthy Nails and Hair are almost always a sign of one's general health. They go hand- in-hand. The Nail root is the equivalent of the Hair bulb. A healthy nutritious Diet is the foundation for nice Hair and Nails. *See DIET caption.* Taking the Hair, Skin and Nail combination Perfectil, Silica or a good Multivitamin tablets can aid nail nutrition. Ask your health food store to provide whatever you require. Nail problems and suggested remedies are;

- Ridges and dips: lack of nuts, seeds, fish and leafy green vegetables. Supplement with Calcium / Magnesium / Vitamin D also Vitamin B Complex.
- Fungal infections: Molkasan or Spilanthes can treat successfully or Acidophilus may be needed if with severe Fungal infection.
- White spots or brittle Nails: Silica.
- To help prevent biting of Nails paint regularly with Tincture of Myrrh, also taking Vitamin B Complex daily.
- Parsley is an excellent Hair and Nail tonic. *Turn to Parsley caption.*

NAPPY RASH

A natural aid is two or three drops of Tea Tree Oil mixed with two teaspoons of Manuka Honey diluted in a little warm water and then applied. Where there is extreme irritation it may be Candida when Acidophilus can be used. Allergenic's Baby Wash of gentle bathing milk is highly recommended, being 100% natural, free from synthetic preservatives.

NAPPIES

The organisation WEN (Women's Environmental Network) tells us that over 3 billion Nappies are used in the UK and Ireland every year, most of which end up in landfill sites. It is estimated that over €700 or £500 can be saved by using Terry towels during the time a single child needs them. Apart from the financial saving the environment would be helped immensely. There are services, which supply them. In the UK the National Association of Nappy Services can advise. Tel 0121 693 4949.

NASAL STUFFINESS

Use Olbas Oil as an inhalant or take Lobelia tablets.

NAT MUR, NAT PHOS, NAT SULPH

See Tissue Salts caption to learn more about these simple excellent remedies.

NATUROPATHY

This Encyclopedia is built around or based on the Naturopathic way to reasonable or better health. Like all who follow this lifestyle, I firmly believe, with unequivocal evidence coming to light: *That we are what we eat and drink, we are as our lifestyle, we are as we exercise and as we sleep'.* **The vast number of everyday ailments, all so prevalent, are mostly as a result of abuse of our bodies, of poor eating and drinking habits, of an inordinate lifestyle. Nature and all things natural hold the remedy for the majority of our health problems.** One of the dictums of Naturopathy is that promoted by Hippocrates - 'The Father of Medicine' - who said: "Food should be our medicine and medicine should be our food". Food was pure when he quoted these words almost 2,500 years ago, not like much of the junk we are offered as 'food' today. Provided it is given a fair opportunity to do so, the natural heals. *One of our greatest herbalists, Thomas Bartram, Editor of the wonderful* 'Grace' *Magazine, states in his* **'Encyclopedia of Herbal Medicine'** *(See Bibliography): "Naturopathy is based on two basic principles. The first is that the body possesses the power to heal itself through its eternal vitality and intelligence. The second is that the body is its own best healer. All the practitioner does is to create the most favourable conditions to stimulate and enhance this healing power of nature. All is based on natural medicine and nature cure".* The Encyclopedia you are now reading points you to the simplicity of *NATUROPATHY.*

NAUSEA

It is important to find the cause and treat accordingly. Aids to settle the stomach are Ginger, either as capsules, tablets or in the form of tea, also Peppermint oil, Blue Flag Root, Camomile Tea or Calamus tablets. Do not eat for two hours after vomiting. Sip as much natural drinks as you can. Sucking ice cubes helps. An old and successful remedy is warm milk or a bowl of milk pudding such as cornflower, flaked brown rice, or the ever-reliable Slippery Elm. The latter is a wonderful healer where there is upset stomach. It can be taken as a drink, served as a creamy liquid or mixed with porridge. It can also be taken in tablet form. Pure Manuka Honey taken with any of these is an invaluable aid to settle the stomach. Medical help should be sought if the sickness persists.

NAVAL FUNGUS

See Umbilicus Fungus Caption.

NEEM

Long looked upon by the people of India as one of the great aids to many health problems. It would be widely used as a non-steroidal treatment but for the fact that the mighty drug companies cannot patent it. Because it is obtained naturally it cannot be allied to their big moneyed ideas. Excellent as a treatment for head lice and other bugs also as an insect repellent. There are no chemical dangers or side effects with Neem. Visit the health food shop where literature is available to explain the diversity of this purely natural remedy. It should not be used in its neat state, but should be diluted before use.

NERVE TONIC

See Nervous Exhaustion Caption.

NERVES (AS FOR EXAMS)

See Exam Nerves Caption.

NERVOUS EXHAUSTION

Nervous exhaustion, tension and emotional imbalance occur where a build-up of pressure, stress and worry comes to the point where it is almost unbearable. Often due to deficiency of Vitamin B Complex, Calcium / Magnesium / Vitamin D or Zinc. I have yet to speak with anybody 'suffering from their nerves' as is often heard to describe the nerve ailments, who when questioned, realised that the cause can very often be a Diet low in nutrition. This can be aided by a tonic such as Floradix, Floravital, Biostrath or Nettle Juice leading to a good Multivitamin tablet to be taken continuously. The natural *DIET* and supplements as suggested under caption, also Pulsatilla or Combination F New Era have all helped aid recovery. Visit your health food shop and ask them about Bach's Rescue Remedy or other simple natural no side effect aids, of which there are several. *Change to Diet as advised under caption* is almost always the medicine required for Nervous Tension and Exhaustion, just as it is for much of our everyday sickness.

NERVOUS TENSION

See Nervous Exhaustion Caption.

NETTLES

This herb, known as a weed, looked upon with disdain by almost everybody including gardeners, is one of nature's gifts to the world. Because it costs nothing nobody wants it. It can be used as a safeguard against colds and flu, to banish children's eczema, and to aid skin diseases. It is a tonic and blood cleanser, helps ward off hay fever, also to cleanse and strengthen the lungs. Assists in preventing nose bleeds, helps lower blood pressure also strengthening the immune system. It is used to help banish hives.

It builds up our natural resistance. *Few know about the goodness of Nettles, certainly not the medical profession, including the almighty drug manufacturers. Imagine them trying to patent the Nettle or prescribing it!*

Armed with a pair of gloves and a strong scissors it should be harvested from March to September, cutting off the top six inches or full young plant. Washed and cut up, it can be either dried and stored in glass jars, or frozen fresh, using it as required as a vegetable by boiling for 15 minutes. The water can be taken as a tonic and the greens mixed with butter, to be eaten like spinach. It can also be infused as tea. Nettle teas and the dried herb are also available from the health food shop. Once cooked Nettles never sting. They are an outstanding medicine, which could not be more natural. The boiled Nettle water when cooled is equal to or perhaps better than many of the off-the-shelf tonics available. It can be kept in the fridge for up to four days.

N

NETTLE RASH

See Hives Caption.

NETTLE STINGS

See Stings Caption.

NEURALGIA – General

This can be extremely painful. Sometimes there is an underlying cause, which must be treated. Often Neuralgia is caused by debility, with the Diet to be improved. *See DIET caption.* Vitamin B Complex and Combination A New Era are good remedies, also take the minerals Zinc with Calcium / Magnesium / Vitamin D long term.

Neuralgia very often comes from cold weather or perhaps from being in a draught such as an open car window. The wearing of hat or cap is often the simple remedy.

NEURITIS

This is a symptom rather than a disease and should be treated accordingly, when the root problem has been diagnosed. In many instances the partaking of Vitamins B Complex and E with extra Panthothenic acid, has banished the illness. Polyneuritis can be as result of lifestyle and inferior Diet, which lead to ill health. *Pure natural DIET as captioned,* into which is incorporated some food supplements including the Minerals and Vitamins recommended, is usually the remedy.

NEW ERA

See Tissue Salts Caption.

NIGHT BLINDNESS

See Eyes Caption.

NIGHTMARES

Use the herb Skull Cap, taken in tincture form or as dried herb, infused as tea, to be taken three times daily or if taken in tincture form follow the instruction shown on the bottle.

NIGHT SWEATS

See Menopause Caption.

NOISE

We live in a world polluted by amongst other things, Noise. It must be repeated again that here we are our own worst enemies. Noise-induced hearing loss is the most prevalent irreversible industrial disease in most countries. You may ask: "Why are you putting this in a Natural Remedies Encyclopedia" The answer may sound censorious but I believe in the slogan so often used in these writings - 'Prevention Is Better Than Cure'.

Where Noise is the cause of deafness there is no cure. People need to be aware of the dangers, especially to children, where it may even affect their mental health. **We should have monitoring of sound levels, also easy access to ear protectors. If we have eye tests, why not hearing tests? One has only to listen to the extremely loud oompa-oompa noise of what is often improperly termed 'music', which the listener endures when he or she is travelling in the confined space of a motor vehicle or which appears to be the norm at discos, dances, night clubs, and where young people gather for entertainment. There appears to be no realisation that the extremely powerful din is harmful to hearing and that those who listen may be effected hearing-wise, especially in later life. The public should be more aware of the hazards of Noise, also not being afraid to complain about it.**

On the Channel Tunnel contract where over 15,000 personnel were employed at one stage or another, no construction personnel were allowed to work without a hearing test. The majority of those who worked underground had defective hearing because of having worked previously in noisy, often confined areas. It was jocularly remarked that: 'If there was no sign of deafness the applicant for work had no tunnel construction experience', because the use of ear muffs and almost all forms of health protection aid in the working area have only come into use in recent years. Even now one can see that in many instances they are not being used where necessary. Because they are mandatory in many industries, one must assume that they are available to those involved; therefore what is set out at the top of this caption about *PREVENTION* is very true.

We have only ourselves to blame for most cases of over exposure to Noise. *If you have to shout to be heard above the noise level you are in the danger area.* Look after your hearing because nobody else will. Like some of our other faculties it is irreplaceable. *Turn to Ears also Hearing captions.*

NOSE

- Boils on edge of nostril: Silica

- Burning in nose: Nat Sulph

- Congested: Olbas Oil

- Ozaena. (Crusted inside with offensive discharge): Combination D New Era, also put smear of Allergenics Emollient Ointment into Nose. Pinch the nostril to close and work the ointment into the effected part. Ozaena is often a sign of being run down and there may be the need for a tonic or a change of Diet.

- Rhinitis; *See Rhinitis caption.*

NOSE BLEEDS

Often acts as a relief valve to blood pressure. There can be many causes. Despite the experts not being in agreement, the oldest remedy is still a worthy one, where cold compresses such as a cloth soaked in cold water, a cold block or piece of metal or steel is placed on the nape of the neck with the patient holding the head back. Nettle tea and Vitamin E helps strengthen the blood vessels.

NUTRITIONAL THERAPY

This is not just another alternative medicine or method of treatment, to attain good health. It has been there for all time. The problem is that most of the medical profession, the drug companies, also the 'food' conglomerates and processors, in their quest to make more and more money, have entrapped us with chemical filled medicines and 'foods'. The many 'foods' and 'drinks', additive-filled, also denatured, which are now being taken, are certainly not therapeutic or nutritious. This Encyclopedia is based on Naturopathy and Nutrition, with everything written about being entirely natural. **The caption on DIET describes and repeatedly sets out the foundation for better health, including lifestyle.** We are informed that from one third to half of some cancers are caused by Diet - what is eaten. This is just cancer alone. What about the hundreds of niggling ailments and sickness we are confronted with daily? What about the serious illness and disease? **On a survey done recently it was found that over 96% of shoppers do not look at, read, or bother about the ingredients label.** This is incredible. *Imagine a concoction, a* *combination of any of the following taken into the most wonderful, the most intricate system in the world, the human body. It can read like this, with thousands more to be added on, with endless permutations, when added to the stuff we are expected to purchase as 'food' or 'drink'. Trisodium Citrate, Artificial Flavours, some toxic as in smoked fish, Aspartame, Saccharin, Potassium Sorbate, Sodium Metabisulphite, Sodium Benzoate, Carboxyl Methyl Cellulose, Emulsifiers, up to 20 types of syrups and sugars, Hydrogenated Oil, Citric Acid, Sodium Alginate, Potassium Hydrogen Carbonate, Lactic Acid, Salt and more salt, Potassium Chloride, Stabilisers, Sulphate Ammonia, Tri Calcium Phosphate, Flavour Enhancers, Mono Sodium Glutamate, Disodium Inosinate, Dehydrated Chicken (where from we will never know!), Chemical Antioxidants, Sodium Phosphates, Sodium Tripolyphosphates. There were little more than 50 additives 70 years ago, all natural, with water, milk, herbs and spices being the basis. Reading the list shown here is startling. Imagine the other 4,000 to 5,000 thousand- plus substances being included here. If people are not interested in what they are eating, they are certainly not interested in being healthy. How can they be?*

I am convinced, being doubtless, that much of the fare dished up, forced on us as 'food' and 'drink', is perverse, unnatural, processed, anything but sustaining or with health giving properties. If only those who scan our food stores or supermarket shelves for the groceries, especially those who purchase them, were to be fastidious also diligent, in both reading the ingredients labels and rejecting everything with additives, their health also the health of the families of the nation would improve dramatically. The doctors incomes would decrease and the profits of the multi national all powerful drug companies would be drastically lowered. Daily, over the years, I have spoken with many who were unwell, as I advised and prescribed. In almost every instance the main cause of their sickness was the DIET. **NUTRITIONAL THERAPY** was the answer, or in simple terms, a change of Diet to pure natural, unprocessed additive-free foods. The return to better health of mind and body was very often beyond belief. *See DIET caption* to help reap the results. It must also be noted that lifestyle must be changed to fit in with the natural Diet or vice versa, also there is the need for Exercise and regular Sleep pattern because all work in conjunction with each other. *Turn to Exercise and Sleep captions also.*

NUTS

All Nuts, except peanuts, mixed with sunflower, safflower or other seeds, raisins and sultanas make excellent snacks. Nuts are extremely nutritious, containing much goodness, including health giving Oils, Vitamins, Minerals and Trace Elements. They must be natural and unsalted. Visit your health food shop, who carry a varied selection of everything natural, including dried fruits and Nuts which are preservative and mineral oil free. Much of the fruit when used with Nuts to make Fruit and Nut mixtures purchased off-the-shelf in food stores or supermarkets have been treated with mineral oils and preservatives. The health food store sells only natural dried fruits and Nuts.

OATS & OATMEAL

Oats is an outstanding natural nutritious food. There is some in muesli and in many processed breakfast cereals. There is nothing except pure Oat flakes in porridge. There are no additives. For some ulterior reason all-too-many are inclined to look scornfully on pure natural porridge, the sole ingredients being Oat flakes and water. With a little milk added in the making the taste is even better. Following the 'quick cook' instructions, it is easily made. Avoid the microwave. *See Microwave caption.*

It is beyond comprehension why so many at breakfast-time reach for the psychedelic package of additive-filled cornflakes or other roasted cereals. They are just fillers, containing little if any nutrition. They invariably contain what was good food before flavour enhancing, sugar coating, processing, toasting and bandying about with, then being sold as breakfast cereals. Reading the ingredients label of many of the packages should in itself be sufficient reason for the partaker, if interested in future good health, to say: **"Lets have porridge or home made muesli in future"**.

Natural Oats whether it is pinhead, rolled or in the form of flour, contains a balance of Carbohydrates, B Complex Vitamins, Calcium, Potassium, Magnesium and other nutrients, all of which are natural and highly beneficial to a healthy system. They also help to control blood sugar and cholesterol levels. Consider the natural prime food value of Oats, which are relatively cheap, an excellent provider of energy and very much which is healthy. Porridge is easily assimilated. One never hears of the ailments heartburn or indigestion when porridge has been eaten.

Oats contain more protein and a better quality than any other cereal apart from Quinoa, also the range of amino acids, so essential to our well being, as present in Oat protein, is outstanding. Oats, as in porridge flakes, is the one major grain proven to lower Cholesterol. The intake of fats, regarded as a danger to our health, are of no consideration with Oats as they are contributed mainly by the neutral fats and phosphatides in the grain, having approximately equal linoelic acid content. Included in the fats referred to are a group of waxes which are specific to Oats, having a decisive bearing on the overall food value of the cereal. It is an extraordinarily valuable fibre. Much more about the good of porridge and the ingredient Oat grain could be written if space permitted.

Oats whether as porridge or natural muesli, taken daily for breakfast - the most important meal of the day - helps increase physical performance and well-being. There is a better attitude of mind and mood. It helps those ill or convalescing, is good for tummy upsets, especially gastro-intestinal disorders in children. **Trials carried out show that mental performances, emotional disorders, mood swings, hyperactivity and the attitudes of school children and adolescents, have all responded favourably to an improved Diet centred on porridge.** Only now are the medical profession and some of the health gurus referring to the good of whole grains, particularly oats, informing us as if this had only come to light recently. All interested in natural food and better health have always promoted its good. *See caption headed Muesli,* which has rolled oats as its base. The mighty 'food' processors who give us the many additive-laden breakfast 'cereals' have almost brain washed both children and adults into accepting their sugarised, over- hyped, unnatural products.

OBESITY
See both Slimming & Dieting Captions.

ODOUR – BODY
See Body Odour Caption.

OEDEMA
See Water Retention Caption.

OFFENSIVE BREATH
See Hallitosis Caption.

OILS
Many herb Oils, as used in Aromatherapy, are referred to as essential Oils, being some of natures aids to well being. These include, amongst others, lemon, fennel, garlic, lime, lavender, and rosemary. They are potent antiseptics. Recently we hear of the successful use of Tea Tree Oil, including that of its effectiveness against antibiotic resistant bacteria. These Oils have many uses including hair, skin, and body treatments, as shampoos, mouth gargles and for massage as in Aromatherapy. Find a supplier of pure Oils and because certain brands are better than others, try to keep to the one most suitable for you. **Assortments of books on the subject of aromatic Oils are available from 'Cygnus' Books.** *See Bibliography for address, etc.*

OILS – COOKING
See both Captions, Cooking Oils also Cooking Oils – How They Are Produced.

OIL OF EVENING PRIMROSE

See Evening Primrose Oil Caption.

OIL – OMEGA

See Omega Oils Caption.

OIL – FISH

See Fish & Fish Oils Caption.

OILY SKIN

See Skin Caption.

OINTMENT

'Allergenics' Non Steroidal Emollient creams and Ointments have been dermatologically tested, being safe to use on Eczema, Psoriasis, Dermatitis and other dry, itchy skin conditions. They are extremely good, being fully natural, available from health food stores or pharmacies.

OLIVE OIL

This is the elixir of cooking oils when virgin, cold pressed and pure. Oils, including those of the Olive Oils on offer, which have been heated or processed, will have lost most if not all of their nutritional benefits. Many of them can be harmful to health, having become hydrogenated. Use pure Olive Oil on salads, either neat, or in salad dressing, with vinegar and other aliments or simply take one dessertspoonful twice daily as a stomach liner and aid to digestion. To help control cholesterol also as a skin tonic, pure Olive Oil is as medicine. Look for the cold pressed virgin Oil. Although it is a fruit juice or oil it has only natural sweeteners. Pure Olive Oil contains pure natural fatty acids having high Oleic Acid content also Vitamins A, D, K and E. *See both captions Cooking Oils, also Cooking Oils - How They Are Produced.*

OMEGA OILS

To the lay person the matter of essential fatty acids can be extremely complicated. In recent years, as if to confuse further, we hear of the amounts necessary for reasonable health. We are told about Omega three and Omega six fatty acids. One of the problems in the past is that there has been doubt about the correct ratio. This has been simplified and made easy by the introduction of Udo's Choice Oil also Organic Choice Omega 3+6+9. They contain a combination of essential fatty acids, including the balanced amounts of Omega three and six, all of which can help to correct where there is a deficiency of Essential Fatty Acids. I have no hesitation in recommending these Oils, although others have endeavoured to imitate the formulation. To learn more about these wonderful health- giving fats and oils *turn to Udo's Choice Oil caption*.

ONIONS

Another vegetable, which being so easily obtained, is given scant thought as to its goodness and health-giving virtues. Before the advent of modern drugs in the past half century, older people relied on the Onion as a preventative and cure, giving it much praise. Little research has been done, which again makes one offer the question: *"Are we going down the right medical road ?"* It contains amongst other things bioflavonoids, silica, and sulphur. It helps relax the bronchial muscles and can also be used as a blood tonic or purifier. It is good for the heart and circulation, also helping to control blood sugar. Halved raw Onions, hanging in the home, have prevented the spread of contagious disease, including colds and flu's. Much more could be written about the nutritional and medicinal values of Onions. Here again the drug companies or medical gurus are not interested. It cannot be patented. It is too natural. Onions will not help them make the millions. They are a prime food and medicine, raw or cooked.

OSTEO ARTHRITIS

See Arthritis Osteo Caption

OSTEOPATHY

Osteopathy is effective for a host of conditions, including back pain, tinnitus, hiatus hernia, irritable bowel syndrome and other ailments, the list being exhaustive. Many link Osteopathy with bone manipulation, which is wrong, not realising that Osteopaths can treat a huge range of ailments. They receive a somewhat similar training to doctors who use conventional or chemical medicines. The treatment of illness is entirely different, being highly beneficial and favourable as they treat the soft tissues, spine and joints, with emphasis placed on treating the nerve fibres. Osteopaths have a high success rate. Find a qualified therapist in the yellow pages, should you require one.

OSTEOPOROSIS

I have been taught that high blood pressure is a silent killer and that Osteoporosis or brittle bone disease is a silent crippler. I have bulging files on the subject, and much written evidence, as if this were needed, that 'Prevention is Better Than Cure', because Osteoporosis is irreversible, incurable. *It is very largely preventable.* There are no symptoms until the disease is well advanced. We are informed that it affects one in three women and one in seven men. The menopause time leaches the calcium from the system, hence the significant difference in ratio in brittle bone disease. *Daily when women of all ages are spoken with about Osteoporosis and its dangers, of the use of Calcium / Magnesium / Vitamin D, or about the prevention of the disease, through eating and drinking natural additive free, nutritious foods and liquids, also how it is brought on because of the leaking of Calcium from the body during and after menopause, it is unbelievable the ignorance displayed. This word is not used lightly, but that is exactly how it appears. The general public need to be educated about osteoporosis.* Today there is not the lack of education amongst women as witnessed in years gone by, and one would expect that the majority would by now understand the dangers and threat of Osteoporosis, that they would have heard or read about it. My feeling is, that the outlook is like that of men regarding heart attack. *'It cannot or will not happen to me'.* Think again, think carefully, because as set out, Osteoporosis is a crippling disease and irreparable. **The medical profession have not long been recommending Calcium, so very necessary for bone health. The health food industry and all interested in natural health have been trying to get the message across for over a century. Our voices were very often not listened to. We were regarded as nutcases in the past but not anymore, because we are - and have all too often been - proved right. Even now one sees drug-company manufactured Calcium on its own, being prescribed, sold and used, when it is a fact that it must be properly formulated and combined with the other minerals Magnesium and Vitamin D. This is how it has been sold in the health food shops for many years, all natural and non-synthetic.** It is never too late to start protecting oneself against Osteoporosis or brittle bones, with the advice being that all men and women over the age of 35 should be taking a balanced tablet of natural Calcium / Magnesium / Vitamin D and equally as important taking a serious look at what they eat, the DIET. Pure natural food is very important in the aim to avoid brittle bone disease, which is Osteoporosis. *Turn to DIET caption.* Read carefully and again it is repeated *'Prevention is better than cure'.* **Exercises with regular and sufficient Sleep pattern are equally important. Remember it is never too late to start, but please and I repeat please, take steps to prevent Osteoporosis now.**

OTITIS

See Ears Caption.

OVERWEIGHT

See Dieting, also Slimming Captions and especially the Hay Diet Caption.

OZAENA

See Nose Caption.

PAINKILLERS

One has only to walk into the filling station, supermarket or retail outlets to purchase any of the hundreds of pills and medicines available. Few if any are cures, being just stoppers of pain. Repeat doses are one of the chief reasons why so many are sold. It is not to be wondered at that we are a sick nation. Thousands of painkillers such as aspirin, paracetamol, codeine, ibuprofen and all-too-many other chemicals are taken daily, without thought of the long-term consequences. They can have detrimental effects to many users, particularly when on other synthetic medicines or if taken before or after drinking alcohol. Natural painkillers are Petasites, Black Cohosh, or Bach Rescue Remedy.

PALPITATION

Often due to worry, stress, smoking or the many symptoms of heart disease, over-active thyroid, or anaemia. Sometimes frequent during pregnancy. A teaspoonful of pure natural honey in a glass of warm water often helps correct. Other remedies are Hawthorn, Lobelia, or Cramp Bark. Herbal remedies should not be taken during pregnancy or if breastfeeding, without consulting your doctor.

PANTOTHENIC ACID

See Vitamins and Minerals Caption.

PARACETAMOL – (Acetaminophen)

Why is there a need to mention this synthetic and highly unnatural analgesic drug in this Encyclopedia? It is because Paracetamol and all-too-many unnatural drugs, with many risks, are freely available over-the-counter, while simple harmless remedies such as St Johns Wort are being placed on prescription. If the doctor's trade unions, the Irish Medical Organisation and the British Medical Association, have their way, all natural remedies will be either banned or on prescription. The latter will mean nothing because the majority of the medical profession are completely ignorant about natural or herbal remedies - neither are they interested - other than to remove what is anathema to many of them.

PARONYCHIA (Whitlow)

Often due to fungal disorder. *See Nails caption.* It is usually a sign of under-nourishment due to poor Diet, which should be corrected. Immediate remedy is the partaking of a tonic such as Floradix, Floravital or Biostrath. Echinacea or Devils Claw will also aid recovery, all in conjunction with natural Diet of pure foods. Soak the infected nail in diluted tea tree oil, massaging the solution into the nail bed. Repeat three times daily until the infection has cleared. Whitlow is a sign of impure blood or of being run-down. *The advice under Diet caption* and the remedies mentioned should quickly correct this health problem.

PARANOIA

This psychotic state of mind, with delusions of being followed, spied on, persecuted, often leading to aggressiveness, has been helped enormously by change to pure, natural, nutritious Diet of additive-free, non-processed foods. Supplement where necessary. *Read the DIET caption,* which is comprehensive, and be guided as to what can be health-giving, often acting as medicine. This also includes much valuable information, health-wise, about vitamins, minerals and food supplements, which can aid return to better health.

PARENTING

This description of bringing up children has only appeared recently. One would imagine it is about bringing children up properly, about control, teaching, answering questions, being in charge, leadership, guidance, loving and much more, including being unpopular when firm decisions have to be made and stood by. Many young people are not being taught the meaning of the word 'No'. I am only concerned with natural remedies and this includes our greatest medicine, natural nutrition, and additive-free, unprocessed foods. How many parents know anything about this in our modern age, where speed and pace of life demand that pure and natural food is the only sustenance to be taken, in order to keep both adults and children healthy, in mind and body? We hear of the increase in children's diseases, including asthma, diabetes, obesity, allergies, and much more, despite the thousands of synthetic tablets and other drugs available. Many are of little or no benefit, blatantly over-prescribed, especially antibiotics, which can be extremely harmful. The over-use at time of birth and during infancy is often uncalled for, unnecessary. **Alternative therapists maintain that the minor illnesses, which occur to children, are strengtheners of the system, allowing more serious illness to be warded off later in life.** It must be repeated that a child's health is the responsibility of the parent or guardian and the advice is, to *turn to captions under DIET, Children's and Teenagers Health, Exercise and Sleep. Change to the natural to realise that pure, unadulterated food is almost always better than any medicine. I write as a parent interested in better health. We had little sickness or illness 20, 30 or 40 years* *ago, with no queuing or waiting for medical attention. Pills and medicines were not handed out like sweets. Food was natural. Exercise was taken. Almost all had to walk and also abide by proper sleep pattern. There was little alternative.*

PARKINSON'S DISEASE

This disease of the central nervous system takes hold gradually. There is no known cure at present, although there are high hopes that the radical new treatment, known as deep brain stimulation and which has shown good results so far, will work to alleviate Parkinson's Disease. Diet of pure natural foods can help slow the illness, also bringing a better state of body and mind health. *Turn to Diet caption.* Supplements which help the brain and nervous system are: Vitamins B complex with extra Vitamin B6 also Coenzyme Q10 and Vitamins E and C. When on medical treatment it is advisable to speak with your doctor before taking herbal or other supplements, although all are compatible. The natural *DIET* as suggested will help enormously.

PAROTITIS

See Mumps Caption.

PARSLEY

This edible evergreen herb is another of nature's pure foods and medicines. It is a diuretic, assists the body during menstruation and menopause, especially when with hot flushes. It is an aid to digestion, helping to eliminate flatulence and colic pains, good for prostate, hair and nails. Parsley contains minerals, including calcium, silica and potassium. It is high in Vitamins C and A. Can be eaten with salads or in fruit purees, also as a herbal tea, which is available in the health food shops. Pluck a handful of fresh parsley, chop and place in a saucepan covering with one pint of water. Bring to boil and simmer for one minute. Strain and when cool drink a cupful after meals. Parsley should not be taken when pregnant, if breastfeeding or if with kidney inflammation.

PEDOMETER

A Pedometer is a gadget, which can be like a friend. As a walking companion it shows the distance traversed. They are comparatively cheap to purchase and can be regulated to give kilometres, miles and steps. The more sophisticated types give calories burned, heartbeat, etc. Obtainable from or will be ordered by any good sports shop.

PEPPERMINT

Oil of peppermint capsules are an excellent aid for indigestion, to relieve catarrh, divirticulitis and other bowel problems, including irritable bowel syndrome.

PEPTIC ULCER

See Ulcers Caption.

PERIODIC SYNDROME

No doubt it has always been with us as an ailment, but only in recent years has it been diagnosed and referred to as Periodic Syndrome. It affects teenagers who suffer pain in the centre of the stomach, often together with vomiting. It can be likened to spasms of the intestinal muscles, lasting up to four or five hours. It is brought on by a complaint, which is becoming all-too-common, even in young people, namely stress, and should be treated as such. *Proper Diet of natural food, change of lifestyle, sufficient sleep with proper sleep pattern also exercise, all work together to ward off Periodic Syndrome.* Slippery Elm drinks also Peppermint Oil capsules are excellent help to relieve the pain. *See Stress caption.*

PERIODONTAL DISEASE

Previously known as Pyorrhoea. This degenerative gum disease usually occurs, like most gum and teeth problems, because of inferior Diet, also from poor mouth hygiene. Rinse mouth three times daily with Menosan or a solution of six to 10 drops of Tea Tree Oil to a glass of water, or use Aloe Vera gel or juice. Complete change of Diet to nutritious foods combined with added supplements, which include a good natural Multivitamin, also extra Vitamins E and C, Zinc and a Devil's Claw tablet will help the gums and mouth to better health. Rutin is a further aid to help banish the problem. *Also see Gums, Teeth and Toothpaste captions.*

PERIODS

See Pre Menstrual Syndrome and Menstruation Caption.

PERIO MENOPAUSE

This occurs as a forerunner of - a warning - that the menopause will follow. Most women experience some of the perio menopause. Many have never heard of it. With hormonal changes taking place within the body there can be mood swings, erratic periods, sudden weight gain, hot flushes, insomnia, fatigue and other upsets. It is simply the start of the menopause and should be treated as such. *Turn to Menopause caption* and be guided by the advice given.

PERSPIRATION SMELL

See Body Odour Caption.

PESTICIDES AND INSECTICIDES

Much evidence is available that imported fruit and vegetables also some of those homegrown, have higher than the recommended traces of the health damaging chemicals. The general public have little if any knowledge about agri-chemicals. Toxicologists are unlearned about the long-term consequences to health, with many of the pesticides used being undetectable in laboratories. There are several ways to avoid much of the risks. Thoroughly wash all fruit and vegetables whether cooking, eating raw or for salads. Peel where possible. Purchase home-produced food, organic if possible. Keep asking for organic; eventually the message will be received. Consider growing your own. If you don't have a garden there may be community allotments in your district. Fresh fruit and vegetables, including greens, are a must for better health.

PHARMACEUTICAL INDUSTRY. The

The drug manufactures continue to mushroom into multinational conglomerates. Frequently we hear and read about takeovers and amalgamation of the various companies, as they become rich through the unrestrained production of chemical medicines, many of them of little use. Many do harm to the body.

An example of the staggering turnover in the industry is to be found in Ireland. They are the largest net exporters of drugs in the world. Last year the figure was over €13 billion with over 21,000 people employed.

We are informed in the trade papers that the Pharmaceutical industry, including the pharmacists, is a lucrative business, with a great future. The pharmacies, which retail these products, enjoy average profits of over 30% on each item sold, a confidential report reveals. It also states that the level of competition is low. We are also told of the excessive costs of generic prescription drugs, many of which are sold for very much less as branded medicines or tablets. It is a fact that some producers have enormous mark up on products supplied directly to the Health Service. Here again the softly, softly approach is apparent, with no complaint or criticism from those who are supposedly in authority. All are part of the 'Foods', 'Drinks', Pharmaceutical Drugs and Health Service Merry-go-Round. Their trade may be healthy but their products do not appear to help the health of the nation. One has only to look at the waiting lists and hear of the Health Service being criticised and lambasted to realise that those who control the drug companies must be laughing all the way to the bank. It is time for those responsible for the health of all to pull the plug. It is very obvious that a mini-dictator is needed to run the Health Service in order to control the almost irresponsible sale and use of pharmaceutical drugs. The obscene profits, the equally senseless and crazy outlay on drugs by the general public and the welfare state, is reflected in the salaries paid to the many 'fat cats' in the Pharmaceutical and drug industry. The Chief Executive of Glaxo Smith Kline saw his salary rise by 13% to almost £2.8million Stg. - almost €4 million last year. Need one comment further? *Turn to The 'Food', 'Drinks', Pharmaceutical Drugs and Health Service Merry-go-Round*, the opening chapter of this Encyclopedia.

PHLEBITIS

This usually occurs when varicose veins are present, where the walls of the veins become inflamed. Often brought on by sedentary lifestyle, with little exercise being taken. Where Diet and lifestyle have been changed there is almost always a vast improvement in health, with proper intake of good food being excellent protection against Phlebitis. Treat as advised under Blood Pressure High caption, when you have spoken with your doctor, because if with phlebitis there is always the danger of thrombosis or clot. *Change of Diet and lifestyle can go a long way towards solving the problem.* Blood Pressure (High) caption gives much good advice to help Phlebitis and to aid circulation problems.

PHYTOTHERAPY

This is the treatment used by our ancestors, before the advent of chemical and synthetic drugs, now so easily obtained. It means the use of plants, herbs and their extracts to treat the various symptoms of the many ailments and disease with which we are plagued. Very often these were 'home made' or made up by the local quack, with no proper control over their content. Now we have sophisticated methods of producing the many phyto medicines available. They are quality assured, laboratory-controlled, properly packaged and labelled, medicinal, herb and plant products. **BIOFORCE** *are one of the leaders in this natural remedy speciality, giving us a wonderful range of herbal products, which are available over the counter from the health food shop and now from the pharmacists. The latter have condescended to acknowledge their efficiency, as many turn to and demand the simple natural remedies, seldom if ever with side effects. Dr. Vogel, who was a marvellous natural health pioneer who founded Bioforce, is mentioned under caption. See Bibliography for details about further reading on the subject of PHYTOTHERAPY, including Alfred Vogel's book* **'The Nature Doctor'.**

PILES

See Haemorrhoids Caption.

PILL

See Contraceptive Pill Caption.

PIMPLES AND SPOTS

Not to be confused with acne. Frequently caused by inferior Diet, including 'junk foods', sugarised, processed products and fizzy 'drinks'. Eating natural additive-free foods, combined with intake of Pulsatilla, Calc Phos, alternated with Calc Sulph or tonic, such as Floradix or Kindervital should result in clear skin also better and energetic health. Combination D New Era has proved an excellent remedy for this problem. The greatest and most successful remedies are the pure foods and drinks taken. *Turn to DIET also Skin captions* to be guided about how to have healthy, clear skin.

PINS AND NEEDLES
See Legs caption.

PLANT ALLERGY
See Allergic To Plants Caption.

PLAQUE
See Teeth Caption.

PLEURISY
Seek medical assistance. As a tonic or pick-me-up to help in recovery from Pleurisy the most natural aid is a Diet of pure non- processed foods. *See DIET caption,* which, also gives recommended natural Vitamins and Minerals, to be alternated every two or three days with the tonic Floravital. This will help ensure a quick return to better health, when recovering from energy sapping or debilitating illnesses such as Pleurisy.

P.M.S.
See Pre-Menstrual Syndrome and Menstruation Caption.

POLLEN
Recent research shows that Pollen is a major aid to ease the symptoms of pre menstrual syndrome. Tension, bloating, weight gain, irritability and state of depression associated with PMS, have been dramatically reduced by the taking of Pollen. The health food store can supply this natural food, which is as medicine. The question can be asked: 'Why have we not heard of this before?' Simply because the drug manufacturers cannot patent Honey, Propolis or Pollen, all from the honeybee. The producers of the natural product have not got the resources, the money to advertise, like the multi-national drug companies do incessantly. Therefore, another natural remedy - an aid to better well-being - is almost unknown. Money is more important than the health of the public. The patenting and registration of synthetic drugs is part of the cash till for the almighty chemical conglomerates. Visit your health food store and ask for further information on Pollen and Propolis, also about their health-giving properties.

POLYNEURITIS - Inflammation of peripheral nerves.
See Neuritis Caption.

POOR CIRCULATION

Treat as High Blood Pressure Caption.

PORRIDGE

Here is one of nature's gifts to us as good food. *Read under Oats and Oatmeal caption* to learn about this purely natural cereal, from which Porridge is made and to discover how much goodness it contains.

POST NATAL DEPRESSION

Depression is just that, whether postnatal or at any other time of life. Many women feel really down after giving birth. The weepiness, anxiety, often with anger or feeling guilty, referred to as 'The Baby Blues', can come to some after what has been an exhaustive and worrying time. **Apart from what your doctor suggests, which is all too often the prescribing of antidepressant tablets, there are many natural aids to help return of energy and well being.** The first thing to look at is the Diet. Is it nutritious, natural, unadulterated and additive-free? Do you have a good breakfast? Are you eating fruit and vegetables? Very often the type of food partaken of is the root cause of the depression or low feeling. Calcium / Magnesium / Vitamin D combination, taken with Zinc and Vitamin B6 can help enormously, or consider taking a natural Multivitamin such as Wellwoman or Pregnacare. Agnus Castus and Milk Thistle help restore the hormones to their natural state. Rhodolia is a great aid to help the mood, also available from the health food store. Regular pattern of sufficient sleep is necessary. Don't bottle things up. Confide in and talk with a friend, off-loading your fears, cares and worries. It is good to talk. This is a time when a kind and considerate partner can do incredible good. **As harped upon in this Encyclopedia, Diet of natural food, Exercise and Sleep are as medicine. Turn to read all three captions, combine them and be amazed at the increased sense of well-being and energy, with that depressing feeling often being a thing of the past.**

POTASSIUM

See Vitamins and Minerals Caption

POTATOES

Not too long ago, and occasionally even now, the Diet and slimming gurus inform us that potatoes are fattening. This is nonsense. They make a valuable contribution to natural Diet, containing no fat, when boiled, steamed, baked or roasted. **As crisps, chipped, sautéed or cooked in oil they should be avoided.** Potatoes are an excellent source of starch, also containing some Vitamin C. What better natural food for an active person than a plate which contains an amount of mashed or boiled potatoes, with either fish, meat, cheese or egg dish, topped off with a knob of pure butter or a spoonful of cold pressed Olive Oil? Potatoes should be removed from plastic bags before storing in a dark, cool place to avoid greening, which is detrimental to health. Protect from frost. Instant potato powder is unnatural, best left on the shelf.

POULTRY MEAT

Because of lack of space the captions in this Encyclopedia in some instances only dwell fleetingly on aspects of the heading. So it is with chicken meat. When chicken is purchased it very often contains more than chicken. It is well known within the trade that the processing of Poultry leaves much to be desired. Many are not aware of this when purchasing this kind of meat. It would take several pages to set out how some of the chicken on offer is far from chicken meat, free from additives. It can include the addition of other meats, especially pork, also water. To find out the frightening facts about the Russian roulette practised when eating chicken, read the best seller 'Not On The Label', by Felicity Lawrence, as detailed in the Bibliography section of this Encyclopedia. *Also turn to Meat caption.*

POT PLANTS

Scientific evidence shows that potted plants in the home or office are capable of absorbing pollution toxins from the air, also providing oxygen.

PRAYER

Evidence is there, if this is needed, that there is a healing power in prayer. It is like a relief valve, as the cares of the day are off-loaded. Many who find it difficult to cope with the mountain of sickness, debt, loneliness or other problems can find comfort and peace of mind by turning to and talking with their GOD. We live in a faithless and perverse generation where we have to almost fight the defeatist attitude of our culture, media, the educational system, health service, the work place and even some of our friends. Andrew Carnegie, the well-known philanthropist, said of his father, that: "He attended various churches. He had discovered that there were many theologians, but religion was one".

In Bibliography section particulars are included of a wonderful inspirational publication, a mind calmer, which gives daily reading. It is titled 'The Word For Today, Your Quiet Time Companion'. It is free of charge from United Christian Broadcasters, P.O. Box 255, Stoke-on-Trent, ST4 8YY, UK, or P.O. Box 5784, Edmondstown, Dublin 16.

PREGNANCY

As with all off the shelf synthetic remedies and medicines, almost all herbs and herbal remedies are best avoided during pregnancy. What is set out here is entirely natural and discretionary. Tell your doctor if you wish to follow the advice and be advised. He most certainly cannot disagree with any advice given here about natural food and its goodness. **From the outset, and at all times, try to adhere to purely natural nutritious food *as set out under DIET caption.* Avoid any of the vitamins, minerals or food supplements mentioned at the end of the DIET caption unless prescribed by your doctor or therapist.** The natural food taken will give that extra zest and vigour needed to help allay stress and anxiety. Take Raspberry Leaf Tea or tablets also Royal Jelly. Two invaluable natural aids are Pregnacare, which is a natural pregnancy supplement and Pregnacare cream. They have been expertly developed. The former contains 16 essential nutrients, including Folic Acid, with the cream formulated from botanical extracts, also Vitamins C and E to moisturise and care for expanding skin during pregnancy.

PRE MENSTRUAL SYNDROME (PMS) and MENSTRUATION

All women, many to their chagrin and discomfort, know how they are affected by this intertwined indisposition. The symptoms are harmless, but to some can be very depressing, tiring and upsetting. *It is only in recent years that women have spoken and written openly about period time, which was referred to in almost hushed tones in the past. Some have little or no problems at this time, others are seriously effected. There must be over 100 particular ailments or disorders, many of them niggling, which can affect those with PMS, or during Menstruation.* Examples are: breast tenderness, headaches, mood swings, bloated-ness, feeling depressed, painful periods, heavy and irregular, with spotting in between, nausea, fluid retention, joint aches and pains, extreme tiredness and lethargy. There is often a craving for sugar, sweets or chocolates, with very many other physical and psychological symptoms. Over the years, I have helped many to ease, banish, and be rid of the often-nightmarish problems of PMS and the discomfort of menstruation. Examples of how husbands have made the approach, seeking help, have led to laughs and good-humoured banter with their wives when they later told of the relief obtained. A letter of thanks in front of me, when change to natural food was advised some years earlier, with instructions to take Agnus Castus, Propolis, Pollen, Black Cohosh, Vitamin B6 and Iron supplement also Calcium / Magnesium / Vitamin D tablet, states how: "This really works wonders" (her words). This lady tells of how there were and are no further distressing problems. Also mentioned is of how Pulsatilla taken with Cramp Bark did away with painful periods. Deficiency of Vitamin B6 leads to imbalance between oestrogen and progesterone.

I am firmly of the opinion that PMS and menstrual problems, like very many ailments, are mainly the result of a Diet low in proper nutritives, also to insufficient Exercise and bad Sleep patterns. Many who took up Yoga speak of its excellent body and mind benefits. It is an extremely good form of Exercise, as is walking. There are natural non side effect supplements, which have, to re-quote the letter writer: "Worked wonders". Agnus Castus is an all-round women's friend at PMS and Menstruation times, as are Raspberry Leaf tea or tablets. The extraordinary elements, which Agnus Castus contain, cannot be over praised in their relation to menstrual ailments. If feeling weepy, with deflated spirits or in pain take the little tablets of Pulsatilla.   Low levels of Calcium, Magnesium also Vitamin B Complex as in Brewer's Yeast and Iron contribute greatly to the problem of PMS. Extra Vitamin B6 is required with the Brewer's Yeast. Studies show that some 10 to 12 days before menstruation the Calcium and Vitamin B levels drop consistently. This is when the ovaries are least active. The elements in the Calcium / Magnesium / Vitamin D supplement work in combination. Essential Fatty Acids are effective to control many of the problems associated with PMS. Evening Primrose Oil or Udo's Choice Oil are two providers of EFA's. Cramp Bark and Spirulina have been spoken of highly by those who use them. The Cramp Bark for period pains, taken with Spiriulina, is a Dietary aid where it is not possible to have regular access to natural food. Black Cohosh, which has been used in Germany for over 40 years, has been clinically tested for it efficacy to control period pain and other PMS symptoms, including irregular periods and depression. Many find Sepia to be the best remedy for period pains. The Calcium, Vitamin B complex and Iron, with Black Cohosh and Agnus Castus taken together with the EFA's, in combination with the DIET suggested, will bring vast improvement, even freedom from what is sometimes regarded as a tormenting affliction. Pollen or Propolis have helped enormously.

With a little discipline, thought and planning, a stress and ailment-free life can be the lot of the majority who have PMS problems. Smoking and alcohol must be avoided. Sometimes when it has reached the stage where there was no relief, despite observing all instructions, the simple remedy has turned out to be gluten free or dairy free Diet, because of untraced allergy or intolerance. Similarly if the problem continues all month, there may be underlying conditions such as under active thyroid or something, which your doctor must diagnose and by whom you must be guided. Tell him what your ideas are. Ask for allergy, blood or other tests. It has been found that many extreme PMS sufferers are highly alert, being well regulated in their work or environment, having sharp memories and good leadership.

Black Cohosh must not be taken long term or if with blood pressure, when taking contraceptive or hormonal pill, when pregnant or if breastfeeding. *See DIET, Exercise and Sleep captions. All three combined can lead to a wonderful improvement in mind and body, where PMS and its niggling or other problems can be, as a woman said recently: "shrugged off"*

PREVENTION OF DISEASE OR ILLNESS

In the UK and Ireland over £78 billion or €116 billion plus will be spent on and in the Health Service in the next year with budgeting for an increase of 50% within four years. The figures are staggering. All the time the call is for even more money. Much of this will be paid out in wages, salaries and to the drug companies, who cream off many billions as they churn out their medicines. *Daily we see headline items such* as: 'Giant Pharmaceutical Company under pressure to deliver more products and profits'; 'Construction work to begin immediately on €100 million plant which will create 220 jobs to manufacture tablets'; 'Turnover passes 1.5 billion euro as profits jump 24%'; 'Healthy outlook for pharmaceutical and chemical sector'; 'There have been no closures in the past 25 years, with most established plants growing rapidly in size and capacity'; 'The largest bio pharmaceutical factory in the world has been established outside Dublin with a 1 billion dollar investment. It will employ 1,300 people'; 'Pharmaceutical giants saw pre tax profits double last year'. The following headlines are in much smaller print: 'We suffer from self-imposed illness as we eat, drink and smoke our way to ill health'; 'Our health service is not doing the business'; 'Health trouble worse than black hole'; 'Our sick health service grows worse'; 'Six hospitals want new drugs vetted'; 'France prescribes clearout of wasteful medicines'; 'Big health squander'; 'US food and drugs body warns of anti depressant and suicide link'. **Not a word about DIET or the 'foods' we put into our bodies. There is not even a line about prevention of disease or sickness. The pharmaceutical and synthetic medicines industry may be in a healthy state, but many of those who depend on their products are not.** You are probably saying: "What has all this information got to do with the heading of this caption PREVENTION OF DISEASE AND ILLNESS?" The headlines set out are a stark reminder that 'Prevention is better that cure'. *Those who are paid handsomely to run our Health Services, those who do not appear to be responsible to anybody, should be bluntly told of their failure to educate or take action to prevent ill health. Last year they allocated for prevention and health education a paltry 0.08% of the many billions spent, the amounts set out at the beginning of this caption. Yes, this meagre amount allotted to PREVENTION, places one of the most important aspects of health care at the bottom of the list. Here is another example of how our health bureaucrats have got their priorities wrong.* All must realise that *'PREVENTION IS BETTER THAN CURE'.* This is highlighted throughout this Guide, with much advice given as to how it can be done. *See The Food, Drinks, Pharmaceutical Drugs and Health Service Merry-go-Round chapter in the introductory part of this Encyclopedia.*

PROBIOTIC 'FOODS'

See Functional Foods.

PROCESSED 'FOODS' AND 'DRINKS'

The word, processed means altered, converted, refined, transformed, treated. This describes much of what we are offered and use today as 'food' and 'drinks'. It has destroyed levels of Vitamins, Minerals and Nutrients due to the processing, much being without fibre and often indigestible. In the health enlightening book **'Let's get well'** by Adele Davis *(See Bibliography)* it is summed up thus: *"The tremendous increase in ill health has paralleled the ever mounting consumption of sweets,* chocolate, refined processed 'foods', soft 'drinks' and confectionery, with the corresponding decreased use of natural foods, including fresh vegetables, wholegrain breads and especially natural cereals. Yet the intake of nutritionally barren 'foods' sky rockets still more each year". The multi billion dollar / pound / euro refined 'food' industry has gained such power that it keeps people in ignorance, literally controlling the health of our nation. It's relentless radio, television, newspaper and magazine advertising reaches like the life crushing tentacles of an octopus into every home. We're expected to accept the mishmash of information written in our newspapers and magazines, clever mixtures of truth, misinformation and propaganda. They depend on their advertising income from the 'foodless' food industry. This is particularly designed to prevent the slightest interest in nutrition from interfering with enormous profits. Where is the nutrition in colours, preservatives, and fillers, the many other chemicals and inedible additives in our 'foods'? There is little good in much of the 5,000 plus substances used as 'food' additives. There is nothing pleasing which can be said about them. *Turn to Additives caption* to read further about the make up of much of what is offered to us as 'food' also read the chapter in opening pages: **'The Story of a Family who Ate their way to Ill Health'**.

PROPOLIS

Like honey and pollen, Propolis is another pure natural food produced by the bee. It is as medicine, being an extremely good antioxidant, which helps strengthen the immune system, being an aid for digestive, respiratory and breathing problems. It can be used to both treat and ward off sore throat, colds and 'flu. Propolis or Pollen are worthy aids for menstrual problems. They are available in either tablet or capsule form from the health food store.

PROSTATE GLAND

There are many with Prostate Gland problem, known as Benign Prostatic Hypertrophy (BPH). Thankfully the percentage of men with Prostate cancer and Prostatitis is relatively low. The latter is quite uncommon, usually occurring in young men. It is not to be confused with the quite common BPH, which, despite what some maintain, is definitely age-related. Some suffer from the condition as early as their 40's. Some have it from their 60's onwards, with up to 80% having it in their 80's. The cause is unclear. *I had, and I suppose still have the ailment. I have helped hundreds to live with Prostate Gland enlargement and resulting urinary problems, including having to visit the toilet several times during the night. It is difficult to pen these words without a feeling of anger, because like many other disorders, here is one which can be treated naturally and simply with enormous success. I have had many men visit me who were on conventional drugs, who had to get out of bed several times during the night, then feeling worn out during the next day. I gave them my advice as to what to use just as has been given to hundreds of others whom I have helped.* Take Saw Palmetto, Lycopene, Zinc/Copper combination, Pulsatilla and Pumpkin Seeds. Grind the Pumpkin Seeds in a liquidiser and store in an airtight container, taking one or two dessertspoonfuls each morning with porridge or natural additive-free cereal at breakfast time. A 5mg supplement of Lycopene, taken daily, gives cartenoid pigments, which are a Prostate cancer fighting combination. Whether with Prostate Gland or urinary problems all over the age of 40, men and women, should be taking Zinc because the body no longer makes it. Zinc must be combined with Copper to work efficiently. Zinc/Copper tablets are usually blended to correct proportions. 'Quest' brand is an example of a proper combination. There are various brands of Saw Palmetto. I have no hesitation in recommending Bioforce Saw Palmetto drops or Kordel's Saw Palmetto Complex. Everything mentioned in this Encyclopedia is available from the health food store. Seek their advice if in doubt. ***The majority of the medical profession do not wish to know about the natural way of treatment for BPH. They would rather experiment with hormone, gene or vaccine treatment, none of which appears to be helpful.***

Avoid fatty foods, also alcohol, which most certainly is an enemy of the prostate. *See DIET caption* and if possible partake of what is advised because natural food is one of our greatest medicines. It must be remembered that there is no cure for the problem, or seldom need for operation, because one can live with it if it is treated properly. I have made the mistake of giving up taking the remedy or aid when the assumption was that all was clear, only for the need to get up at night, as before. Not alone is one able to rest, but the inflammation or extreme enlargement, which leads to cancer, can be kept under control. *As well as the natural remedies advised, with abstention from alcohol as already mentioned, which is hugely responsible for the problem in the first instance, there is a need to study the DIET and Exercise captions and be guided by the advice given.* This includes the recommendation to drink up to eight glasses of water daily. If with Prostate inflammation do not drink for at least three hours before bedtime.

P

PROZAC

This antidepressant chemical, which is Fluoxetine, is mentioned because of its unnatural features. Side effects include vomiting, diarrhoea, fever, skin problems, insomnia, convulsions, dizziness and others. The long- term consequences, as with the use of many unproved drugs, is unknown. The manufacturers have the audacity to inform us that it is safe; while those who know otherwise tell us it is not. *Prozac should be avoided if at all possible.* There are natural remedies such as Skullcap, Damiana or Valerian, for the treatment of depression, equally good, but side effect free. *Turn to Depression caption* or seek further advice from the Health Food Store personnel.

PRUNES

Prunes, which are dried plums, are another of nature's gifts. They contain higher concentrates of most Vitamins, except C, than does fresh fruit. Wash and strain before soaking overnight in boiling water, even if the package states 'Ready for eating'. Prune juice or the water in which the fruit was steeped is equally good. Prunes are fat- free, also being a good source of dietary fibre, excellent to aid where there is constipation or lazy bowel movement.

PRURITIS

See Itching Caption.

PSORIASIS

This very common skin condition affects well over 1.5million people in the United Kingdom and Ireland. It does not appear to be that prevalent, probably because there are so many with the ailments that are embarrassed to speak about it or bring it to the notice of others. I have helped many to a pleasant change in health by the relief of Psoriasis, also being annoyed by those who during the time after vast improvement of the problem, had not the courage and discipline to continue the treatment. They returned to their old habits of taking alcohol, inferior Diet or bad lifestyle. There are many who are irresponsible when it comes to better health and well-being.

Change of Diet to pure, natural unprocessed, additive-free food is the first and most important step. It is vital to eliminate alcohol, caffeine, citrus fruits, tomatoes, peppers, aubergines and spicy foods. They are inflammatory to the cause. In many cases the good foods mentioned under Diet, when partaken of, have led to much success in the elimination of Psoriasis. By going further and entering into a gluten free, dairy free Diet the results have been amazing, with the Psoriasis often banished, certainly very much improved, with a greater feeling of health; zest and energy.

Many within the medical profession will tell you that there is no cure. This is not so. Natural food will not be mentioned. Psoriasis is dietary, stress and/or nerve-related, in my opinion. It is often not realised that almost all with Psoriasis have abnormal cholesterol count. If this can be normalised and there is seldom reason why it cannot, then by choosing natural Diet and lifestyle, the clearance of the skin problem is extremely quick. Supplement natural Diet by taking daily: Zinc / Copper combination, Vitamin A, Lecithin Granules, Milk Thistle, Udo's Choice Oil and Manuka Honey. These when combined with nutritious food have brought sterling results. Other aids, which have helped immensely, are Kali Sulph and Aloe Vera Oil, also the partaking of fish oil and the eating of fish regularly. Manuka honey when mixed with Cod Liver Oil and smeared over Psoriasis has often banished the scaliness. After the de-scaling this remedy must be used on the skin for some weeks to help eliminate the redness. Find out what suits you best, do not deviate from it and hopefully be Psoriasis free. If all cannot be free from Psoriasis it can certainly be largely controlled. Watch the improvement of skin and health when disciplined enough to accept the advice given. As mentioned it may even mean turning to dairy or gluten free foods, but if all are natural, unprocessed, additive-free, they could prove to be the medicine required. *See Cholesterol, Allergy and DIET captions.*

PYSCHOTROPIC DRUGS

These stimulants, sedatives, antidepressants and tranquillisers have a high tendency to side effects and dependency. It is desirable that all, especially the elderly, be weaned off them if at all possible. There are many natural remedies to replace them, all non- addictive. Those, which I have found to be the most suitable are mentioned under relevant nerve and mind-related captions in this Guide. Natural food is one of the best medicines known. Seek the help of the health food store personnel and be advised further.

PULSATILLA

Available in tablet form or as a tincture, Pulsatilla is one of the most versatile all round herbs available. Its excellence is little known, because again, there is no money in it for the drug companies. It is too simple a remedy. It is one of the earth's gifts for the prostate gland and the reproductive organs, male and female. Helps relieve nervous tension and associated headaches, asthma, respiratory problems and to calm the mind. It is good for insomnia. Being anti-bacterial, when used in tincture form it can relieve earache. As a blood tonic it combines extremely well with Echinacea to eliminate boils, spots and pimples also being used to treat acne, in conjunction with pure natural Diet. Combined with Cramp Bark it helps relieve painful periods.

Pulsatilla, Zinc/ Copper, Ground Pumpkin seeds and Saw Palmetto have all brought immense help for prostate problems eliminating the need to urinate frequently, so helping the sleep pattern at night. Pulsatilla is also good for sinusitis. Combined with Hawthorn it is an aid to restoring temporary hearing loss. As already stated its health-giving qualities are unknown to the majority.

PUMPKIN SEEDS

These health-giving seeds contain vitamins, minerals and trace elements which are extremely good for prostate problems, cystitis and kidney health. In order to partake of easily, with little chewing, it is suggested they be ground in a liquidiser then stored in an airtight container, taking a dessertspoonful or more with porridge or natural cereal at breakfast time.

PYORRHOEA

See Periodontal Disease Caption.

IF ALL WITHIN THE HEALTH SERVICE AND MANY WHO COMPLAIN ABOUT ITS
SHORTCOMINGS WERE TO ADOPT THE ADAGE 'DON'T FIND FAULT, FIND A REMEDY', A
SOLUTION MIGHT EASIER COME ABOUT.

QUINOA.

Can rightly be called the 'Mother and Father' of all grains. It is unique because it is also a fruit and a herb. Here is the perfect food or as near perfect as one can find. All-too-few in the Western world know of its goodness and nutritional qualities. Its protein properties are better than that of meat, being natural. It contains calcium of a high quality, vitamins and other minerals, is very low in fat, with essential fatty acids. One could fill pages to write about this master food, including its goodness when sprouted also of its need in the Diet of vegetarians. We read much drivel about 'superfoods', where the writers are of the opinion that food containing additives can be included. Quinoa would be the top of my list of SUPERFOODS whether sprouted or cooked as a milk pudding. It is a natural living nutriment. See Sprouting of Seeds and Pulses caption. Quinoa and many other health giving grains, seeds, pulses, dried fruits also milk pudding bases such as semolina, tapioca, ground and flaked rices, sago and whole wheat macaroni are available at the health food store.

RASH

This word can cover a wide range of skin problems. Included are nappy rash, shingles, infectious diseases of children, sunburn, food or other allergies, psoriasis, rosacea, acne and others. *See under various captions, also skin.* All will advise pure natural *DIET,* which is the fundamental basis for all skin and health problems. There will, of course, be need for change where there are allergies or need to avoid certain edibles such as citrus fruits, gluten, dairy or other types of food.

RAW FOOD

The excuse of not having time to cook and so resorting to fast, junk or additive-filled, off-the-shelf prepared meals, cannot be accepted. If properly organised it takes little time to prepare good nutritious food, including Raw Foods. A liquidiser and sharp knife can be a huge asset. A meal of sliced or pureed mixed raw fruit and vegetables or perhaps vegetable and pure fruit juices, gives the enzymes, vitamins and minerals, which are so vital to digestion and better health. Mixed with whole-wheat pasta, boiled potatoes, or salads they are highly nutritious. A little foresight and planning can be the forerunner of better health. Many raw foods are full of goodness and combined with fruit are excellent as snacks. Meat or meat products are not to be regarded as suitable for eating raw.

RAYNAUD'S DISEASE

This little understood problem, which must be regarded as a circulatory disorder, although this is debatable, results in white, frozen-like, stiff fingers or toes, with ears and nose also affected when the weather is cold. It is often chronic. Sometimes there is an underlying cause when the combined problem is referred to as Raynaud's Phenomenon, where the affected parts can turn blue, often swelling. Most sufferers are women and it is often coupled with migraine. Again Diet comes into account. Where there has been change to natural additive-free, gluten-free Diet and the partaking of suggested vitamins and supplements, there has been a dramatic change to better and warmer feeling. Wrap up extremely well, wear gloves and warm headgear, take exercise and do not neglect the problem. It can lead to further complications if left unchecked. These include damage to the blood vessels, veins and artery walls. Take Calcium / Magnesium / Vitamin D supplement continuously, also Vitamins A, C & E, Lecithin and Udo's Choice Oil. The most important supplement to take is Ginkgo Biloba, which combined with those mentioned, especially Vitamin E 400IU, taken daily long-term, has brought marvellous results. If on blood thinning medication consult your doctor if considering taking Ginkgo Biloba. *Turn to DIET and Gluten-Free Diet captions* and be further guided. Assistance and advice from the Raynaud's and Scleroderma Society, 112 Crewe Road, Alsager, Cheshire ST7 2JA or PO Box 2958 Foxrock, Dublin 18.

RDA's

These letters, which are associated with vitamins and minerals, mean Recommended Daily Allowances. The figures, which usually appear opposite the ingredients listed in the supplements, are highly questionable. We are now told that they are far too low. It appears as if the numbers were rounded, plucked almost at random. In many cases they bear no relation to the daily allowance required. Some are up to 10 times too low. Except for Vitamin A, Niacin, Selenium and Iron there is no danger of overusing what is signified in the *RDA's,* unless one sets out to do so purposely. Seldom if ever is there a report of side effects from any vitamins, minerals or food supplements. There are many, all-too-many of these incidents with chemical drugs, which are in an entirely different category from what is being written about.

READING

The therapeutic effects of this wonderful pastime are known only to those who do so. It relaxes one and helps calm the mind. There is a wonderful selection of books in our underused libraries, making it a cheap or often costless hobby. It is a good way to help form a child's character, compared to say Television, an enemy of all that is good, including our health. All children should be encouraged to Read. Literary problems, including spelling, are extremely high, with the art of both conversation and Reading at a low point. This is more than coincidence. Books should be left where those who wish to read can conveniently pick them up.

RED CLOVER

Highly praised by many who use it, especially for treatment of eczema and certain skin diseases, also for coughs and bronchitis.

REFLEXOLOGY

Reflexology therapy can help to relieve many conditions. It entails the use of pressure on points of hands and feet to pinpoint and treat ailments. The pressure points refer to where energy channels meet. It works on the principal that reflex points on the feet correspond with, or to, every part of the body. By working on these areas, the Reflexologist can detect and correct blockages in the energy pathway, so allowing for them to be released or cleared. It is now available as a treatment in some hospitals, being well established as a top complementary therapy, all due to the change of attitude by the medical profession. Because of the demand for Reflexology treatment they have come to recognise its natural help to well being. I was very impressed with the use of Reflexology, especially the vast numbers of ailments, which can be remedied. The relief of thyroid problems are an example of the goodness of Reflexology. It has also helped enormously with stress relief, back pain, circulation, arthritis, hay fever, obesity, quitting smoking and many other less serious niggling ailments. Reflexology has been of great benefit for children, especially those with weight problems.

REIKI

The word means 'Universal Life Energy', being a simple technique, which enhances health and energy, including one's general outlook or sense of purpose. It is a very old form of Japanese spiritual healing, brought West in the late 19th century. Practitioners draw on Reiki energy, in turn channelling it to those in need. It is a simple form of *'Hands on healing'* with courses run regularly where one can, if so inclined, learn over a week-end all the rudiments required to get started. Reiki, which is simple, safe and effective, with no doctor, no special belief or system needed, has had very favourable results and reports. It is based on principles far removed from the sphere of conventional science. Again the medical profession would look on this kind of treatment as alien to their orthodox chemical medicines. Like other things alternative, Reiki has its advocates and devotees, being highly praised. Qualified Reiki therapy practitioners are listed in the yellow pages.

R

RELAXATION

Here is a wonderful, entirely free therapy, an invaluable aid to health, well being, mood, mind and emotions. *If you have a busy lifestyle, constantly on the go, under pressure, rushing around, with extremely active mind, under stress or tension, it is essential to both make and take time to relax.* Sensible people realise the necessity to take a break, especially at weekends. The yearly holiday is just not enough. Find a hobby or other interest. Read, spend time with relatives or friends. Yoga, golf, meditation or walking are wonderful revivers. A change of scenery, doing something different, will help. S*it and relax at meal times, finding a quiet environment, avoiding eating hastily. Give your digestive system time to settle down after food, because eating on the run plays havoc with the body.* Healthy people pace themselves in daily life, just like the long-distance runner when in competition. Learn to relax and enjoy each day and resultant better health. *Also see Leisure caption.* **It is wonderful to relax, do nothing and have somebody to help you do nothing!**

REPETITIVE STRAIN INJURY (RSI)

Virtually unheard of until recent times, now in the top 10 complaints treated by doctors. It was usually found where there was continuous production by on-line workers, who often worked on what was termed 'piecework', entailing production bonus. This resulted in RSI, with pain in hands and arms also sometimes in neck or back. Now we see a huge increase of the problem in both adults and children, because they are continuously stooped and tensed over computer keyboards, games consoles, also with extreme repetitive use of thumb or hand, especially when text messaging. It results in severe pain, where carrying out mundane tasks can be agonising. Pain can be relieved by taking balanced Calcium / Magnesium / Vitamin D supplement also Vitamins E, C and B complex. Osteopathy has given relief quickly. Advice from RSI Association, Chapel House, 152 High Street, Yiewsley, West Drayton, Middlesex UB7 7BE, UK

RESPIRATORY HEALTH

Despite the health, safety and environmental administration officials increasing in numbers in recent years, we have an enormous upsurge in respiratory, pulmonary and lung-related diseases and ailments. We cannot hide the issue of high levels of environmental pollutants such as carbon monoxide gases, chemicals and smoke, also the overuse of antibiotics and other chemical medicines, many no better than placebos, some harmful to the human body. Heart, circulation, digestion, kidneys, bowel, lungs and breathing are dependent on each other for good Respiratory and breathing health. Contaminated air must be avoided. Smoking is certainly alien to good Respiration and breathing, with passive smoking equally so. The packet containing the drug states 'Smoking Kills'. Many ignore the message, at their peril. All interested in good health need to keep their natural defences in top condition. Proper breathing must be practised, with correct and complete inhalation and exhalation of pure air to the lungs. Exercise is very important. Again we come back to the best weapon in defence of better health, a pure natural whole food Diet. This, combined with proper lifestyle, aided by antioxidants such as Quest Cell Life also Vitamins A, C & E, Pulsatilla and Garlic capsules all combine to give better Respiratory health. Lobelia is an excellent aid, highly recommended. The nose, mouth and, of course, the lungs, extract the vital oxygen from the air we breathe and if healthy expel carbon dioxide. We all need the so necessary energy to enable us cope with everyday problems, health and otherwise. *This can be provided in abundance by the intake of pure natural Diet or supplements as suggested here and under DIET caption. Also turn to Buteyko Breathing Therapy and Exercise captions.*

RESTLESS LEG SYNDROME

See Legs Caption.

RHEUMATIC FEVER

Seek medical attention. Aids to recovery are a Diet high in seafoods, vegetables and other purely natural nutritives. Vitamin E with 200mg Vitamin C taken twice daily helps prevent the formation of scar tissue. Consult your doctor and ascertain if these can be used as complementary aids. **See DIET caption, the goodness of which no GP can dispute.** Many of them are not knowledgeable of, or conversant with, this simple natural treatment. Be guided by the information and advice given under that caption, which can only lead to better health.

RHEUMATISM

To single out this affliction of joints, muscles and bones is practically impossible. It includes up to 20 disorders, including arthritis. Responds extremely well to a dietary change. *See Arthritis DIET caption* which is equally good for Rheumatism. The following are notably good aids to bone and joint pains: oily fish, turnip, celery, cabbage and broccoli. Eliminate peppers and aubergines. Pepper and salt are to be avoided. The ever reliable Devils Claw (Pagosid), Runo or Aloe Vera Joint Complex are invaluable aids for joint pains. Some extol the good of the former; others use Runo or the Joint Complex.   Evening Primrose Oil, Udo's Choice Oil, Activ Juice or the combined supplement Jointace have helped restore to pain free health. Again it is necessary to stress the need for Calcium / Magnesium / Vitamin D balanced combined supplement, to be taken long-term. All natural products mentioned are available from the health food shop or they will order them. *Also see Bone Health caption.* Advice given there also helps to alleviate Rheumatism.

RHEUMATOID ARTHRITIS

See Arthritis Rheumatoid Caption.

RHINITIS

Molkasan, Coenzyme Q10 and Immunace help to strengthen the immune system, which in turn controls Rhinitis. If with allergy the reason must be discovered in order to treat.   Combination H New Era is recommended for allergic Rhinitis. *If necessary see Allergy caption.*

RHODIOLA

This little publicised herbal aid to body and mind has an amazing list of health benefits. Tests show of its positive influence on memory, mental alertness and to help concentration. It has been shown to improve sleep pattern, to relieve depression, migraine and to reduce fatigue levels, also having aphrodisiac qualities. It raises serotonin levels so making the partaker feel happier. It provides a boost in energy levels also having a positive affect on the heart. There are no known side effects and it is best taken in 250mg capsule form. Rosea herbal tea, made from the roots of Rhodiola, is also available. Visit your health food shop and be advised further about this wonderful remedy and the many others available. ` `

RHUBARB

Contains Vitamin C and Calcium, also being high in fibre. Sweeten with pure honey when cooked. This once Springtime fruit is now grown all year round. Good for skin, hair and nail health.

RIBOFLAVIN

See Vitamin B Complex Caption.

RICE

Brown Rice, which has not been de-husked to give us the easily cooked much less nutritious white Rice, is an excellent food, on a par with potatoes or wholemeal bread. White Rice is better for bowel or stomach problems including irritable bowel syndrome. To enable to cook easily soak the brown grains overnight, or from the health food shop obtain flaked or ground brown Rice, which are also ideal for milk puddings. The latter do not need soaking and can be used to produce a purely natural, quickly cooked, rice pudding.

RINGING OR NOISES IN EARS

See Tinnitus Caption.

RINGWORM (TINEA)

This contagious skin disease is often picked up from those who have been in contact with animals, being caused by a fungus. Melissa taken as tea or in tablet form, Echinacea, Clivers or Thuja taken internally, with external use of diluted Tea Tree Oil dabbed on the affected area three to four times daily, will take only a few days to have effect. Add eight to 10 drops of Tea Tree Oil to the bath water as additional treatment. The diluted oil can also be used to disinfect clothes, bedding, brushes or combs. Tisserand brand of Tea Tree Oil, blended with Manuka Honey also Tea Tree Oil cream are recommended.

RITALIN

Mentioned simply because here is another synthetic unnatural narcotic, a brain drug, a psycho stimulant, which is so strong that it has to be prescribed under strict control by the medical profession. It is used to repress ADHD, better known as

Hyperactivity. If only those responsible for the affected young person would turn to natural DIET caption advice as in this Encyclopedia, with everything mentioned being natural, non processed, additive free, considering it as medicine, there would be little or no need for this unsafe, all too powerful stimulant, which has no proven record, only that of side effects. It should only be used as a last resort, if at all. *Tackling the food manufacturers, especially those who churn out the thousands of additives also the giant drug companies, who turn out equally as serious, health drugs, is vital to help solve our health problems, including hyperactivity.*

The natural remedies Efalex and Eye Q Oils contain Omega three and six oils also Evening Primrose Oils, which have proved remarkable, with a calming effect on overactive or hyperactive children, when combined with intake of *natural foods*. They are a hand, eye and brain co-ordinator, certainly an alternative to Ritalin, with no side effects. These are available from the health food store. *Also turn to ADHD caption.*

ROSACEA 'Also referred to as adult acne'

It appears as small lumpy, red pimples, some with puss. The face is usually persistently red. The condition has been linked to alcoholism, which is best avoided, but there is no proof of this. Avoid exposure to sunlight. Do not rub or massage the face. Exercise, which is important, should be taken when or where it is cool. Avoid sweating or overheat. Do not use cosmetics or makeup. Do not self-diagnose. There are many natural complementary remedies to aid, subdue or banish the problem. Avoid all dairy products, eliminate coffee, spicy foods, chocolate or sugarised products. Note the following to use in conjunction with the advice given. Drink weak tea. Eat raw or pureed vegetables such as carrots, cabbage, broccoli or other greens. Take Brewer's Yeast, a good Multivitamin tablet, Efamol 500iu daily, Agnus Castus, Udo's Choice Oil and Zinc. Early diagnosis and treatment plus the discipline to follow what is prescribed, can result in Rosacea being eliminated. *Nutritious, natural, additive-free DIET is the all-important remedy.* Pure natural foods are as medicine for Rosacea. *Turn to DIET caption.*

ROUGHAGE

See Fibre Caption.

ROYAL JELLY

This is a secretion from the queen bee. It is recognised for its energy and health-giving properties, being good for the immune and digestive systems. It is a natural antibiotic. Helps slow ageing process, fights stress, also good for skin, hair and nails. It is a member of the honey, propolis and pollen group. If the mighty drug companies could patent or register these pure natural products they would be at

R

the top of health giving aids lists. All are available from the health food store in their natural form. The general public have little if any realisation of their aid to better health.

RUBELLA

This infectious, mild viral illness was seldom serious in children, being much more so during pregnancy. Now we are told of its danger as an illness. This can perhaps be attributed to the fact that because of the overuse of antibiotics and other chemical medicines, children's and even adults systems are unable to fight disease, including Rubella. Children are given far too many of the drugs, which are prescribed whether desired or not. In the circumstances it is very important to consult a medical practitioner. As an aid to recovery nutritious Diet of natural food is as medicine. *Turn to DIET caption.* Children's tonics such as Kindervital or Junior Multivitamins are available from the health food store, all being natural. If seeking aid from a pharmacy demand the natural remedy, which in all probability they will know very little about.

RUNDOWN

This leads to lethargy, being without energy, susceptible to all too many niggling ailments, which the debilitated are prone to pick up, with frequent colds or feeling unwell. The person concerned is often described as being 'Run Down'. If you feel under the weather, Run Down, exhausted or need revitalising *see Tonic caption also turn to nature's greatest medicines, which are described under DIET caption.*

RUTIN

This marvellous bioflavonid, which used to be included in the old Vitamin B, is now available separately, as Rutin, in tablet form. It is amazing that this little-heralded natural remedy is seldom recognised for its worth as an aid to better health. There are amounts of it in buckwheat but more especially in the eucalyptus tree. Must be taken with Vitamins C and E to reap the full benefits. It is an aid to bleeding gums and to strengthen capillaries and walls of veins and arteries. As a tea it is a strong antiviral, especially for colds, coughs, 'flu, and chest complaints. I have witnessed its efficiency when prescribed for blood pressure, Buergher's disease, angina, varicose veins, hardening of the arteries, and haemorrhoids and as a cholesterol aid. Here again is another invaluable remedy, which cannot be patented by the multinationals, therefore almost unknown except in the natural health circle. *See Heart also Blood Pressure High captions.*

S.A.D.S.

Seasonal Affective Disorder, better known by the short word SADS, is a form of depression known also as 'Winter Blues', because it occurs during the short, often dark- like days of November to March. Lack of daylight and, more especially sunshine, are the root of the problem. Insufficient light levels cause us to produce high amounts of the sleep-inducing hormone called melatonin, which can lead to SADS. Symptoms include depression, fatigue, and despondency, with a huge tendency to complain and nag. Sugar cravings are a common symptom. Sugary foods will make you energetic but this will be short-lived, because after taking this undesirable commodity, it means that when the sugar clears from the blood, one will feel even worse. *Unfortunately, those who suffer from SADS receive little sympathy, being perceived as complaining, nagging, self- centred, oversleeping, and anxious, along with a host of other signs of this energy- draining disease, because this is what it is - an illness.* It was only discovered in the 1970's when Herb Kern came to the conclusion that he felt so much better in the Summer months as compared to the Winter. Yes, there are many of us who can say this and not relate to SADS.

In 1982 a description of Seasonal Affective Disorder was published by way of a paper. All this is only recent, despite having being informed through writings and poetry, some sad and melancholy, about short, dark, gloomy days with little light – all, of course, in Autumn or Winter. Hippocrates, the father of medicine some 400 years BC, made mention of patients with Winter depression.

Few, if any, realise or admit to having the ailment, not being aware of their problem, which is obvious to others, especially those close to the person with the SADS. It is very difficult to deal with, because the victim of the illness does not, and will not, recognise that they are suffering, except on the odd occasion. This, allied to the fact that although there is an undeniable attitude about the sufferer, those intimate very often do not realise the problem, knowing little or nothing about the symptoms. This can partly be attributed to the reality that it has not been recognised as a disease until quite recently, and even now difficult to accept. Many affected persons tend to have an unhealthy immune system, suffering from colds, often flu-like. People who work in offices with little natural light, or

S

perhaps in buildings with few windows, are prone to the sickness. The symptoms usually disappear in Spring, as daylight hours get longer. *It is notable that the seasonal variation in suicide rates coincides with the time of year when Seasonal Affective Disorder is prevalent.*

The remedy is simple: if the sufferer can be convinced or persuaded to follow the advice given here, which if put into practice in early Autumn and throughout the Winter months, is a preventative. Light is the all-important factor. Waking at daybreak, walking in daylight for 30 minutes or longer, a trip to the sunshine if possible, also exercise or aerobics in daylight, all help to prevent the disorder. It is a good aid to open the door or window at commencement of daylight hours, to breathe deeply and hold for several seconds, also to do gentle loosening exercise. A light box which is specially designed for the complaint has given good results. The SADS patient sits in front of the light each day for 15-30 minutes. Be guided here by your doctor, although some know nothing about this therapy, or even about Seasonal Affective Disorder, or contact one of the several suppliers as listed in Natural Health magazines. Proper Diet of pure natural foods, including salads, also lots of green vegetables, is necessary. *What is recommended under that caption will help lead to vibrant health, which enables the person concerned to be free from SADS. The Diet will also recommend certain supplements which will also help. Be disciplined about sleep, with eight hours or more at regular times.*

Mention has been made of nagging, which is all-too-often as a result of undiagnosed SADS. Marriage guidance counsellors have completed many surveys. The results , which have received publicity, are truly astounding. Over one quarter of husbands when asked about their wives: "Would you marry the same woman again?" replied: "No". It was not because of their being bad housekeepers, being extravagant, with no common interests, lack of disloyalty or unfaithfulness. No, the big threat is nagging. The woman seldom lets up, especially when with SADS, like one with a chip on the shoulder, the one who is always right, always finding fault. In front of me is the result of one of these surveys. It was compiled by a women's group, who set out, as they thought, to put the lie to what they believed was nonsense. They admit that: "Their eyes were opened" - their words.

The stories told of the bad-tempered, unhappy, dissatisfied, ungrateful, discontented and abusing nagging women are numerous, as well as being sad. *Doctors will tell of husbands visiting them when unwell, often being diagnosed with ulcers. When questioned about their lifestyle they let it be known of their anguish of home life, with nagging being regularly referred to. This fault is high up on the list of worries which lead to ulcers or other men's ailments.*

As mentioned regarding SADS and the person with the disease, the tragedy is that few are aware of nagging and its affects. On being told that this applied to them they would not be shocked, always disagreeing. They would certainly not believe that they were turning the lives of others into a mini-hell. For, as long as the writer remembers, and even today, the nagging wife is a: 'Concert Hall joke'. Now we have counsellors and survey teams studying the problem, trying to put into practise methods to try and improve the differences between husband and wife or partner. The nagging wife is certainly a problem. Many should stop and think of nagging and the SADS relationship, with SEASONAL AFFECTIVE DISORDER when undiagnosed, being very much the cause of dissention or discord. Being run-down, anaemic, eating inferior foods, are like fuel to the problem, because they make the SADS ailment worse. A blood check can often be necessary to discover if anaemic. Good food, supplements where necessary or a tonic can very often correct the imbalance. *Turn to DIET, Exercise and Sleep captions* for further advice and help. Combined with light, they are to me the remedy and preventative of SADS.

SAGE

Sage is an extremely good aid to reduce hot flushes and night sweats at time of menopause, because it contains phytoestrogens, that is if oestrogen levels are high. It can also be used as a mouthwash or gargle to relieve laryngitis, tonsillitis or sore throat, also if with mouth or gum ulcers. It is obtainable made up as Menosan from health food store or some chemists. If with Diabetes or prone to Epilepsy consult your doctor before taking. Avoid during pregnancy or if breastfeeding.

ST ANTHONY'S FIRE

See Erysipelas Caption.

SALADS

See DIET caption which gives list of ingredients for nutritious, delicious salads, the advice being to *EAT SALADS REGULARLY.*

SALMON

Sad to relate that what we are offered now, which should be regarded as a delicacy - the King of fish - is seldom natural. Despite the denial and counter-denial there is much evidence to show that Salmon feeds and the chemicals used to turn the grey flesh to pink, are not safe. None are aware of the long-term consequences of the use of unnatural substances such as Canthaxinthin, which as an additive is overused in food for human consumption. There are many other chemicals used too, including vaccines, disinfectants and antibiotics. Battery-farmed Salmon, as it is offered now, is not pure food, and is best avoided until fish farmers get their act right. This will be extremely difficult for them to do. *Turn to Fish and Fish Oils caption.*

SALT

We are continually being advised to cut down on Salt. How can we if in some

instances there is over 10 times the recommended amount in the sophisticated, over-processed, manufactured 'foods', offered for sale. The Western Diet contains much more Salt than we require, which can lead to a multitude of ailments, with circulation and high blood pressure being at the top of the list. We are reliably informed that if everybody in the U.K. and Ireland reduced their Salt intake by just a half a teaspoon daily, it could prevent over 11,000 deaths annually.

In front of me are two containers, each of which is supposed to contain Salt. One is from the health food shop and contains Pure Salt, the other is one of the best-known brands of Salt as sold by supermarkets or food stores. *The label reads: Sodium Chloride, Potassium Chloride, Flavour Enhancers, (B621, B635), L-lysine Hydrochloride, Anti Caking Agents; Magnesium Carbonate, Potassium Hexacyanoferrate 11, Sodium Hexacyanoferrate 11. The purchaser will no doubt accept the exceptionally well-presented container for what is says: 'Low Salt' without giving the chemical additives a thought. It pays health-wise to read the ingredients label.*

The Food Safety Authority has just issued a report calling for a 'radical reduction' in Salt intake. There are several recommendations as to what *'should be done'*. Nobody in control says what *'must be done'*. The half-hearted approach by the Authority to their friends in the food industry reads 'The food industry should reduce Salt content by one third over the next five years or so'. This could be five years, ten years or whatever! What a carry-on in relation to our health. *Food manufacturers have been warned by the Government to cut down on the use of Salt. What of warnings about some of the other hundreds of substances, some equally dangerous to our well-being, which they use to manufacture 'food'? Who will enforce or regulate the warnings?* Leaving the Salt cellar or container off the table would still leave us with too much of the product.

SANDWICHES

Do you know what was in the makeup of the last Sandwich which you purchased?

Frequently many like myself drop into the food store or the Sandwich bar, even the restaurant, for a Sandwich. I have always felt trustful, fool that I have been, that a Sandwich was nutritional fresh food, unadulterated, additive-free. Not any more. Much of what is in the Sandwich is additive-laden whether it be cheese, meat, spread, salad ingredients or what ever. Because of my trust in the supplier I could not believe it recently when I read the ingredients label on a takeaway sandwich, which had the words 'Fresh Sandwich' printed on the label. Because it was bought in packaged, the ingredients had to be displayed. Buy it made-up in a restaurant, café, or Sandwich bar to find out that this law does not apply. The make-up, the components are very often the same, additive-laden. All are apparently ensnared in this food 'merry-go-round', which you can read about in the introductory part of this 'Encyclopedia. Investing in a thermostatically-controlled Sandwich toaster, then using wholemeal bread and chosen additive-free filling, leads to eating purely natural Sandwiches, especially if feeling like a snack meal. At least one will know what is in the make-up of the Sandwich.

SATURATED FATS

These are the undesirable or hard Fats found in meat and some dairy products. They are not essential to the body, being harmful. Fried foods are to be avoided. *See Fat caption for further explanation.*

SAW PALMETTO

This herb can be added to the list of 'nature's gifts to all'. An aid to the male reproductive system, also to bladder efficiency, but especially to treat Benign Prostatic Hypertrophy (BPT). It can and does reduce enlargement of the prostate gland, thereby helping to eliminate the need for frequent nightly visits to the toilet, resulting in interference with proper sleep pattern. It has been the subject of many successful trials, having no side effects. Despite the goodness of this natural remedy, few doctors, if any - other than those interested in natural remedies, will mention it, the result being that it's efficiency is little known. *Oh why, oh why, can't the natural and the synthetic be brought together for the sake of the health of all?* Fortunately or lamentably, whichever view is taken, there is no money in Saw Palmetto for the pharmaceutical industry. It cannot be licensed as one of their products. It is too natural. *Also see Prostate caption* to be guided further about Saw Palmetto and its use.

S

SCIATICA

Caused by irritation of the Sciatic nerve in the lumbar spine. Often combined with low back pain, or can follow on from this as the pain moves about. There can be an underlying cause, which can be linked to stress, worry, and state of mind or inferior Diet. It can be brought on by 'slipped disc', osteoarthritis, osteoporosis, kidney or bowel problems, which should be treated after diagnosis in order to gain relief. Sciatica often leads to a feeling of being under the weather, with little zest for life. It can seriously affect not only the mobility, but also the body and mind of the sufferer. It is often a pain, which comes and goes, sometimes absent for weeks before recurring. Given proper attention the majority can eliminate the problem, often within a day or two. Exercise is very important. *See Exercise caption.* The Alexandra Technique Therapy gives almost 100% success. Combination A New Era, Black Cohosh, Devil's Claw (Pagosid) also Prickly Ash Bark have brought relief or restoration. *See Alexander Technique also DIET captions.*

SCALDS

See Burns & Scalds Caption.

SCHIZOPHRENIA

This disturbing, almost dementia-like condition can be due to a metabolism change, which affects the way of thought, taste, smell and where the effected person is totally disorientated, paranoid and continually complaining. The chemical drugs prescribed, such as dopamine, certainly do no good. I have experienced and watched Schizophrenia sufferers return to normal health by their being looked after and fed a pure natural Diet of additive-free food, but with the elimination of both gluten and dairy products. There was a need for natural Multivitamin supplement or Vitamins, as suggested under DIET caption, also the use of fish oils long-term. Now with the advent of Udo's Choice Oil or Organic Choice 3+6+9 which gives the required balance of Omega three and six, plus much else that is good, especially for mental health, the task of finding proper nutrition is made easier. *See the advice under Coeliac, Gluten Free also Dairy Free Diet captions, combining these with what is suggested here.*

SCHOOLBAGS AND RUCKSACKS

Very often little thought is given to their design. They are seldom, examined by the purchaser, parents, guardians or teachers. Very often they are over filled, sometimes with unnecessary material. Parents seldom realise the burden of the bag, which can lead to back problems, in later years. As in every-day life, our youth need guidance about much, including the often ill-fitting Bag or Rucksack.

SCHÜESSLER DR

See Tissue Salts Caption.

SEA SICKNESS

See Travel Sickness Caption.

SEBORRHOEA

Can be traced to inferior Diet and lifestyle, where there is a deficiency of Fatty Acids, Vitamin B Complex also the Minerals Zinc and Selenium. These, taken in conjunction with pure food Diet and Udo's Choice Oil, all combine to eliminate the problem, as well as a return to better health. There may be a need for Fatty Acid supplement. Udo's Choice Oil is an excellent combination of omega and other oils which helps correct fatty acid deficiency. This is much of the cause of Seborrhoea. *See DIET caption* to read about one of the greatest remedies for skin and blood problems. This is pure, natural unprocessed food, with supplements where advised.

SELENIUM

We've only heard of the need for the trace mineral Selenium in recent years. Increasing research tells us of its relevance to disease prevention, with dietary lack, especially in the UK and Ireland. This is allegedly because of over farming, with excessive use of artificial fertilizers, also to acid rain. **An equally more serious aspect is the overuse of food additives, which when processed eliminate much nutritive good, including trace elements such as Selenium.** It has an important role in the thyroid metabolism, sperm, and proper reproductive performance. It is an aid to ward off cancer, to strengthen the immune system and to enhance the mood. It has recently been proved to have a role in the fight against Aids. Sources include garlic, kelp, liver, seafood, lean meat, Brazil and walnuts also whole grains. Despite all the warning about lack of Selenium, excess intake can be dangerous, therefore a supplement such as Bio Selenium and Zinc which also contains other Vitamins, will be well within the advised requirements. There are various other brands available from the health food store. Selenium taken with an apple gives a combined boost to flavonoids, providing much goodness. Flavonoids, are found in fruit, especially apples.

SEPTICAEMIA (BLOOD POISIONING)

See your doctor. Almost always occurs because of low resistance due to inferior Diet or lifestyle. *To aid recovery and protect against further blood poisoning refer to and be advised by DIET caption.* An aid to correct impure blood is Floradix, which contains Iron also take Vitamin B Complex or Brewer's Yeast.

S

SEX DRIVE (LACK OF)

This is a complex and wide-ranging subject. Can be caused by underlying complaint, such as heart, thyroid, or hormonal. Cholesterol levels can affect the desire. Often due to inferior Diet with lack of Vitamins B Complex, C and E, low calorie-intake or protein deficiency. This can all lead to stress, fatigue and other ailments, also that lack of get-up-and-go attitude so necessary to help arousal. Penelope Sachs, in that inspirational little book: **'Take care of yourself'** *(See Bibliography)*, gives excellent advice about increasing your Sex drive. "Getting adequate sleep, exercising in fresh air and enjoying a balanced Diet will all help to increase your Sex drive. Limit your caffeine and alcohol intake. But aside from this don't forget to wear Sexy clothes that make you want to have SEX". *Also turn to Aphrodisiacs and Erectile Dysfunction captions.* Note what Penelope said about DIET and you are advised to read under that caption about good *FOOD*, which can lead to a zest for life.

SHAMPOOS

The majority of Shampoos are soap, detergent-based, chemical, compounds, with many doing little to improve the health of the hair or scalp. I often look with scepticism at the various Shampoos displayed. Just like the word natural, where less than 1% of the ingredients can be so, with the Shampoo then described as natural, is the use of the words – 'For dandruff treatment'. Dandruff can only be cleared from the inside by intake of the minerals that are lacking, usually found in natural and nutritious food. *Turn to Dandruff caption.* There are purely natural soaps and Shampoos available from the health food store or specialist shops, which are genuinely good as hair Shampoos. Allergenic brand Shampoo is certainly in this category. *See Cosmetics caption* which gives list of brands of hair and skin care products, all purely natural or visit the health food store.

SHINGLES (Herpes Zoster)

Any person who has had chickenpox is liable in later life to be affected by Shingles. The virus can remain dormant in a nerve in the body. Often when very much older, especially in middle or old age, the virus will reactivate itself. This can occur as a result of inferior Diet or lifestyle, when the resistance is low, with the herpes virus being reactivated, not as chickenpox but as shingles, when it follows the nerve system where it has been inactive for years. Unless treated properly it can be extremely painful, lasting for some considerable time, even for up to 12 months after diagnosis. *Several of my doctor friends agree that orthodox medicine, including the drug Idoxuridine, gives little or no relief for Shingles. In the words of one Doctor: "A complete waste of money".* There are natural remedies, which have certainly helped. Some good results have been witnessed. Number one is a change of Diet to pure, nutritious, natural unprocessed foods, with the addition of Vitamins B Complex, C and E and the supplement L-lycine. Taking 200IU of Vitamin E daily for 30 days and then 400 IU daily has helped clear Shingles. Almond Oil dabbed on the blisters has given relief, but my favourite remedy is to apply the juice of fresh pears. It has not worked for all but has certainly cleared the skin and nerve problem for many. From time to time one hears of somebody having a 'cure'. I know several and would have complete confidence in many of them. One person I know, pricks his finger, says a prayer, smears some of the blood on the affected part of the body and expects three visits. The 'cure', and I use this word blatantly, has never failed. He asks for no money, can be called a quack, but to the many who know him he has been a saviour. Many whom he has cured, including those whom I have sent to him, regard him as a friend.

SIDE EFFECTS OF ANTIBIOTICS

Antidotes are Devils Claw (Pagosid) or Reiki therapy.

SILICA (Silicea)

Silicea is good for skin, hair and nail health. It is available in powder form or as tablets. *See Tissue Salts caption* to read about Silica uses.

SINUSITIS

Inflamed or blocked Sinuses can be painful and irritating. Sinusitis can be the aftermath of flu or cold, sometimes combined with smoke-polluted air, or even allergy. Try not to partake of milk or dairy products. There is no proof that this is a problem but it has proved beneficial where there was allergy, which the person with Sinusitis was not even aware of. When the problem clears it is often possible to return dairy foods to the Diet. Plantago, Iceland Moss, Pulsatilla, Echinacea or Lobelia have all brought relief. Golden Seal tablets of 500mg daily have proved exceptionally good. What works for one may not work for another. Find out which works best. All are natural with no after effects. Very often with chemical medicines the remedy is worse than the ailment. All of the remedies listed can be obtained from the health food store.

SKINCARE

The manufacture of Skin, hair, and beauty products is something with which I am familiar, having gained an amount of knowledge about their formulation. Chemical and natural are in their make-up with many being of little aid to better Skin. The word NATURAL, as stated elsewhere in this Encyclopedia, is often a misnomer. This is certainly so with Skincare products. *Any operator or company can put Natural on the product even if it contains as little as 1% Natural ingredients. This is disgraceful to say the least. One sees rows of so-called Skincare aids, with the word Natural, where 99% of it is not. Few know this. The Skincare business can in many ways be likened to a license to print money, dare one use the words: 'All too often a rip off' The container or packaging often costs more than the ingredients, with astronomical mark-ups in the pricing.* **Perfume is an example of much that is inferior and harmful to Skin. Many of the ingredients come from the 'distillation column' being mineral oil-based. Of the thousands of chemicals used, less than one sixth have been tested for human safety, indeed many are hazardous, to be avoided.**

Set out here are a few of the lessons learned, both from being in the Skincare business and more especially from those with Skin problems. Using old, past their 'use by date' Skin products, often causes the latter. Many of them contain chemicals, which are incompatible to the Skin. Irritation is often caused by wearing clothes, which have been washed in certain detergents or powders, often not rinsed thoroughly. Seek out and use mild and natural washing powders, adding only the minimum necessary. Wearing cotton next to the skin is best.

There is no such thing as a miracle cream or lotion. Skin, hair and nails can give one the answer as to how healthy a person is, and to me indelible skin can only be obtained or result from treating from the inside. Good wholesome nutritious, additive-free Diet as repeated and harped upon in this Encyclopedia, is the foundation for good health and resultant perfect Skin. See Nettles caption to read about the goodness of nettles as a Skin tonic. Silica, which is available in tablet or powder form, is a good Skin food. It is a cleanser and eliminator for hair, nails and Skin health. Many Skin products contain fats or oils, which can lead to or result in Acne.

The Hay Diet is an example of what is good for Skin, also being a healthy slimming aid. Take Udo's Choice Oil or Organic Choice 3+6+9 Omega Oils. These contain the essential fatty acids so necessary for good Skin health. Even in their 80's women have soft smooth Skin when they take this combination. **Drink copious amounts of water because dehydration affects the Skin before being noticed elsewhere. Up to eight or more glasses daily is as medicine for the Skin. Mixed in a glass of warm water 2 teaspoons each, of Aspells Cider Vinegar and Pure Honey, as sold by health food shops, is a wonder tonic for Skin and health, including the figure, when taken three times daily. A Vitamin- enriched product for external beauty is Perfectil, which is a combination of many health-giving properties, being highly recommended.**

It is not realised that most of the weight-losing Diets we are beset or pestered with are in conflict with better health and most certainly will not lead to good Skin or personal well being.

Women are very trusting. They seldom if ever read the ingredients labels on food and when it comes to chemicals in cosmetics and toiletries they treat them similarly. *Some of the chemicals used in cosmetics, including skin products, can be harmful. Many of the so-called Skincare products are synthetic-based, having little natural ingredients. These can do harm in the long-term.* All Skincare products sold in the health food shop are natural. They have a range of pure chemical-free aids, including Tisserand, Jason, Avida, Anika, Dead Sea Magik, Weleda, Neals Yard and others. These are all purely natural and entitled to be termed so. *See Diet, Exercise, Sleep and Hay Diet captions.* Think NATURAL for all products whether for body or skin health.

SKIN PROBLEMS

See under various captions as Acne, Eczema, Dermatitis, Impetigo, Cold sores, Warts, Itching or others. The health food store and some chemists can supply the all-natural, preservative or steroid-free range of ointments and creams such as Allergenics, also face and shower gels. There are lotions, including baby washes, specially formulated for those with irritating Skin or sensitive scalp. Allergenics products are a natural and extremely good alternative to hydrocortisone creams, which are usually prescribed for Skin disease. If there is fungal infection there may be a need for Acidophilus. Confide in the health food store personnel who have much experience of natural treatment for Skin problems. **The Tissue Salts described under caption in this Encyclopedia are almost unknown for Skin health. I strongly recommend their excellence.** *Also see Nettles caption.*

SLEEP AND SLEEPLESSNESS

Natural Sleep is as natural medicine. Here is one of our greatest remedies. All need regular Sleep, which is so necessary for good health. Sleep at regular times and hours is a must. The old adages are relevant: 'Two hours before midnight is worth four after'; 'Early to bed and early to rise makes one healthy, wealthy and wise'. Laugh at these at your peril. Some people only go to bed when they feel they must, not following a regular pattern. The younger you are the more Sleep is required. Many are governed by what others do, not realising that requirements vary greatly from person to person. Before the advent of television there was a much more regular pattern to Sleep than of late. Almost all need a minimum of seven hours or more of good sleep but it must be regular as far as possible (i.e. going to bed and rising at the same time). Every seven to 10 days it is a good idea to have an extra early night, or a lie-in, giving an extra hour or two of rest.

Often I have spoken to people who are tired, lethargic, or suffering from a worn-out feeling. On questioning them about Sleep they admit having had only a few hours nightly. Further questioning leads to the fact that they don't have regular times for retiring to bed. Some almost regard having to go to bed as a chore, being of the opinion that it is time to go when feeling sleepy or exceptionally tired. This is wrong. We need to recharge our bodies so that we can feel active and sprightly.

Good Sleep is as necessary as good food. Lack of Sleep may not appear to many as serious, but it affects the quality of life, the ability to think and make decisions, often leading to drowsiness. It can impair our immune system, even bringing on blood pressure and diabetes. It leads to drivers nodding off, where even a fraction of a second can be fatal. It is one of the highest causes of driver-related accidents, with very serious consequences.

Few are aware that there are Sleep patterns and stages. The first three stages, nodding off, losing consciousness, then deep Sleep, all occur within 15 minutes of falling asleep. Stage four lasts for four to five hours and stage five is known as our dream Sleep, averaging two to three hours. This changes as we get older, as we get less of stages four and five, when the tendency is to Sleep less and to wake earlier, to have more broken Sleep. Often this is brought on by the need to visit the toilet because of arthritic pain, prostate or other health problem. Despite this we should stick to a regular pattern of seven to 10 hours Sleep as outlined. When dozing and waking, just lying in bed, one can be assured that at least they are getting rest.

Sleeplessness can be caused by problems, which appear serious in the mind of the person. Worry is the big one. Many, when questioned, admit that when awake they worry, having what seems is an over-active brain. But that is not the case, with problems about money, work and family being to the fore. This can be taken so seriously that it leads to all kinds of complications, mostly because of lack of Sleep. All affected like this should learn to control their fears, shutting them out of the mind, and concentrating on getting the all-so-necessary Sleep and rest.

Throughout this Encyclopedia the message repeated constantly is that: 'We are what we eat, how we exercise and Sleep'. Call it lifestyle if you wish. If prone to insomnia, Sleepless nights or Sleeplessness, which are all the same when placed together like this, the question will be posed: 'What has this to do with my Sleep pattern' The answer is: 'Very much'. In a state of general well being, which can be obtained by proper eating habits, the partaking of good, natural, wholesome, unadulterated food, including drinking pure water, combined with daily exercise, one will find that Sleep comes naturally. Even then there may be times when because of the pace of life, sometimes excitement or other enjoyment, distraction, or perhaps work before bedtime, it may be difficult to fall asleep. Learn to switch off, to relax, and to close the mind to the all too many distractions, such as television or computer. *This is where simple, natural remedies can help. None better than a cup of warm milk or water, if you can take just warm water, to which is added a teaspoonful or two of pure natural Honey to be taken before bedtime. Take with this a balanced Calcium / Magnesium / Vitamin D tablet. Pulsatilla or Bio force Night Essence are also good for insomnia. Very often a simple solution to the problem is to use some drops of Lavender Oil on the pillow or to purchase a hop pillow. Rhodolia taken one hour before bedtime has brought continuous Sleep and rest.*

Many times it has been discovered on discussing the matter of beds, that the mattress or pillows are the cause of Sleeplessness. A reasonably hard mattress, with natural down or feather pillows, can be the answer to Sleep problems. It is recommended that mattresses should not be used when more than six years old. They should be turned regularly. Sleeping with head to the North has helped. An excellent Sleep inducer is gruel. This is made as porridge, adding extra water or milk to make it more liquid or drinkable. Sweeten with Honey. Recently there was an article in a daily newspaper, where a young scribe or hack referred to gruel. His remarks were derogatory, referring to it as being used by the poor in days long gone by. My family was not poor, but like Dwight Eisenhower said: "We just had no money". I drank gruel. It was as natural medicine, extremely good.

Beware of falling into the trap of taking Sleeping pills. They are highly unnatural, being addictive. Over a period of time they can cause irreparable brain and other serious health damage. Continuous use of

sedatives, even the so-called mild over-the-counter tranquillizers, all result in dependency. Soon they become a must, an addiction, often resulting in horrible side effects. Nothing good can be said or written about these evil, synthetic substances. The full evidence of their dangerous affects will never come to light. The manufacturers, the gigantic multi national pharmaceutical pill pushers, moneyed, all-powerful, will see to that. Many within the medical profession, the doctors, also have much to answer for in respect of these barbiturates as they continue to dole them out. *Seldom is the patient told that to mix any synthetic tranquillizer or sedative with alcohol is highly dangerous. There should be a legal requirement that all synthetic medicines whether liquid, tablet or capsule, have a danger notice printed on to stipulate this serious matter. This to include prescription medicines and the many non-prescription medicines so easily purchased over the counter.*

Sleep or the lack of it need not be a worry if one practices the simple instructions and makes use of all things natural, as written about in this Encyclopedia. Find out what suits you best. This is usually done by trying the various remedies or suggestions, but it is important to take long-term, when retiring to bed, the Calcium / Magnesium / Vitamin D tablet. *Turn to Exercise and DIET captions*, which are relevant to Sleep, Sleeplessness and resultant better health.

SLEEP – CHILDRENS LOSS OF

A poll shows that many children are getting insufficient Sleep. This can be put down to Television, Computers, Games machines and the Mobile phone. The consequences, mentally and physically, can only be guessed at, because the present generation is the first in this plethora of diversions. Children do not, as in the past, go to bed in a relaxed, calming environment. They read less and are read even less to. Some get very much less sleep than their parents. This must affect their educational ability, school results and more especially their health, because sufficient and proper Sleep and Sleep pattern is as food and medicine to a young person. **There is an urgent need for stricter discipline, if the dire affects are not to be borne later.**

SLEEPINESS

This comes about almost always because of inadequate Sleep or improper Sleep pattern. Sometimes it is caused by lack of fresh air as in smoking or hot atmosphere. If feeling drowsy when driving, the advice is not to fight it but to pull in somewhere and have a snooze. Some 10 to 15 minutes is often sufficient. Better to get to the end of the journey safe and sound than not at all. The lives of others may be put at serious risk too.

SLEEPWALKING - IN CHILDREN

Remedies are Silicea 30c or half to one cup of Artemisia / Mugwort, sweetened with Pure Honey, taken at bedtime. Pour boiling water over the herb and infuse for ten minutes. All remedies mentioned in this Encyclopedia are available from the health food store or some chemists.

SLIMMERS DISEASE

See Anorexia Caption.

SLIMMING- *(also see Dieting caption)*

Slimming, dieting, obesity, overweight are words we hear and read of daily, with the word detoxing having being added quite recently. All, which are interlinked, are regarded by too many as problems. Advice on Slimming, how to reduce weight, the problem of obesity, including detoxing, is churned out at an enormous rate. They are all moneymaking words, which make up the Dieting industry. Some of the would-be experts are lining their pockets, as those who think they have a problem join in the headlong rush to lose weight. *We are all built differently, also our metabolisms are dissimilar.* For those who don't understand about the metabolism it involves the breakdown of constituents of the bodily intake, liberating energy and other complex substances, so vital for our well-being. It breaks down and distributes those so necessary nutrients as well as what is stored within the body. This is a brief explanation.

There is an obsession with the look of the body. Certainly there are those who are too fat - even obese - there are others too thin, if this is possible to some. There are those who are plump, almost always well built, who consider themselves overweight. There are a vast number normal but here again many of them think otherwise. *If only those who have reasonable good health would stop worrying about their looks or figure and enjoy themselves, they would be much happier. There is no need for the vast majority to Slim, because as stated here, if healthy and well built they should accept this and carry on.*

Those who decide to journey on a Slimming or weight-reducing course, are offered, almost always: *'A sure and certain formula'!*

Seldom if ever is there mention that when the menopause stage of one's life is reached, or sometimes after hysterectomy, there is a big tendency to put on weight. This can be attributed largely to impaired functioning of the endocrine glands or the hormones. Being thin, obese or overweight can be caused by their under or over performing, their unbalanced state. Here again the endocrine system, unless there is some underlying ailment or disease, will function properly if the discipline is there to accept and put into practise the advice given in the captions of this Encyclopedia regarding Diet, Exercise and Sleep.

My experience of the subject of weight consciousness, from speaking with those who do have a problem, also with many who believe they have and do not, could fill books. Slimming books are always among the best-sellers lists.

Losing weight successfully is not a case of just eating less. It is about combining healthy eating and drinking with exercise and sleep, with the addition of some other things essential and beneficial to breakdown of healthy nutritional and natural food. I reiterate, emphasise and make no apologies for repeating myself when it comes to the words slimming, losing weight, weight loss, or call it the battle of the bulge, that the vast majority of those who think about their weight, including their figure, have not got a problem. Much of it is all in the mind. Again I say: "If in good health, being reasonably well built, even plump, accept it and carry on, remembering to eat healthy foods and take regular exercise with proper sleep pattern".

Throughout this Encyclopedia I have referred frequently to the Hay Diet. Again I am being verbose when I describe it as the best health-giving formula ever presented and more especially as an aid to a Slim, trim figure. This thing about Slimming or weight-loss is something that can be regarded as a phobia with many. It is most annoying because, except in cases of the very thin or of those who are genuinely fat, there is usually no problem with all-too-many who think they need to lose weight. They are often just of large bone structure. ***It is the make- up of the individual that must be considered, before embarking upon what can all-too-often rightly be referred to as a faddist Diet.***

'We are what we eat' and to this can be added how we exercise. Take a look at what you eat and be honest. Yes, be honest, and you will end up being surprised. Keep a diary for several weeks, showing the food, which you have partaken. List and write down everything you eat and drink, including alcohol, coffee, fizzy 'drinks', snacks or fast 'foods'. *There will be no need to cut down on foods, on what you eat, provided that it is natural, sugar and additive-free, unprocessed. Eat Healthy Foods. Many do not realise the difference between healthy foods and the highly sugarised, processed additive-filled, overheated or micro waved convenience 'foods' we are offered daily. Turn to Diet caption to learn how to live well and to Hay Diet caption to find out how to use that Diet, which as I have stated is the greatest health-giving slimming Diet devised.*

An amount of drivel is written about the need to detox. The dictionary definition is: *'To remove poisonous substances from'.* Detoxing has only been heard of recently in connection with our health. Before this detoxing was done by the liver, or it referred to the drying-out of a person suffering from alcoholism. The question can be asked: *"Why should any person eating healthy natural foods as defined in these writings need to detox"* What poison or badness is there to eliminate? The answer is: *Natural, unprocessed, additive-food is a detoxant in itself.* To me detoxing is a fad. Short-term detox can be a shock to the system.

One person who came to me feeling unwell, with headaches, skin and other problems, none of which she had in the past, confessed to having been on a detoxing Diet. The whole thing came as a shock to her system, not alone had she been advised by a pharmacist to detox, but nothing was said about the need to change her Diet, which was extreme, to say the least. Before being advised to detox almost all this woman ate was processed, additive-filled, unnatural 'food', much of it microwaved. Her main meal consisted of fried stuff. *Big change was needed in her Diet, detoxing was not the answer.* As well as this she was taking the contraceptive pill and other medication from her doctor. Most of the medical profession fail to ask about Diet, which seems to be of little consequence to doctors. It stands to reason, that just like trying to give up cigarettes or to conquer other habits or bad lifestyle: before detoxing, a properly- planned nourishing Diet must be adhered to for some time previous. When asked had she consulted her doctor about detoxing the answer was "No". *Instead of advising detoxing for loss of weight or other wise, far better to change the Diet to pure natural foods as written about. These are sufficient detoxant.*

To ensure feeling of good health, also to help keep trim, take Lecithin also Milk Thistle. The latter is regarded as excellent for protection of the liver. Helix Slim is another natural detoxifier, a slimming aid, also having a host of other health-giving benefits. A healthy liver goes far to ensure a healthy and full-of-vitality feeling. An extremely good and little-known aid to help attain desired weight is the purely natural Slimming formula Antifat. It helps reduce the rate of conversion of carbohydrates to fat. Another old reliable with health-giving virtues, a detoxifier, an aid to control weight, to Slim and good for skin and hair is Pure Cider Vinegar such as Aspells, obtainable from the health food store. Mix two teaspoons of each Cider Vinegar and Pure Natural Honey in warm water, to be taken two or three times daily. Lecithin granules - do not be fobbed off with tablets - act as an emulsifier, keeping fats in suspension. They are invaluable to help lose weight, being an aid to better health, also being a brain food, because they contain the nutrient Choline. Lecithin has been described as a liver protector, being recommended as a help in times of mental stress, also excellent as an aid to weight control and loss of pounds. Turn to Lecithin caption. A balanced Calcium / Magnesium / Vitamin D supplement, plus a slow release Multivitamin will aid further. To help the suggested supplements, which must be taken in conjunction with pure natural additive free Diet and Exercise, an effective way to reduce excess weight is to take Helianthus drops and Dandelion. These are herbal

remedies and as such are entirely natural, as is everything written ~~in this~~
Encyclopedia. All are obtainable at the health food store, which also ~~have a~~
selection of pure natural foods, drinks and much more which is nutritious ~~and~~
fat- free. Half a grapefruit at each meal has always proved good to help control
weight. Sweeten with pure honey, not sugar or other sweetener. Natural is best.
Some people have the idea that lemon juice will help them lose excess weight. It
may be of some help but this has not been proven. It can leach calcium and other
minerals from the body. Coming in contact with teeth it can destroy the enamel.

I repeat chew your food properly; don't rush your meals, because good food is
there to be enjoyed. All suggested, combined with natural Diet, would work
wonders for health also weight-wise. **Don't expect it all to happen in a day or
a week. It is much better to reduce excess weight slowly and surely. Be
patient. It will take time to bring the resultant feel-good factor.** Exercise,
which is shunned by many to their detriment, is of the utmost importance in the
quest to fight the flab and to be healthy. *Turn to Walking and Yoga captions* in this
Encyclopedia and study carefully. No need for strenuous, repetitive, laborious
exertion. Learn how to enjoy yourself.

You have been asked to keep a diary and to list all you eat and drink. Eliminate the
unnatural, the sugary, the fizzy and the additive-filled products. In other words start
by looking at your eating habits. Forget about crash diets, cutting down on food.
This is a mistake. *Starving your body leaves you with a craving for fat and sweet
foods.* It also affects the metabolism, something I have explained. Many think that
eating just one meal daily is the right thing to do. This is wrong. Eating three four
or more times daily and regularly is much better for the system and to help lose
weight.

The word discipline also enters in. This is especially important when it comes to
drinking coffee or strong tea, the need to avoid snacks, biscuits, sweets,
chocolates and all forms of confectionery. A slice or two of wholemeal bread, a
piece of raw vegetable such as carrot, or better still some fruit, are ideal snacks.
Turn to Snack Food caption.

If you don't begin each day with a good natural breakfast you are a loser and will
remain so. There is nothing better than a bowl of porridge or natural sugar-free
muesli, taken with some fruit, to set one up for the day. The feel-good factor will
come. *Turn to Breakfast caption.*

*Often one can follow a strict Diet, almost starve, feel bad and lose little or no
weight. It is much better to feel good, to be healthy and to carry the extra few
pounds. The majority of men speak of how they prefer a happy, healthy, buxom
woman with a laugh and a good sense of humour, a feel-good factor. I repeat See
DIET, Exercise, Sleep, Hay Diet and Dieting captions..*

S

inable in powdered form or as tablets, being an excellent
.h after illness, also if with gastro enteritis, stomach ulcers,
el syndrome. Helps to relieve hangover. It is an excellent
cing or recovering from illness. Here is a natural remedy,
e's gifts to us. The medical profession and the drug companies
.t is just too natural. Your health food store can supply.

SMELL – LOSS OF SENSE OF

Take Zinc/Copper combination and Nat Mur. It may take six/eight weeks to recover the smell, but from my experience this always solves the problem.

SMELLY FEET

See Feet Caption.

SMOKING – Including How I Stopped Smoking and Have Helped Many to Do So.

So much has been written about the dangers of Smoking that the question could be asked: "What more is there to say or write about the horrible habit?" From my experience as a Smoker who was able to give up, as one who has advised hundreds on how to stop, as one who has suffered the death of a loved one, a young woman, who as the doctor said: "If she had not been a Smoker, she would have been alive today", I feel that there is much to be said and written. I have seen some of my best friends, all Smokers, die of cancer in their 30's, 40's and 50's. I have had those with emphysema visit me, to ask if I could suggest a remedy. The results of smoking are to be seen daily in so many ways that it is entirely stupid to continue the habit.

Immediately on meeting a person who Smokes, especially a woman, one can tell by the texture of the skin if the person does so. *It Is Tragic How Little One Learns From Another's Experience.*

Females who Smoke are at risk if pregnant. It is linked to cervical cancer, osteoporosis, early menopause, stroke, heart diseases and premature death. All, including non-Smokers, who inhale the obnoxious fumes are in danger in so many ways, that the only advice to be given is STOP. The question is: 'How?' I have seen many cease who took my advice. **It is my contention that if a person is strong enough physically, being healthy, the addict is a long way towards winning the battle. Having being warned of the consequences of continuing the use of the weed, then reorganising my life and lifestyle, especially the Diet, I was able to stop smoking.**

In Britain, the United States and Ireland SMOKING causes nine out of 10 deaths from lung cancer, the most common cancer in these countries. It is a major cause of heart disease and stroke, also other lung diseases such as bronchitis and emphysema. It causes many other diseases, all documented. Smokers not only tend to die earlier than non-smokers, they suffer much more from ill-health first. They take more time off work through illness. Those who are killed by Smoking are losing an average of 10/15 years of life, often suffering - sometimes tragically for years - before they actually die.

In what is written and said about Smoking or when speaking with a person who seeks a remedy, I have yet to hear of or see mentioned the astronomical cost of Smoking, monetary-wise. When one considers the price of just 10 or 20 of the weed, it is beyond belief that no matter how much the cost, cigarettes remain an evil necessity, because of the addiction.

Amongst my kin there have been many rows in the past due to a family member being a heavy Smoker. Sometimes the atmosphere was almost unbearable. This was not because of the Smoke. It was because of the Smoking!   I used say: "When this young lady took a pull of the drug, one almost expected the Smoke to come out from the toes". This is mentioned to show how much this lovely person was hooked on the 'fags'. Some years ago Budget Day came. Cigarette prices were increased. My daughter has not Smoked since that day over six years ago. If she could give them up, then anybody can, if they are prepared to take the advice given here and what is advised under Diet caption. **Putting cigarettes out of her life can partly be attributed to the advice I gave her. She was reluctant to do anything at first, far from being convinced that a natural, unprocessed, additive-free food Diet would do anything to help her. But the Diet was then followed fairly rigidly, leading to better health, improved state of mind and the determination, which comes from this - all of which combined to enable her to *STOP SMOKING*. Not only that but she lost excess weight, just abiding by the pure food Diet advised and now looks slim and shapely, with a hugely improved personality. There is no more grumpiness or complaining attitude as when Smoking.**

Medical experts, independent and otherwise, around the world, are in agreement that prolonged exposure to other peoples tobacco smoke, *'passive smoking'*, not only irritates eyes and nose of others, it smells - one could say stinks - hair and clothes, with the most damning indictment being that it is also the cause of serious health problems, including cancer as already pointed out. Suffice to say that Smoking causes more unnecessary diseases than all other factors put together, within Britain and Ireland, also over four times more premature deaths than the total caused by road, fire and all other preventable accidents.

At last the mighty 'tobacco barons' have been stopped in their tracks. *The Irish Government must be congratulated on being the first to take firm steps to keep pubs, restaurants and other places where the public gather, Smoke free. The fact that the smoker ignores warnings such as: 'Smoking Kills'; 'Smoking can cause a slow and painful death'; and other omens of its fatal consequences, points to the terrible addiction of nicotine.* The UK Government propose to bring in similar measures in 2006, with many other countries arranging to do so in the near future.

In my daily life as I Smoked and ate my way to ill-health, I was taken aside and into the confidence of my relative - a doctor - and told that if I did not change my way of living, my lifestyle, my life on this earth would not be for too long. All this unasked for advice was not accepted lightly, or without some argument or debate. I resented being told that I was a workaholic, an alcoholic, also it appears I was a cigaretteaholic. The advice given then has proved to be invaluable. *Not only did this person change my outlook on life, my health, give me assistance to stop smoking, but over the years he told me all he knew and had learned about natural remedies, alternative medicines, also about adhering to and championing simple, plain, unadulterated foods and lifestyle.* This was far removed from how I treated my body then, with irregular meals, sometimes just a huge one daily, sometimes nothing, just snacks, chocolates, sweets and chewing gum. The frying pan was indispensable, with little vegetables and no breakfast. There was no breakfast as I reached for the cigarette, the drug. I did as almost all smokers do. I have not even mentioned alcohol, another failing.

Here is how I stopped smoking and have helped many to do so. I disciplined myself to have three regular, full-of-goodness, additive-free, meals daily. The breakfast was, and still is, the most important meal of the day. Since then, almost 40 years ago, I have put many on the road to recovery by advising a morning meal of porridge with fruit, then wholemeal bread, pure honey and weak tea. Forget coffee. It has no goodness. *Turn to Coffee caption.* The porridge is made with skimmed or semi skimmed milk and water, with no salt or sugar. This breakfast has never been deviated from except on the odd occasion when shredded wheat or sugar-free muesli was eaten. *The reader must be asking almost impatiently: 'When are we being told how to stop smoking?'. Listen carefully. You are being told. Read on, do not falter.* This advice works, I know, many know.

Proper, natural, regular meals provide the main help and discipline to STOP. The smoker reaches for a cigarette first thing in the morning. Some 98 out of 100 smokers do not partake of breakfast - the most important meal of the day. This must be emphasised because the smokers are too weak-willed, unhealthy, when reaching for the fag, the nicotinic carcinogenic drug. Yes, do ask the question: "Why do you almost harp or labour on about proper eating, natural food Diet? What has this to do with giving up cigarettes?". *The answer is: "Because if the smokers who are interested in giving up the coffin nail, the cancer stick, obey the advice given, partake of the foods suggested and discipline themselves, then in the weeks following the start of this DIET, the willpower, the determination and especially the strength and feel-good factor will allow them Stop".* I know. This is how I did it. I can introduce you to many others who did it this way when they took my advice.

Regularly I have telephone calls from people who ring to say: "Thank You". Every Christmas day I have a call from a man in the North of England who says words to this effect "I have never touched a cigarette since you put me off them". This was over 20 years ago.

Sadly from a health point of view, the nutritional value, the vitamins, minerals, the sustenance so badly required in our present-day climate of fast and processed 'foods' is very often lacking. Much of the junk 'foods', fries, chips, crisps, fizzy 'drinks', burgers, micro waved 'foods', most of which are fast 'foods', cannot be regarded as natural, pure, wholesome, nutritious food. Much of its sustenance value is nil. *This is why natural food is recommended, but even then there is often the need for a good Multivitamin, preferably slow-release, also extra Vitamins E, C and the minerals Zinc/Copper. Reading the DIET caption explains fully about this and what is needed to attain better health, with increased strength of body and mind, so necessary to STOP SMOKING.*

Visit the health shop and ask questions about the genuine, simple things, which you are advised to use. The need for three regular meals of nutritious food daily is emphasised, and if the need for a snack arises, *be guided by the advice given under Snacks caption.* No matter what way you set about stopping SMOKING there must be the desire to do so and remember this demands willpower. *No use saying: "I'll cut down on them". It does not work. One pull daily is one too many.* By eating properly, having regular meals of natural, nutritious foods, cutting out cups of coffee and inferior food snacks, by disciplining oneself to do all this, I can sincerely confirm that within a short time the improvement of health and well-being will be such that you will do as I did, when I put cigarettes, tobacco and four pipes into the front pocket of the car, disposing of them in the garbage bin some 12 months later. *Two or three things you must also understand. The longing for a pull of the nicotinic poison, one gasp, will be there for a very, very long time.*

The dangers of the early, first thing in the morning, cigarette must be avoided at all costs or indeed at any time. *These last words from my experience may sound sanctimonious. Often in the past I have felt like starting again. At the same time I have helped many to stop and have given advice freely, often ridiculing whenever necessary. My family have instilled into me the fact that I would be a proper hypocrite, letting down all those whom I have helped and for this reason I will never touch the horrible weed.* I STOPPED, MANY OTHERS STOPPED, AND YOU CAN STOP. *See Reflexology also Hypnotherapy captions.* I can vouch for both being excellent therapies **but the SMOKER must whole-heartedly co-operate.** There is no point visiting them if not prepared to give up smoking by simply STOPPING. Good food, additive-free is as medicine. **It can also help you STOP SMOKING, as already verbosely repeated.**

S

SNACK FOOD

There are bad 'Snacks' and Snacks. Washed fresh fruit or vegetables in bite-sized pieces are good. Use carrots, tomatoes, melons, grapes, bananas, apples and celery. One could list many things which could be kept in the fridge overnight or even for days. Include nuts, seeds, raisins, currants, plain popcorn or others. Natural Snacks are also available from the health food store. Keep a bowl of fresh fruit where you can see it and dip in when feeling like a Snack. The difference between these and sugarised or other 'Snacks', health-wise, is unimaginable. Investing in a good thermostatically controlled sandwich toaster enables one to have delicious Snack meals which can be purely, natural food.

SNEEZING – PROLONGED

Take Vitamin C, up to one gram daily, also Lobelia.

SNORING

Often linked to high blood pressure, circulation problems, allergy or alcohol before bedtime, or being overweight. Taking Ginger capsule or L-cysetine which is an Amino Acid, also Snoreeze have helped to eliminate snoring. Before retiring to bed blow the nose thoroughly and clear catarrh or mucous from the throat or nose. This has helped many who carried out the simple exercise. Spouses have thanked me for the advice. Further help is available from British Snoring and Sleep Apnoea Association on 'www.britishsnoring.co.uk.'

SOUPS

Every 'Soup' displayed on the food store or supermarket shelf must list the additives. *Here is an example of what some of the top sellers contain: Lactose, Potato Starch, Hydrogenated Vegetable Oil, Onion Powder, Salt, Maltodextrin, Rice Flour, Flavour Enhancers, Monosodium Glutamate, Disodium Inosinate, Disodium Guanyate, Colours, Plain Caramel, Paprika Extract, Yeast Extract, Tomato Powder, Dehydrated Beef, Flavouring, Soya Sauce Powder, Vitamins C, E, A, D & B12, Niacin, Thiamin, Folic Acid, Sugar, Spices And Herbs. All this for a bowl of 'soup', much not being nutritious. It could be harmful in the long-term. Here is an example of additives and processing at its worst. The manufacturers even add synthetic vitamins, as if these would enhance the other elements. Why put these in? Either Soup is pure Soup or it should be illegal to refer to this kind of stuff as 'soup', which should be left on the shelf of the food seller.* There are some pure or organic Soups, additive-free, containing much that is nutritious. It just means searching the shelves for them, just as one has to do to find additive-free pure natural yoghurts. They are more expensive. Why? Because one of the reasons for additives, man-made or synthetic, is to cheapen the 'foods', including 'Soups', to make more profits for the processor and the seller. Your health is way down the chart. It stands to reason that the pure, unadulterated must cost more.

What better than a bowl of nutritious homemade Soup? It is easy to make, can be done in bulk, then put in required serving portions and frozen, to be used as required. Get organised, using a good cookery book to ascertain the ingredients. The water costs little. The liquidiser is the all-important gadget. This can turn out to be an enjoyable pastime and certainly so when the fruits of the labour are viewed, having followed the instructions given. It is natural food in every way. Much of what is offered as 'soup' contains everything except Soup. Next time you buy SOUP, or indeed anything supposed to be edible, study the ingredients label. Leave the additive-filled stuff on the shelf.

SORE THROAT
See Throat Caption.

SORE THROAT – PERSISTENT
See Doctor.

SPASTIC COLON
See Irritable Bowel Syndrome Caption.

SPEECH THERAPY

Despite all of the modern conveniences, apparent affluence, improved communications, including constant use of mobile phones, we are faced with literacy problems as never before. We have more, whatever about better, education. Despite or because of all this it is now widely publicised that there is a grave shortage of Speech Therapists who are needed to help correct the manner of Speech and talk. Spelling, grammar and punctuation are appalling even in newspapers, especially the tabloids. Text messaging is certainly no aid to Speech or literacy. Since the advent of Television, the art - if that is the word to use - of conversation, has diminished, with reading by the young almost forgotten about in many homes. Where once we viewed rows of books, even newspapers and magazines, there are few to be seen now, only the Television, seldom switched off, which is an ever-present, unsociable companion. It is certainly no help to conversation or Speech. Our libraries, which are free to all, are little used. *Turn to Reading caption.*

SPINA BIFIDA

The need for Folic Acid and Vitamin B12 before and after conceiving is highlighted. Folic Acid can be found in green vegetables, wholemeal bread, potatoes, beans and oranges. To be sure of obtaining proper amount, supplementation is best. The medical profession have only recently become aware of this natural remedy or requirement, with Folic Acid now being manufactured by the drug companies. The health food store and those like myself who know of its natural goodness to counter neural tube defects, have been promoting its necessity and goodness for many years. Even now, all too many women are either unaware of or not interested in the need for Folic Acid. A multivitamin, such as Pregnacare, will provide Folic Acid and much else good for before conception and when pregnant.

SPIRULINA

Sports men and women, walkers, cyclists, mountaineers and workers use this little known, all-round whole-food supplement. It is the nearest thing yet to being a natural meal in tablet form. Spirulina is a blue / green micro algae that grows naturally in mineral rich lakes. It boosts energy, strengthens the immune system, improves skin tone, hair and nail growth and provides every day high-level nutrition, with almost no calories. It satisfies hunger, reduces cravings and supports both vegetarian and vegan diets. It contains more protein than any other natural food, except quinoa or dates. Included are the eight essential amino acids and 10 non-essential amino acids. Xynergy health products, who produce New Generation Life Stream Spirulina, have done much to pioneer and research this beyond ordinary, nutritional supplement, which helps fortify the body. If detoxing it helps because of its non-calorie content. It is an invaluable aid to recovery where there is Anorexia.

SPOTS AND PIMPLES

See Pimples and Spots Caption.

SPROUTING OF SEEDS & PULSES

Sprouted seeds, beans and peas are a source of enzymes, vitamins, minerals and much that is health giving. Here are green foods at their best. Partaking of Sprouted Seeds regularly can lead to dramatic improvement of immune system and general well being. Easy to Sprout Seeds or Pulses are Alfalfa, Peas, Lentils, Wheat, Mung beans, and Chick Peas, with Quinoa being one of the best, high in natural protein. Millet and Sunflower seeds are also very good.

You can start by buying a Sprouting kit or by using my out-dated but equally good method. Thirty years ago when I started Sprouting barley, chickpeas and quinoa, the seeds were soaked overnight in a glass jar, sealing the top. Next day they were put into a colander and covered with muslin. I do the same thing now using a screw top jam jar, which I almost half fill with the seeds or pulses, then filling with water. I cover the colander with a polythene bag. Rinse under the tap two or three times daily for two days, when seeds or pulses will have sprouted. Place in a bowel, where they can be kept in a fridge for up to five days. Eat when the urge is there for pure sustaining, natural good food. Use as a salad ingredient or as a snack food. Sprouted Seeds or Pulses are excellent for those slimming or trying to lose weight.

STENT

See Heart Bypass Caption.

STERILITY

See Infertility Caption.

STIFF JOINTS

See Joints and Joint health Caption.

STINGS

Bach Rescue Remedy is an aid to settle a child who has received a sting.

Bee:	Mix bicarbonate of soda to a paste by adding milk or water and apply, or smear with crushed Garlic.Remove Bee Sting as quickly as possible by scraping out, not pulling out.
Wasp:	Pure Malt or Cider Vinegar dabbed on.
Nettles:	Dab on Lemon juice or rub on Arnica.
Midge & Insect:	As a preventative against Midge and insect stings, especially if going abroad, take Thiamine tablets for three to four weeks before travelling. This never fails. Midge bites can be relieved by the use of Honey and Bicarbonate of Soda mixed and smeared on. *See Insect Repellent caption.*

S

STOMACH

Acidity:	*See Acidity caption*
Bloated:	Treat as Flatulence
Cramps:	Devils Claw, Indian Brandee or Mag Phos. If persistent seek medical aid
Flatulence:	*See Flatulence caption.*
Gastric:	*See Gastroenteritis caption.*
Gastritis:	*See Gastritis caption.*
Ulcer:	*See Ulcers caption.*
Upset:	It is important to find the cause and treat accordingly. Slippery Elm, Calamus, Udo's Choice Oil or Combination S New Era have all proved remedial. When the vomiting ceases return to eating and drinking carefully, taking Slippery Elm, milk puddings, natural soups and foods gentle on the digestive system. I cannot understand why antacid tablets or medicines are used when the vital hydrochloric acid is so necessary for stomach health. Stomach and bowel

problems can be brought on when taking contraceptive pill, being very difficult to diagnose.

STOMATITIS

This is inflamed and sore mucus lining of the mouth, sometimes with ulcers. There is usually an underlying problem, which should be treated. Often brought on by inferior Diet and lifestyle, resulting in becoming rundown. Bad dental hygiene is an aggravation. Visit to dentist can help. It is an ailment which almost always responds to change to natural Diet, also taking of tonic such as Floradix, Floravital or Biostrath for two weeks and then with continuous use of natural Multivitamin tablet. The excellent Sage-based remedy Menosan used as a mouthwash three times daily is recommended. Acidophilus capsule kept in the mouth for as long as possible has proved good. Change to pure natural food Diet has been the best medicine. *Turn to DIET and be guided.*

STONES IN KIDNEY

See Kidneys Caption.

STRESS

I have bulging files on this subject. It is as the eminent herbalist Thomas Bartram, editor of '**Grace**' magazine states: "A 20th. century disease". Previous to the 1960s stress and strain had to do with metallurgy, shear, modulus and construction materials. Now Stress means worry, very much of it unnecessary. *The medical profession inform us that Stress-related problems now make up the bulk of complaints from patients.*

Those prone to Stress are the ever busy, competitive, often impatient, who worry unduly. The consequences of Stress are far-reaching. The constant pressures, with life's often illusory and infatuating worries, also irregular pattern of sleep, can lead to serious health problems. These include heart, digestion, stomach and other disorders, even to bringing about a change in the hormones of the body, with the immune system becoming suppressed. Negative thoughts and emotions, which are present when overstressed, play a major part in the lead-up to most diseases. Positive thinking is beneficial to health. We need to be able to laugh at ourselves including our mistakes. STRESS IS OFTEN BROUGHT ON BY TRYING TO DO SOMETHING ABOUT SOMETHING YOU CANNOT DO ANYTHING ABOUT.

If energetic and feeling well, Stress is easily brushed aside. As with all ailments, mental and physical, natural additive free **FOOD** is as medicine. When speaking about depression it is easy to offer advice, but many Stress sufferers are not for accepting it or change of lifestyle. *One can list aids to help fight Stress, but it is a waste of time doing so if the person has not got the foundation on which to base the remedies. The bedrock of better health comes about by the partaking of pure* *natural Diet of nutritious food, free from additives, colour, preservatives, sweeteners, etc. No apology is made for the repetitive advice given in this respect.* In this Encyclopedia there are over 1,000 ailments listed. The cause of most of them is nearly always inferior Diet of processed 'foods' - therefore duplication and recurrence of theme is necessary.

I have ample evidence to prove, if this is required, that rejuvenation of health and therefore oneself, by combining proper Diet, Exercise, Sleep and Sleep Pattern, is the premier remedy in helping all to cope with Stress. We must also learn to balance work, relaxation, rest and leisure. Unwind and talk, two great medicines. Don't bottle up the emotions.

Talk to somebody, a friend or relative. Often we think we have problems or worries until we hear those of others, then realizing we have none. Learn to say: 'NO', even if some, especially children, do not appear to understand the meaning of the word. Learn to pace yourself, one of the best pieces of advice given to me. Slow down and live.

Last year a woman came to me worried about her daughter, saying how Stressed she was. The young student was sharing a house in the city, far away from home. We discovered that her Diet and Lifestyle were deplorable. The mother said that it would be very difficult to get the daughter to change her habits. She was given the various articles on DIET, Exercise, Sleep, Yoga and Supplements, also a sheet of A4 paper on which I printed: 'THERE IS ONLY ONE WAY TO CHANGE YOUR LIFE, CHANGE YOUR WAY OF THINKING'. It worked and I had a 'Thank You' card from the mother of a now healthy daughter.

You, the reader, if dealing with Stress or Stress-related problems, is asked to read caption on Diet which includes suggestions regarding Supplements, Exercise, Yoga and Sleep, all of which lead to well-being, resulting in Stress being almost unknown.

Udo's Choice Oil and Rhodolia tables are both excellent aids to help Stress problems. Reflexology Therapy has proved wonderful for Stress treatment. The doctor will certainly not prescribe this natural remedy.

It is not the work but the worry, that causes the Stress and the strain,

If only all would remember that with worry there is nothing to gain.

It is not the work but the worry, which leads to an early grave,

So change the way you are living,

You'll be surprised at your strength for being brave.

(Acknowledgement to 'Grace' Magazine)

STRESS – INCONTINENCE

This sensitive or uncomfortable problem can be overcome. It happens when the pelvic muscles, which control the flow of urine, become lax, often after pregnancy

1g or after menopause. Men are also affected. Take pure unsweetened rry Juice or Kordel's Cranberry 10,000 which also contains Uva Ursi and . Drink the herbal teas Lady's Mantle or American Cranesbill. The latter, which is an excellent remedy, can also be taken in either capsule or tablet form. All, including pure, unsweetened juices, are available from the health food store. Avoid coffee, alcohol and fizzy 'drinks'. *See DIET caption* and be guided about the need for abstention from these. Exercises are needed to improve pelvic floor muscles. Stopping and starting several times when urinating is one exercise. Stop urinating half way through to find where the muscles are. When bladder is empty, do the exercises by contracting the pelvic muscles while counting to 10 about 25 or 30 times. This to be done several times daily until the problem is rectified.

STROKE

This occurs when the blood supply to the brain is disrupted. There are several natural ways to help those who are recovering from Stroke or to help in its prevention. Body warmth is a must. Keep well wrapped-up, wearing warm clothing. It is advisable to warm up the car before getting in to drive off. Constant and regular blood pressure checks are vital, with steps taken to lower where necessary. If overweight try to lose some of the excess. Avoid smoking and smoky atmosphere, also alcohol. There is a need for gentle exercise, even just keeping the muscles active, also regular sleep and proper sleep pattern. Include with Diet recommended the antioxidants Vitamins E and C also Lecithin granules, with Hawthorn and Rutin being further aids. *As well as reading the DIET caption, which extols the good of pure, natural foods, other captions which help in prevention of stroke and perhaps those recovering are Exercise, Sleep, Blood Pressure and Yoga.* The latter is an easy, gentle form of exercise for both mind and body. WARNING: BEFORE PUTTING ANY OF THIS ADVICE INTO PRACTICE SPEAK WITH YOUR DOCTOR. TELL HIM WHAT YOU ARE DOING OR INTEND TO DO. THIS IS MOST IMPORTANT ESPECIALLY WITH REGARD TO EXERCISE. This is not an alternative to your GPs advice, being only complementary. In speaking with Stroke patients I have found that where others have given nutritional advice, much of it includes the use of processed foods containing additives and non-edible products. This is not conversant with better health. The food must be natural to be nutritious.

STYE

This is infection at the base of the eyelash. Almost always occurs as a result of impure blood, being rundown. Bathe the eye with Manuka Honey diluted with tepid water or with warm Camomile Tea. Change your Diet to pure foods and a tonic such as Floradix or Salusan. This will help prevent future similar infection. Kindervital is recommended for children. *Turn to DIET caption* to be advised about how to have better health and how to eliminate impure blood problems.

SUGAR

Our Government and those responsible for our Health Services - or should one say the ill- health of our people - should take on the mighty, all-too-plausible 'food' manufacturers. This to include the ingredients processors, who suavely tell us that what they offer is safe, despite being without proof of the integrated use of the additives in relation to our bodies. The legislators, who talk loud and often - many of them with the voters in mind, some with vested interests - should also call a halt to the indiscriminate use of one of our greatest health hazards, namely SUGAR. It is not a food. If we are what we eat, how can the use of this 'As fat' product be condoned? *One can almost hear the defensive hackles rise to shout: "Sugar is not fat". It might as well be, because the body turns Sugar into the same hard fats that make platelets more sticky, interfering with insulin and essential fatty acids functions. Unused sugar in the body is converted into and stored as fat, highly detrimental to all.* It rots and damages teeth, also feeds bacteria, yeast, fungus and cancer cells. It interferes with Vitamin C, therefore with our immune system. It speeds up ageing, pulls Calcium and other Minerals from the body and much more which is damaging to our health and well being.

Sugar is an enemy of good health. The Sugar barons have much to answer for, when it is brought to the attentions of all who regard good health as wealth, that the amount of Sugar used annually, including that of the food industry, was approximately 1kg (2lbs per head) in the year 1900 whereas it was approximately 60kg (130lbs per head) in the year 2000. This manifestation is an incriminating allegation against the Sugar processors as we eat our way to ill health. The reader is probably thinking: 'I do not use this amount of sugar'. Because so much sugar is used for food, drink and commercial manufacturing processes there is little realisation of the vast quantities consumed.

The Sugar industry tells us that there has been a decrease in the sales of Sugar for culinary or home purposes. What they don't tell us is of the explosive or gross overuse of their products by the food and drinks industry, especially in the processed 'foods' and 'drinks' referred to. They also inform us that it is the most natural sweetener in the world. I beg to differ. Pure Honey is the only natural sweetener. Sugar is processed.

High Sugar intake is being blamed for the huge increase in diabetes, obesity and other ailments. We need only minimal amounts. It is in processed, additive-filled, 'foods', including junk, fast and convenience nosh, sweets, breakfast cereals, bread, confectionary, fizzy and alcoholic 'drinks', which are all-too-much of what we drink and eat. The majority give little thought to the harmful substance of Sugar or the consequences of eating it, especially with regard to that of young people. They do not seem to be aware of or realise the relationship between Sugar and teeth, obesity, heart and circulation problems, osteoporosis, mental health or the very many other

S

ailments caused by intake of sugar.

Dr Fredrick Grant Banting, who discovered insulin, warned in 1929 that diabetes had increased proportionately with the per capita consumption of white Sugar. He called refined Sugar a: 'Dangerous foodstuff'. What would he say if he were alive today? Recently a well-known professor described sugar as: 'Pure, white and deadly'. *Sugar is equally as dangerous as smoking, perhaps more so now. Even when taking into consideration the increase in the world population, the production rate of Sugar is mind-bending. Today it stands at over 120,000,000 tons. Since the 1970's, which is not so very long ago, the production has increased by over 50%.* **Add to this the millions of tons of artificial Sweeteners used and referred to under that caption.** *Consider that there was no call for them until recent years. This makes the per capita use of Sugar and sweeteners extremely startling. Being verbose again, I repeat; "Sugar is one of our greatest health foes".*

The Government, in a highhanded, undemocratic manner, foisted the toxic Fluoride on us, stating that it is a must for the health of our teeth. At the same time they allow the Sugar purveyors, also the 'food' and fizzy 'drinks' manufacturers, to provide Sugar and Sugar foods and liquids without constraint. This is typical of political logic. *It is blatantly obvious to all except those with vested interests, of whom there are many, that if Fluoride was banned, as it should be and the use of Sugar and food additives strictly curtailed, the health of all would improve so much that the enhancement and improvement to our lives would be indescribable.* Our teeth health is poorer than ever, with most dentists extolling the virtues of Fluoride. This fact alone sets them up as having little pride in their profession, other than monetary gain. It is not in their interests to promote better dental care and health, other than by insisting on our visiting their surgeries. They will tell one not to eat sweets between meals and to regularly brush our teeth, using Fluoride toothpaste of course. *Turn to Toothpaste, also Fluoride captions,* to be aware of the dangers, especially to children, where Fluoride is not to be used by those under the age of two.

As a voluntary organiser for one of our largest health charities I would like to submit these questions about what can only be seen as a hypocritical attitude. Why is it that when one calls to the offices of, or attends functions or meetings, run by professional health organisations or charities, which can include medical, dental and other health- orientated personnel or society, the food offered usually consists of coffee or tea, with biscuits or other confectionery? Why is it that in hospitals, waiting rooms and other places where many congregate to seek medical aid, also schools and colleges, we are faced with dispensers or even shops where Sugarised products including fizzy 'drinks', sweets, chocolates and other confectionery are for sale? At the same time we are told that steps are being taken to inform us about Diet, obesity and the need to cut down on fats and Sugary products. The hypocrisy and timid advice is such that the Sugar, Food Additive, Food Industry, Medical

Profession, Pharmaceutical and Drug industries gurus can laugh all the way to the bank. If the tobacco industry can be dictated to, surely many other health problems, equally as serious, can be faced up to.

SUICIDE

Why do I write about Suicide in an 'Encyclopedia of Over the Counter Natural Remedies' which extols the use of good food, alternative or complementary remedies and resultant better health? It is done simply because there is a link between the three when I think of this mortal problem. All are aware of the huge increase in Suicide, A.D.H.D., Depression, Stress and other mind or brain-related illness. World Health experts have warned of an: 'Alarming level of mental health problems in the Western world'. In this Encyclopedia there are captions on these subjects. There are increased incidences of Suicide in Winter months, the time when people suffer most from 'Winter Blues', which is SADS.

Those left behind to mourn, including friends and comrades, ask the question: "Why"? Nobody can give the answer.

Is it coincidental or is there correlation that, during the past few years, when we witnessed the increase in Suicide and Suicidal tendencies there has been the huge increase in output of synthetic medicines and food-additive chemicals? The factory-made 'food' is laden with many of the over 5,000 food substances used. At the same time we witness the inordinate production, sale and over-prescribing of medical drugs. The Pharmaceutical Associations openly admit that an amount of it is out of control.

Regularly I meet those who are almost in awe of the doctor. Some cherish the anti-depressants, tranquillizers and other pills or potions prescribed, many of them dangerous and to be avoided. The same people and many others visit the supermarket to buy chemical- filled 'food' off the shelves. They would never think of enquiring about what is in the make-up of the manufactured drugs or so called 'foods'. Being all too trusting, they do not bother to either ask for explanation or to look at the ingredients lists.

Young and those not so young listen to music - which to my ear is anything but melodic - which holds a powerful influence over many. Some of it provokes negative and dangerous thoughts or reaction.

We have an alcohol crisis, as our legislators, those who supposedly govern, bow to the whims of the drinks trade by over-liberalising the drink laws. Many, especially younger people, have not got the necessary money to enter into the present-day culture of drinking alcohol. There is peer pressure as never before.

My firm belief is that, as with SADS, so with Suicide. If a person eats and drinks that which is pure, taking only natural sustenance and nutritious foods into the body he or she can withstand the rigours and pressure of this life. Pure natural FOOD is as medicine to the body. They will have a feel-good factor, being better and stronger

S

in mind and bodily systems. Nothing will be too much for them. Suicide will be far from their minds. *Turn to DIET caption* to help understand what I write about.

All, each and everyone, must grasp the message that: "There probably has never been a period in human history, when the value of pure foods and drinks, including additive-free, nutritional Diet, one could add natural remedies, was more essential than now".

Most illnesses do not, as is generally thought, come on suddenly. The groundwork is done over the years, through faulty Diet - smoking, excess alcohol, overwork or mental conflicts. These and other factors slowly wear down the person's energy, strength and mental abilities. It is extremely difficult to put it this way when writing about the sad trauma of Suicide, but it must be said: *"Men and women do not die, they kill themselves".*

SUPPLEMENTS

See Vitamins, Minerals & Supplements Captions.

SWEETENERS

Artificial Sweeteners are additives, all used to help attract and be alluring to the taste buds of the unsuspecting who consume 'processed foods', with 'bad foods' often made to taste good. Children and our youth are usually the people enticed. From a health point of view sugar - bad as it - is better than any of the permitted synthetic Sweeteners, except where diabetics are concerned. We have been told that the safety of these Sweeteners cannot be guaranteed. How are people to know these things are no health asset, maybe harmful? The propaganda of the 'food' and 'drinks' industry frequently highlights many items which contain additives, including Sweeteners which are unproven, some of them unhealthy, such as the toxic Aspartame. *Turn to Aspartame caption.* People are trusting, not understanding the dangers, or worst of all they do not read the ingredients labels. The advertising or write-up may even contain the words dietary, where these chemicals are included in the additives, where the 'food' has little if any nutrients. Very often we see the words sugar-free on 'food' or 'drink' packaging, only to read the ingredients label to discover there is worse than sugar, because synthetic Sweeteners are used instead. Some Sweeteners, not permitted in ice cream, can be legally added to reduce the use of sugar - i.e. as in jam. They are additives and are not natural. Artificial Sweeteners are best avoided. Sugar used sparingly or honeys are alternatives. *Also see Sugar caption.*

SWEATING – EXCESSIVELY

Not to be confused with night sweats. If not due to hot surroundings or after exercise or exertion, there may be an underlying problem to treat. Therefore seek medical advice. Menosan or Milk Thistle are good aids. Avoid hot spicy foods and alcohol. Inferior Diet is very often the problem. *Turn to DIET caption.*

SWOLLEN ANKLES

See Ankles Caption.

SYNOVITIS

This is puffiness of the Synovial membrane, better known as fluid on the joint, such as knee, elbow or hip. Almost always due to knock, bang or an injury. Vitamin E combined with Prickly Ash Bark and or Devil's Claw have removed the swelling and discomfort within 72 hours.

S

THIS ENCYCLOPEDIA HAS BEEN COMPILED BECAUSE I HAVE SEEN THE BENEFITS OF
COMPLEMENTARY MEDICINE, WITH THE HEALTH OF EVEN THE MOST SCEPTICAL
IMPROVED.
MANY WHO WERE DOUBTFUL ARE NOW ARDENT SUPPORTERS OF THE NATURAL WAY
OF LIVING AND REMEDIES.
THERE IS NO PROMISE OF 'CURE', ONLY REFERRING TO WHAT HAS WORKED FOR
OTHERS AND ADVISING ACCORDINGLY.

TACHYCARDIA

This above normal heart rate is usually due to underlying cause, therefore have diagnosis carried out. It can be as a result of drugs, alcohol, coffee intake, or if with circulatory or heart problems. Turning to proper nutritional Diet, supplemented with Vitamin E, also taking Poke Root and Blue Flag Root can help normalise the heart. *It is important to consult with your doctor before commencing any form of treatment.*

TAPE WORMS

See Worms Caption.

TASTE – LOSS OF SENSE OF

Take Vitamin A also Nat Mur or Combination Q New Era. Sometimes it has taken several weeks of the treatment before returning to normal.

TEAS – HERBAL & OTHERS

I am partial to weak tea every two hours until early evening. There are various Herbal Teas, with most of them being good for different health problems, whether as a drink or otherwise.

Black Tea	as a mouth-wash or gargle is antibacterial. It is also an aid to sore or cracked nipples after breastfeeding.
Calendula Tea bags	treat thrush, both genital and mouth
Camomile Tea bags	placed on puffy eyes help reduce the swelling
Elder Flower Tea	for colds, coughs or sore throat.
Ginger Tea bags	soaked and placed in a tissue help nausea.
Green Tea	is rich in antioxidants, helping to prevent ageing, also being an aid to brain and memory. It has now been discovered that a chemical being extracted from Green Tea may be used to

	provide the starting point for a new family of anti- cancer drugs.
Lemon Tea	helps normalise greasy hair when two teabags placed in washing water.
Mint Tea bags	soaked and placed on tissue is a traditional remedy for hay fever relief.
Nettle Tea bags	are used when washing hair or as an all-round aid to hair lustre.

Two Elder Flower Tea bags soaked in the rinsing water helps to rejuvenate dry hair. Visit your health food store if you wish to learn more about these and other health giving herbal TEAS. *See Coffee caption* to help realise the goodness of TEA as a drink.

TEA TREE OIL

This is a natural antiseptic, which can be used by all. It is for external use only, and has long shelf life. It has aided acne sufferers, soothes bites, stings and helps in treatment of abrasions and cuts. It is safe for children, being natural. It has proved better than some antibiotics. It is regarded in surgery as: 'The finest antiseptic known to man'. Ask your health food store or the chemists who stock Tea Tree Oil for other relevant information. It must be diluted and used as instructed on the container. Optima brand 'Thursday Plantation' range of Tea Tree products are exceptionally good.

TEENAGERS & HEALTH

See Children's & Teenage Health Caption.

TEETH - GRINDING

See Teeth Caption.

TEETH

Mouth, Teeth and gums are a pointer to our health. Good Teeth are one of our most valuable assets, which if cared for will be almost trouble free. Dental hygiene, with proper brushing, using a medium to soft textured brush, is very important. Some use an old or improper brush, with many not being taught how to brush properly. Ask your dentist to show you the correct method. Failure to clean Teeth properly allows plaque to build up, when gums can become infected, inflamed and even receding. This can lead to the Teeth becoming loose in the sockets, or to the enamel being attacked, resulting in sensitive Teeth. Proper brushing removes plaque or it may have to be taken off by flossing by your dentist.

There are two main reasons for bad Teeth and gums, apart from inferior dental hygiene. They are the consumption of fizzy 'drinks', processed 'foods', which are mostly sugarised also fruit 'juices' and other items which contain sugar. Inferior Diet also leads to ill-health and resultant troubles with mouth, Teeth and gums. *The refined starches and sugars found in the 'fizzy drinks' and 'processed foods' are mostly the cause of rotting Teeth, infected by the bacteria they feed.* Pure natural foods with little or no sugar are necessary for good health, including that of Teeth, gums and mouth. *See DIET caption* and be guided by the suggestions, including the partaking of Vitamins and Minerals.

As well as change of Diet, aids to better Teeth health are:

Teeth loose in sockets -	Calc Fluor
Grinding during sleep -	Nat Phos
Bleeding gums -	*See Periodontal Disease*
Sensitive Teeth -	Calc Phos & Mag Phos
To help maintain enamel -	Calc Fluor
Teething problem with infants -	Nat Mur or Combination R New Era
Aid to children's Teeth health -	Calc Phos.

All are natural, suitable for children, with no side effects. The milk infancy Teeth should be cared for as well as the permanent ones. The quality and position of the latter depend on the temporary Teeth all being sound and in place, until being pushed out by the eruption of the permanent set. For adults, Coenzyme Q10 is an all-round supplement to maintain Teeth and gums in a healthy state. *It is not generally known that it is important to brush teeth before eating, in order to remove the bacteria or plaque, which thrives on sugar or starches. Turn to Gums, Mouth and Toothpaste captions* for further helpful advice.

TELEVISION

What has this to do with natural health? It has nothing to do with anything natural, only having an enormous amount to do with ill-health of mind, body and soul. TELEVISION is responsible for glazed eyes, bored expressions, false imaginations, diminished reasoning, obesity, a need for speech therapy, social isolation, fragmentation of long life, couch potato children and young people, with all too apparent laziness of mind and body. *Many whom we would not consider inviting into our homes, supposedly entertain us.* It is an enemy of good health, as many lie about or snooze in front of the goggle box, with young people especially at risk.

Exercise, as in the past, has now turned to inactivity of both body and mind. Except for news, weather, sport and the odd topical item or documentary we are best without Television. The off button is one of its best features.

It is no coincidence that the upsurge in thuggery, rape, murder, robbery and much of the evil we see today, has only occurred since the advent of COMMERCIAL TELEVISION. *We know that a child's character is formed between the ages of two and eight. This is when they are most vulnerable, when they learn the difference between right and wrong, good and bad. The foundation for the individual's traits, mannerisms and outlook on life was, and should be, properly laid down by the parents. Now it is all too often formed in front of the box, where shooting, killing, maiming, and very much more, alien to a child, is colourfully transmitted. The adverts are sometimes more deranged than the other, very often being nasty programmes, which children look on as being the real thing. Children in their formative years need nurturing, training, instructing, disciplining and providing for - all to be combined with an amount of loving.*

Do you remember when children could roam safely or went to school by themselves? All could walk our streets fearlessly. House doors could be left open. You saw policemen walking or cycling in the neighbourhood. There were no rowdies. Football matches were carefree fun games, with sport being sport, not business as it is now. Senior citizens, teachers and others in authority were respected. We took regular exercise, ate properly- cooked food and made our own enjoyment. There was little need for medicine and less for the doctor. *THERE WAS NO TELEVISION*

TENDONITIS

This is inflammation of a Tendon, as with tennis or golfer's elbow. Comes from overuse of the Tendon or is brought on by Rheumatic or other bone inflammation. Natural remedies include Prickly Ash Bark, Magnesium, Zinc, Calc Fluor, Devil's Claw or Glucosamine. Arnica Gel, rubbed on, is a useful external application.

TENNIS ELBOW

Treat as Tendonitis. If swollen or puffed on point of elbow it may by Synovitis and to be treated as such.

TENSION - NERVOUS

See Nervous Exhaustion Caption.

TENSION – PRE MENSTRUAL

See Pre Menstrual Syndrome and Menstruation Caption.

THIAMIN

See Vitamins and Minerals Caption.

THIRST

Most people make the mistake of waiting until Thirsty before drinking water. This is wrong. All need eight, 10 or more glasses of pure water daily. It is as medicine to the body. *See Water caption.*

THORSONS

Thorsons are, and have been for many years, major publishers of natural health, self-help, mind, body and spirit books. Not so many years ago, when natural food and health and the visiting of the health food shop was being promoted by people like myself, we were looked upon suspiciously, being freaks, as we tried to steer people towards the natural. Thorsons were then, and still are, to the forefront in promoting the use of everything natural. They are now an imprint of Harper Collins Publishers, 77-85 Fulham Palace Road, London W6 8JB and publish much that is advisory and educational regarding natural foods and health. Their books are widely available from bookshops, many health food stores or they can be ordered. They will send booklist on application.

THREADWORMS

See Worms Caption.

THROAT

Sore Throat can very often be the forerunner of a cold, or it can be an underlying cause of something more serious. If it persists, seek medical aid. Your doctor should have the experience to know whether it is viral or bacterial. Natural treatments are:

Throat Sore - gargle with the sage based remedy Menosan, which should be in all medicine cabinets, or another remedy is to add three to six drops of Tea Tree Oil to warm water and gargle. Repeat up to three times daily.

Relaxed Throat - Poke Root or Calc Fluor

Tickling Larynx - Calc Fluor

Loss of voice by singers or speakers - Ferr Phos or two teaspoons of each Cider Vinegar and Pure Honey mixed in some tepid water, to be taken every hour for eight hours.

Constant hoarseness Calc Phos

Raw feeling Nat Phos

Stinging when swallowing - Silica

Laryngitis *See Laryngitis caption.*

Mensosan is an all round Throat Tonic, a natural remedy.

THROMBOSIS – DEEP VEIN

See Deep Vein Thrombosis Caption.

THRUSH - MOUTH

The ulcer and painful itching or burning sensation in throat and mouth can be treated naturally. Antibiotics have been linked to increased risk, killing beneficial bacteria also causing upset of the mucous membrane system. Inferior Diet, resulting in weakened immune system, is often the root of the problem. *Turn to DIET caption* and be advised. This can be aided by the taking of natural remedies such as Udo's Choice Super 8s combined with Vitamin B Complex, Acidophilus, Echinacea or Spilanthes. These are all available from your health food shop whose personnel will assist if further advice is required.

THRUSH – VAGINAL

This itching, burning feeling which is candida albicans can be caused by many factors including hormonal imbalance, the wearing of synthetic fibres against the skin, the use of antibiotics which destroy the good and the bad, if using contraceptive pill or if with diabetes. *If Diabetic consult your doctor before taking any remedy natural or otherwise.* The main cause is very often a Diet inferior in nutrients, which can lead to a host of health problems including a weakened immune system.

Wear cotton underwear and avoid wearing tights. Use pure natural soap to wash. Many deodorants, including sprays and tampons, contain chemicals, which should be avoided.

Although one of the most common ailments of our time, few will discuss if with Vaginal Thrush problems, feeling embarrassed to disclose the often distressing condition. It should be treated immediately, because if allowed to continue it can become debilitating, leading to tiredness and other forms of physical illness. As already stated the all-important remedy is the intake of proper nutritious natural food. *See DIET caption.* When the candida is gone, having been banished by proper nutritive intake aided by the natural remedies listed, an amount of other unrelated symptoms and problems go too. The following natural remedies when included with pure natural Diet, have helped eliminate Thrush: Acidophilus, Garlic capsules or tablets, Golden Seal, Udo's Choice Super 8's or Spilanthes. A good natural Multivitamin should be taken continuously, even when the Thrush is eliminated. There may be the need to look at the possibility of allergy if the Thrush problem persists. *See Allergy caption.*

THYROID

If with Thyroid problem read this advice and before deciding to use natural remedies, except of course the partaking of the very important aid to good health, the suggested DIET, speak with your doctor. If on medication, do not change to complementary remedies, especially if with Thyroid problem, without his being acquainted. homeopathic doctors have treated Thyroid problems very successfully. Few realise that Reflexology is highly commended as a remedy for Thyroid gland disease or ailment, including Goitre. Many praise its goodness in this respect.

Over Active - (Hyperthyroidism) There are natural remedies to complement the doctor's advice. Proper nutritious Diet has been found to be the chief remedy to help control the over-active Thyroid. All-too-many are not obtaining sufficient necessary nutrients. Intake of Vitamins A, B, C & E also the Minerals Calcium and Magnesium are necessary. A good Multivitamin, which will contain the vitamins listed here, is desirable to augment the Diet. The Calcium Complex tablet is to be taken at bedtime. Spirulina is a well-balanced collection of nutrients to replace those so vital elements missing from much of today's foods. All these are available from the health food store. *See DIET, Exercise and Sleep captions.*

Under Active – (Hypothyroidism) Certain natural remedies and supplements, added to pure natural Diet, combined with exercise, can help enormously. From the Diet omit the following, which can have adverse effect on under-active Thyroid gland: cabbage, kale, cauliflower, spinach, Brussels sprouts, soya and other greens. A Multivitamin tablet as suggested for over-active thyroid also extra Kelp and Zinc combine to aid the natural Diet. *See DIET, Exercise and Sleep captions.*

Goitre – (Enlargement of the thyroid) This can arise from iodine deficiency or over- consumption of Calcium. Blue Flag Root, Poke Root, Selenium, Magnesium and Vitamin B Complex combined with Diet of natural food have helped alleviate Goitre. Where better health is expected it is very necessary to take exercise in some form. *Turn to DIET and Exercise captions.* I have seen the excellent results obtained through the use of Reflexology for thyroid problems including Goitre, as set out at the top of this caption. If on medication, before engaging in any form of strenuous exercise, speak with your doctor.

TIMED RELEASE VITAMINS

See Vitamins & Minerals Captions.

TINNITUS

The ringing, buzzing, hissing, or other signals in ears or head can drive one almost to distraction. In the past, noise at work was blamed. Now, as the chronic condition has increased enormously, it has been put down to personal stress, high volume

speakers and amplification, noisy gatherings including sports
continuous exposure to noise frequently. Therefore, prevention is a mu
our young people this.

We are told there is no cure, that the problem is a mystery. This is only p
Those with Tinnitus maintain they receive little therapeutic help from t
but one can look elsewhere for assistance. Several natural remedies have helped,
cleared, or banished the aggravation. *See DIET caption* and adhere as far as possible
to what is recommended, all being purely natural, because certain food additives are
now associated with the ailment. Need for nutritious food is very important to avoid
and help rid one of Tinnitus. Following have helped sufferers.

- Feverfew Oil or essence on back of ears or head also taken internally.

- Ginkgo Biloba has proved exceptionally good, but is not to be taken if on
  beta blockers, aspirin or heart medication.

- Plantain and Buchu tablets have helped. They should be taken with a
  good Multivitamin tablet because Vitamins and Minerals are an aid to
  better health including the elimination of Tinnitus.

- Six to eight drops of castor oil taken daily, followed by a glass of tepid
  water which contains two teaspoons of each Cider Vinegar and Pure
  Natural Honey, should be taken for five to six weeks.

- Drink copious amounts of pure water, making sure that it is free from
  the toxic Fluoride which is now added in excess to so much of our
  drinking water.

- A Vitamin E capsule pierced, with drops placed in the ears, has been a
  successful remedy.

TIREDNESS

See Lethargy Caption.

TISSUE SALTS

One of the first homeopathic or natural medicines or remedies I learned about was
Biochemic Tissue Salts or Schüssler Salts. They are both homeopathic and
nutritional medicine, a combination of both. Dr Willhelm Schüssler, who was an
eminent German homeopathic doctor, developed them in the late 1890's. He
claimed that many ailments were, as they are now, due to a lack of essential minerals
in the body. He has been proved right over and over again. **An example of this
thinking of well over a century ago is the use today of Calcium in the fight to
prevent Osteoporosis. Only in the recent past have some of the medical
profession come to realise that the natural way is right, as they have now
condescended to prescribe Calcium and Magnesium. All this, despite their value**

density and strength of bone being advocated for years, by those who understood natural medicine and the need for these minerals.

Rudolph Virchow, who became one of the most esteemed medical professors of all time, laid the foundation of biochemistry almost 150 years ago. His theories led Dr Schüssler, whose scientific vision was far ahead of his time, to put his carefully worked out hypothesis to the test. The brilliant results he achieved enabled him to formulate his unique system, to which he gave the name, Biochemistry. The 12 Mineral or Tissue Salts are harmless, not being drugs in any sense of the word. No remedy could be more natural. They simply provide for the system the efficient inorganic elements, prepared homeopathically, in extremely fine form, which ensures their easy assimilation with resultant restoration to better health.

I have used and prescribed Tissue Salts for many years. They cannot be praised sufficiently. What is most annoying is that so few, especially those in need of minor medication, know little about these excellent remedies. *When permutated by adding the various mineral-salts together they give many pure but different natural treatments.* Here is an example of something being so good, yet so simple because they are in such tiny amounts and so harmless, that research is well nigh impossible, therefore the medical profession cannot reach scientific conclusions. *They are too simple for the almighty money-orientated multi-national drug companies to bother about. These natural remedies would do nothing to enhance their profits, despite their efficiency and goodness to our health.* Only minute amounts are needed.

There are hundreds of niggling health problems encountered daily, many of which can be banished, sometimes within a matter of hours of partaking of the Salts. They can truthfully be called *'The Salts of the Earth'*. They are recommended as remedies for various ailments captioned and written about in this Encyclopedia. All have proved extremely good. **I am convinced that there is a cure for almost every ailment if the Tissue Salts are permutated correctly.** Listed here are the 12 Tissue Salts, sold mostly under the brand names of Weleda and New Era. You will note that they are sold singly or as made up by New Era in Combination form. Taken with Diet of natural additive free food they have an even better chance of successful treatment. *The remedies set out here against the Salts are only a very small list taken from the hundreds of minor or niggling ailments, which Tissue Salts can be used to cure or alleviate.*

Calc Fluor   Calcium Fluoride : For Tissue elasticity, Strengthens veins and arteries, Helps circulation, Helps prevent teeth becoming loose.

Calc Phos   Calcium Phosphate : For Indigestion, Teething problems, Chilblains, Good for children's bones, Teeth, Anaemia, Is a restorative.

Calc Sulph   Calcium Sulphate: For Blood impurity, Spots and pimples, Slow healing skin,

Sore lips, Catarrh.

Ferr Phos	Iron Phosphate : For Respiratory and bronchial problems, Coughs, Colds, Chills, A good aid for the elderly. (It is not an Iron Tonic, being entirely nutritional).
Kali Mur	Potassium Chloride : For Relief of mucous membrane, Good for children's ailments, Aids digestion where Diet is inferior.
Kali Phos	Potassium Phosphate : For Nervous headaches, Tenseness or stress due to worry or over excitement, Excellent for children with school worries.
Kali Sulph	Potassium Sulphate : Works in conjunction with Ferr Phos for lung health, It acts as a lubricant to all parts of the body, Good for scaly and dry skin.
Mag Phos	Magnesium Phosphate : For Cramps, Flatulence, Minor stomach and nerve pains including neuralgia and sciatica, Helps those with menstrual pain.
Nat Mur	Sodium Chloride : For loss of smell, Watery head colds, Helps if with low spirits, constipation, heartburn, hay fever or sleeplessness, It is a water distributor.
Nat Phos	Sodium Phosphate : For acid neutralising, Dissolves uric acid, Settles the stomach, Helps joint pains.
Nat Sulph	Sodium Sulphate : For Body water balance, Flu symptoms, Is a liver aid, Restores liveliness in humid conditions.
Silica	Silicon Dioxide : Helps cleanse body systems. Good for skin, hair nails and as a blood purifier.

As well as what is set out above there are 18 New Era Combination remedies, which may be used for a variety of minor illnesses as indicated on the packs. A Combination remedy is just what it says, it is – a Combination of several of the single Tissue Salts-, which have been chosen for their suitability in treating certain conditions when combined together. Again, because of space limitation, only a brief guide is possible with regard to the many ailments for which these combinations can be taken. The following is a résumé;

Combination A:	For sciatica. Neuritis Neuralgia and allied conditions
Combination B:	Nerviness, stress and during convalescence
Combination C:	Acidity, heartburn, dyspepsia and allied conditions
Combination D:	Minor skin ailments, scalp eruption, eczema, acne etc.
Combination E:	Indigestion, colicky pain, flatulence
Combination F:	Migraine, nervous headache and allied conditions
Combination G:	Backache, lumbago, piles, loss of elasticity in tissues

Combination H:	Hay fever, allergic rhinitis
Combination I:	Fibrositis, muscular pain and allied conditions
Combination J:	Coughs, colds, chestiness, catarrh
Combination K:	Brittle nails, lack lustre hair
Combination L:	Sedentary lifestyle, to help veins and arteries
Combination M:	Rheumatic pain and allied conditions
Combination N:	Menstrual pain
Combination P:	Aching feet and legs, poor circulation, chilblains
Combination Q:	Catarrh, sinus disorders
Combination R:	Infants teething pains, to aid teeth
Combination S:	Sick headache, stomach upsets, biliousness

Each remedy is clearly marked with the indications for which it may be used. Before you start a course of Tissue Salts, please read the label and if your condition persists seek professional advice, because there may be an underlying cause to be diagnosed. *See Bibliography caption for Tissue Salt reading matter, which also gives list of ailments and the relevant Salts remedies.*

TOMATOES

The ever popular Tomato, which contains the powerful antioxidant carotenoid Lycopene, is one of our best foods. It is good whether raw, fried, grilled, in soups or stews, while research tells us it is even better when taken as puree, ketchup or as paste. It has been suggested that Lycopene is even more effective at fighting cancer than other vitamins and minerals. If with kidney stones avoid tomatoes. Lycopene is helpful for Prostate and Cardiovascular disease taken as 5mg supplement, which is the equivalent of 100ml of tomato paste.

TONGUE

Doctors, mothers and all who try to find the root cause of an ailment, myself included, frequently make the request: "Put out your tongue". It is a guide to the state of ones health.

- **Where there are pimples, blisters or sores the Tongue food or remedy is Vitamin B complex.**

Added to this can be:

- Blisters - Calc Phos
- Blisters on tip of Tongue - Nat Mur
- Tongue swollen - Calc Fluor

- Dry in morning - Kali Phos
- Pimples on Tongue especially the tip - Calc Phos.
- Ulcers - Silica, or may be due to gluten allergy

If Tongue is coated this usually relates to digestion, stomach or constipation and should be treated accordingly.

TONICS

Often one becomes run-down, feeling low, with little energy, perhaps with weak immune system. As a result the body is wide open to infection with little resistance. This is when a Tonic can work wonders. The health food shop can provide excellent, natural full of goodness sustenance, such as Floradix, Salusan, Comvita Propolis Herbal Elixir, Floravital or Biostrath. There is Kindervital for the young. They are available yeast and sugar-free if requested. These are pure and natural, all to be recommended, containing herbs, vitamins and minerals all of which lead to vitality and better well-being. 'Wonder of wonders' many pharmacies are now stocking many of these natural products. They ignored and decried everything natural until recent years, but now find that people have turned to non-chemical tonics and supplements, demanding them. *Turn to Nettle caption*, to read about the purely natural, extremely health giving, green tonic.

TOOTHPASTE AND THE BRUSHING OF TEETH

Under Skin caption I wrote of some of my experience in the skincare trade. This also concerns Toothpaste. With the exception of the small number of purely natural Toothpastes available, particularly from the health food shop, including those with Aloe Vera, there are little or none without added chemicals. If with 1% of natural ingredients they can be labelled '**natural**' - Yes 1%. *Toothpaste is one of the most hyped-up toiletry products. Many contain astringents, antiseptics, sugar, abrasives, fillers and other chemicals, with the majority having the toxic compound Fluoride added. This is certainly no aid to better health despite the propaganda about the hazardous industrial waste, which is Fluoride. Very little Toothpaste is natural, being just another money-spinner in the toiletry industry.* ***In a EU Directive, but indirectly, we have been warned of the dangers of Fluoride, where children under the age of two should not use Toothpaste containing the chemical. As a result of this, our health bureaucrats have now advertised that children must not use Toothpaste. No mention of the word Fluoride. They know of its dangers, but if the instructions were that children must not use Toothpaste containing Fluoride, this would be an admission of liability on their part. What an underhand way to deal with something so serious?*** *Adults too should be concerned, because there is a big question mark as to the Fluoride content added, with this also being investigated. Very much of these kind of problems, which are serious, are kept low*

key, with the user, the person most at risk, seldom if ever being informed.
It is a good idea to once weekly dip a wet toothbrush in bicarbonate of soda, then brushing the teeth to obtain a shiny white finish. Aloe Dent is a natural Toothpaste, one of the best available from the health food store. As the name signifies it contains Aloe Vera, which is very good for teeth, mouth cleansing and hygiene. A good toothbrush should have a small head so that it can easily be guided up, down and about the teeth. *It is not realised that the best time to brush teeth is before meals. This will remove the bacteria or plaque, which thrives on starches and sugars. There will then be no bacteria to start the teeth decay course of action.* There is a certain way to brush the teeth properly and next time you visit the dentist ask him to explain the correct procedure. **As set out, the health food store where everything is natural will have a variety of pure Toothpastes.** *Turn to Fluoride caption* to read of the deception, the scandal, how this harmful chemical is forced on us. *Also see the two captions Teeth and Gums.*

TRACE ELEMENTS
See Vitamins and Minerals Caption.

TRANSCENDENTAL MEDITATION
See Meditation Caption.

TRAVEL AND HOLIDAY HEALTH
If prone to Travel or motion sickness, don't worry, there are natural aids to help. Eat lightly before Travelling with just toast or a slice or two of wholemeal bread. Either sit up properly or lie down. Do not read. Avoid looking out to side. All this will help, but the main aid is Ginger. Take Ginger tablets or capsules half hour before journey and every 1-2 hours after. These are available from health food stores or some chemists. Culpeper travel sickness tablets are ginger-based and excellent. Avoid alcohol and smoking. If with fear of Travel take Bioforce Avena Sativa or Bach's Mimulus Remedy for fourteen days prior to Travel and on day of journey take Bach's Rescue Remedy. Milk Thistle Complex and Garlic capsule, taken for 14 days prior to and during holiday, help to guard against bacteria and stomach ailments, especially those so frequently picked up abroad. *Also see Insect Repellent and Deep Vein Thrombosis captions,* with relevant advice, to help one enjoy better Travel and Holiday Health.

TRIGEMINAL NEURALGIA
See Neuralgia Caption.

UDO'S CHOICE OIL

Most people have the false idea that all fats are to be avoided. This is not so. Doctor Udo Erasmus has become a world authority on fats, oils, cholesterol and human health. Also be grateful to this man for his pioneering work in relation to Essential Fatty Acids (E.F.A.'s). Natural, unrefined Udo's Choice Oil contains an ideal balance of the Essential Fatty Acids, Omega 3 (alpha – linolenic) and Omega 6 (linoleic). These E.F.A.'s are so called because they are essential to life itself. They cannot be created by the body and must be obtained through Diet. Refined hydrogenated oils such as in much of the cooking oils and margarines, which are processed, turn EFA's into harmful trans fatty acids. Studies show that most contemporary Western Diets are lacking in Omega 3. To compensate for this many consumers have turned to unrefined Flax Oil, high in Omega 3, but having the right balance between Omega 3 and Omega 6 is extremely important. *Too much of one will cause a deficiency of the other. Over the long term Flax Oil alone can lead to a shortage of Omega 6, just as Cod Liver Oil, which is high in the vital Omega 6 may lead to an uneven balance of Omegas 3 and 6. Udo's Choice Oil was developed to adjust the need for food oil that provides EFA's in the correct amounts.*

As with all discoveries, we find others jumping on the bandwagon, who are offering various blends of oils, but none apparently similar or equally good, apart from Organic Choice 3+6+9 Balanced Oil Blend of Fatty Acids. The 2:1 ratio of Omega 3, Omega 6, in Udo's Choice Ultimate Oil Blends, plus the other added nutrients, offer the solution to EFA needs, in a healthy balance. *We need more Essential Fatty Acids every day than any other necessary nutrient.* They help us attain energy, give stamina, aid kidneys, elevate mood, assist the brain, also where there are learning problems, dyslexia and hyperactivity. Heart, Circulation, Immune System, Skin, Hair and Nails also Digestive System all benefit from these essential fats. They are as antioxidants and anti-inflammatory agents, also helping to lower cholesterol. The huge amount of Udo's Oil and Organic Choice Blend Oils sold points to its almost limitless health-giving goodness. This is manifest, with those who use it acclaiming the properties for skin, stomach, digestion, mood and general well being. *See Bibliography* for details of books published on the subject. *Turn to Fat also Fatty Acids captions.*

U

ULCERS

Ulcers are caused by a multitude of things, which are foes of good health. All should be avoided including alcohol, smoking, stress, worry, over the counter drugs, tranquillizers and extremely hot food and drink. When some of these are combined with irregular meals and inferior Diet of additive-filled 'food' it can only lead to digestive, stomach and other ailment or disease. A weak immune system, which is brought about by inferior Diet and lack of nutrients leads to Ulcers. A big change of lifestyle is number one remedy. This includes change to pure natural unprocessed foods. To help correct the problem, small meals frequently at the outset, with little or no fibre or roughage are needed. Avoid spicy or hot foods. Do not drink with meals. *Milk puddings, gruel or porridge made with half milk and water also Slippery Elm drinks will help to heal the stomach lining.* Take Calamus, Aloe Vera or Udo's Choice Oil with Manuka Honey, which is a wonderful food and antibacterial medicine. These have proved to be excellent aids to recovery when combined with natural Diet also lifestyle change. Mastika has proved to be very good. All will help any stomach Ulcers. Milk and milk puddings are excellent, helping to renew the stomach lining.

For Peptic Ulcers take green vegetables, especially broccoli, and garlic. Drink copious amounts of pure water between meals. Water is an aid to clear peptic Ulcers and cannot be praised sufficiently. Supplement with Zinc tablet also Aloe Vera Gel. The aid of any remedy may not be a requirement if proper Diet is abided by. Other Ulcer remedies are:

- Tongue - *See Tongue caption*
- Mouth - *See Mouth caption*
- Varicose (Leg Ulcer) - Take Manuka honey internally also applying externally. It has antibacterial properties, being in many instances better than antibiotics. When applied externally smear over the open Ulcer. Try to leave the leg unbandaged. Cover loosely at night and apply more honey next morning. Treat for 3-4 mornings. A crust should form, with the leg healing within 21 days. At the same time take Echinacea tablets and Vitamins E and C. All are available from the health food store.

For any form of Ulcer *see DIET caption* to be informed further by the advice given.

UMBILICUS FUNGUS

Always thoroughly dry after bath or shower. Insert smear of Allergenics cream to avoid itchiness and discomfort. Acidophilus or Thursday Plantation Anti Fungal Gel, obtainable from the health food store, will help control or clear Fungal problems.

UPSET STOMACH

See Stomach Caption.

URINARY PROBLEMS

Many persistent Urinary problems have been eliminated by change of Diet to pure unprocessed natural foods. *Turn to DIET caption.* In some cases the need arises to avoid milk and dairy products because of allergy, with diagnosis having being missed out. *See Allergy caption.* All Urinary problems are helped by the intake of copious amounts of pure water. Drink eight to 10 glasses daily. Avoid that which is Fluoridated or with Chlorine. Do not allow the bladder to become too full. When taking certain vitamins or supplements the urine turns yellow or green. This is normal.

* Dribbling or leaking - *See stress incontinence caption.*
* Prostate gland problems - *See prostate caption.*
* Urinary problem due to kidney or cystitis infection - *See Kidneys or Cystitis captions.*
* Blood in Urine - *See your Doctor.*
* Dysuria - The underlying cause must be found and treated, according to what is diagnosed

For Urinary tract health take Zinc/Copper supplement and Kordel's Cranberry 10,000, which contains Uva Ursi and Buchu. This is a very good aid to relieve and eliminate pain and burning sensation associated with Urinary Infections. Drink pure unsweetened cranberry juice as sold by health food store. They specialise in the pure juice. Tinned cranberries are also good when liquidised with plain natural yoghurt.

Boldo is an excellent remedy for certain Urinary problems including cystitis.

U

URTICARIA

See Hives Caption.

VACCINATION & VACCINES

At the outset let it be stated that the inoculation against Meningitis C has proved highly successful, which is excellent news. Joined with this are smallpox and diphtheria jabs, which have also been wonderful preventatives. With other Vaccines there is a huge question mark, including the controversial Mumps Measles Rubella (MMR). Many answers are being sought. *Why are we now told that measles is a deadly disease?* Could it be that children's immune systems and resistance to disease have been endangered because of the overuse of antibiotics, synthetic pills and medicines, from before, at time of and after birth? Can all doctors honestly say that inoculation will only be given if the child is in good health, being with strong immune system and able to absorb 3 in 1 vaccine? *When I was a child, measles was just another form of illness. Few died as a result. We had little if any medication. Then all placed complete trust in the medical profession. Sad to relate this cannot be said now.* If a parent wishes to have one or other of MMR Vaccines surely this will be much easier for the child to absorb. As regards flu vaccination I am told by doctor friends that it is about 25% effective, while the health authorities say 40%. As with many medicines, who knows the long-term consequences of their use? I'm not suggesting that Vaccines are unnecessary, but relying on so-called miracle remedies has not led to good health. *As verbosely repeated, in these writings, there needs to be a vast reassessment of the gross over-prescribing of drugs, including vaccines. Moreover serious thought must be given to, and questions asked, 'Why the need for all this medication, considering it was not required in the past?'* Much of today's rampant illness can be put down to over-prescribing, easily obtained and used, synthetic, so-called medicines. Throughout this Encyclopedia I have advocated and repeated, I hope not overly much so, the basic principles of good health, *'With pure food being the medicine and medicine being pure food'.* Combined with exercise, drinking plenty of pure water, and a good sleep pattern, there comes strength, energy and better health to prevent and fight disease. *Turn to DIET, Exercise and Sleep captions.* Where there has been reaction brought on by Vaccination or antibiotics a visit to a homeopathic doctor will help solve the problems through use of natural antidote. *Also see Antibiotics caption.*

VAGINAL DRYNESS

Black Cohosh is a natural remedy. I have no hesitation in recommending KY Jelly, obtainable from the pharmacy.

VAGINAL THRUSH

See Thrush Caption.

VAGINITIS

Often caused by use of certain brands of tampons, therefore a change to better quality is suggested. This is an ailment, which is also due to either inferior Diet or poor hygiene. *See DIET caption* which includes advice about Vitamins and Minerals, all to help restore to better health and freedom from ailments such as Vaginitis. *If due to the menopause see that caption.* Take Agnus Castus, Black Cohosh or if with smelly discharge take Pulsatilla or Echinacea.

VALERIAN

This non-addictive, purely natural, good relaxant and sedative, is one of nature's greatest aids to calm. It is excellent if trying to withdraw from dependence on chemical medicines such as the harmful Valium, Librium or similar addictive drugs, including sleeping tablets. Valerian must not be taken with orthodox medicines or alcohol. Addictive drugs or alcohol can harm the systems and also kill the natural Valerian.

VARICOSE ULCER

See Ulcers Caption.

VARICOSE VEINS

Can be controlled to the point where they are insignificant. Strengthening of the veins, proper cholesterol level, better circulation and normalising of blood pressure, all lead to better health and well being, with veins giving little if any trouble. *All of this can come from the advice set out under Blood Pressure High caption.* Kordel's Horse Chestnut and Butchers Broom Complex are good for control of venous problems. Bilberries, pure Bilberry juice or Bilberry tablets or capsules are excellent aids for the veins also helping to improve circulation. *If with Varicose Ulcers turn to Ulcers caption.*

VEGAN DIET

Vegan Diet excludes meat, fish and other protein foods, which vegetarians sometimes use, also excluding eggs, dairy products and honey. Asthma, Rheumatoid Arthritis, and those with heart and circulation problems have been treated successfully by adhering to this Diet. For those who wish to follow this health-giving path they can be called the supreme Vegetarian. There are certain things, which the partaker should learn before taking up this Diet. *See Vegetarian caption* regarding danger of Vitamin B 12 deficiency, which can be overcome by partaking of the Vitamin as a supplement. Vegans are advised to take Quinoa either sprouted or cooked. This contains much natural protein, especially when sprouted.

VEGETARIAN

Many have turned away from meat because of the scandals about Mad Cow Disease (BSE), when the processors were foolish enough to allow offal into the bovine food chain, despite being warned of the consequences. There have been other instances, like the addition of angel dust or the over use of many animal medicines. Vegetarianism is a healthy way of living with very much in its favour. It is not just a case of giving up meat, because plans for future foods needed should be made regarding varied Diet, in order to obtain the Vitamins, Minerals and other nutritives so necessary. It is not usually known to those taking up a meat free Diet, of the need for Vitamin B 12, available from the health food store in supplement form. Lack of this Vitamin can lead to pernicious anaemia, which can only be treated by constant injection of the Vitamin. Some become Vegetarians because of animal concerns, many do so with little thought given to the discipline needed, while others do it for cultural reasons. All must be aware that it takes a wide range or variety of pure unprocessed natural foods to replace the nutrients found in meat, fish or other foods, which are being avoided. It is advisable to include in the Diet, supplements containing Zinc, Calcium, Vitamins C and D, Iron and especially Vitamin B 12 as already mentioned. Limit the intake of fats and replace with Udo's Choice Oil, which gives the required Essential Fatty Acids. Sprouted Quinoa is high in natural protein, being better than that which is obtained from meat. *Turn to DIET caption,* leaving out meat, fish, eggs or whatever you wish.

VEGETABLES

See Fruit and Vegetables Caption.

VEIN THROMBOSIS – DEEP (DVT)

See Deep Vein Thrombosis Caption.

VEINS – Thread

Take Vitamins A, C & E to strengthen the veins and so help eliminate the thin thread like marks. *Following the advice given in Blood Pressure High caption will help immensely.*

VERTIGO

This spinning sensation is not to be confused with dizziness. There is a tendency to fall sideways, sometimes feeling sick or disorientated. Can be brought on by Meniere's disease, ear problems, blood pressure, migraine or exceptional emotion or stress. If possible treat the cause, which may be any of above. *See DIET caption* because this is the best medicine available and can lead to return to better health and elimination of Vertigo. Iridology has led to diagnosis and resultant successful treatment. Take Ginger capsules or tablets with food, also Biostrath tonic, both obtainable from the health food store.

VERRUCAE

They are contagious, being picked up mostly in community-shared showers, swimming pools and cubicles, in which others have walked and where flip flops should be worn. *See Warts caption* and treat similarly.

VINEGAR

See Cider Vinegar and Honey captions.

VIRILITY

See Sex Drive. (Lack of) caption.

VIRUS

This is the 'I don't know' answer for illness, when something is undiagnosable. How can one prescribe for a virus without knowing the cause? A friend brought an infected garden plant to the garden centre. They told her it was a virus, but she was not convinced, replying: "I have a friend who is a doctor and he says that when doctors say you have a virus it means your guess is as good as theirs". It would be fair to all that if instead of suggesting a virus one be told "I don't know". Prescribing certain medicines, especially antibiotics, for what is called a Virus, can be extremely dangerous.

V

VITALITY

Without Vitality there is this depressed and drained feeling. A good many who are being treated psychologically and physically are not in need of chemical or synthetic medicine. Physicians, psychologists and many in the home fail to recognise that those who feel as if without energy are often suffering because of complications brought on by poor nutrition, lifestyle, including lack of exercise, or if with bad sleep pattern. One of our big ailments is that of low blood sugar count, which is controlled mostly by proper nutrition and resolving the problems mentioned.

Being anaemic is very often the cause of lethargy, tiredness or lack of vitality. A blood test will give an immediate answer. How many know about or even give this a thought. Here is one of the chief causes of depression, tiredness and feeling low, all of which means a lack of Vitality. Like most of the health problems we have today pure additive-free food is the medicine, aided by exercise and proper rest. It is our greatest remedy. *Turn to DIET, Exercise and Sleep captions* to be guided as to how to help regain energy, reasonable good health and Vitality. *The DIET caption* also gives valuable information about energy giving Vitamins, Minerals and Supplements. *Turn to Fatigue also Lethargy and Tiredness captions.*

VITAMINS, MINERALS AND FOOD SUPPLEMENTS

Less than a century ago, little was known about this subject. There was not the same need for them. Our food was pure and natural, none factory-made. Every day medical science is discovering more about what herbalists, the natural health practitioners, also those living by these rules, knew many, many years ago.

Much of the foods and drinks we are offered are lacking in nutritives, with many of them containing a mixture of the over 5,000 substances which are added to the highly processed products. Combinations of these, very often taken with chemical medicines or pills, make us a sick nation To be aware of this and for excellent advice about natural unadulterated, unprocessed foods, *turn to and read under Diet caption.* **Frequently we read of doctors saying that there is no need for Vitamins, Minerals or Food Supplements because there is sufficient in the Diet. It is foolish to make such absurd suggestions, because all should be aware that our factory-made 'food' is often not FOOD. Most doctors, like the majority of their patients, do not realise what is in much of the foodless 'food' consumed. Properly balanced Diet is impossible, unless we are prepared to be extremely diligent and careful, in what is chosen.**

There is no doubting the fact that Vitamins, Minerals and Food Supplements can be panacea, remedy or invaluable aid to illness, better health or prevention of illness. Most of our present-day health problems are referred to in this Encyclopedia, with the remedies being given. *No apologies are made for the recurring theme of natural Diet, which is our best medicine.*

Don't be alarmed or put off by the seemingly large amount of Vitamins, Minerals and Food Supplements which are displayed on the shelves or written about. This subject is easily understood. In this simple Guide, I have tried to make it just that - SIMPLE. Very often a Multivitamin or Tonic as described under the relevant captions is sufficient.

Many books, which cover natural remedies, health or associated subjects, are available from the library, health food shops or bookshops. The library usually has a very varied selection on Natural Health. All those outlined in the Bibliography section have been chosen specially because of their excellence, health wise.

Some people have the idea that by taking Vitamins, Minerals or Food Supplements with junk and processed foods, the deficiency or health problems will easily be solved. They may help, with this being debatable, but certainly nowhere near the extent of doing so when eating pure natural additive free foods.

Vitamins, Minerals and Food Supplements should not be taken if there is a danger of overtaxing the body, including the stomach. This can happen, with them being of little use, where there is extreme illness, if on an inferior Diet or if taking an amount of chemical drugs or medicines.

Although this Encyclopedia gives much advice about the use of natural remedies, including food supplements, there may be some who require further help and guidance. If in doubt ask a homeopathic doctor, nutritionist, or be advised by the health food store personnel, who are extremely knowledgeable. I have found some pharmacists who have been very helpful about natural and herbal remedies.

The all too obvious 'Pills For All Ills' line of thought does not apply to Natural Vitamins, Minerals and Supplements. When using these take what is absolutely necessary, no more.

IN MANY INSTANCES WHERE THERE IS ILLNESS OR IF FEELING UNWELL,
A SIMPLE CHANGE TO NATURAL FOOD AND DRINKS CAN BE EXCELLENT
MEDICINE AND MAY NOT NECESSITATE THE USE OF SUPPLEMENTS

Here Is A Guide To Vitamins, Minerals And Other Supplements.

VITAMINS	
PRINCIPAL FOOD SOURCE	**MAJOR BODY FUNCTIONS**
VITAMIN A	
• green and yellow vegetables (spinach, cabbage, carrots) • also broccoli • eggs • fish oil • liver	• night vision • bone growth and health • healthy skin and eyes • sexual functioning and reproduction • anti anaemic function • protects against infection • anti-oxidant • anti-ageing
THIAMIN (B1)	
• whole cereal grains • liver • fresh green vegetables • potatoes • brewer's yeast • wheat germ	• converting glucose to energy in muscles and nerves.• body growth • carbohydrate metabolism • nervous system • appetite
RIBOFLAVIN (B2)	
• Brewer's yeast • wheat germ • eggs • green leafy vegetables • peas • green beans • liver	• healthy skin, eyes, hair, nails and liver • converts protein, fats and sugars to energy

PRINCIPAL FOOD SOURCE	MAJOR BODY FUNCTIONS
NIACIN (B3)	
• yeast • liver, kidney • chicken • fish • wheat germ • nuts • soya beans • brewer's yeast • Diabetes, Low Blood Pressure, Liver problems, Gout or Ulcers can all be irritated by over use of Niacin	• synthesis of fatty acids and steroids including sex hormones • health of nerves and digestive system • skin and tongue • co-enzyme for fat-soluble vitamins • involved in function of thyroid and insulin production.
VITAMIN B6	
• liver • lean meats • fish • whole grains • walnuts • sunflower seeds • buckwheat • soya beans • wheat germ • bananas	• fat metabolism • hormone production (adrenaline and insulin) • immune system health • healthy nervous system • skin health • brain aid • formation of haemoglobin
VITAMIN B 12	
• wheat germ • liver • milk • eggs • meat • cheese	• red blood cell formation • healthy nervous system required for normal growth • carbohydrate metabolism • female reproduction process (including foetal health) • bone marrow health • skin condition
B Complex	
This contains all of the B Vitamins also choline, insositol, pangamic acid, folic acid and biotin	
FOLIC ACID	
• liver • wheat bran • asparagus • green vegetables • kale • spinach • turnips	red blood cell formation • healthy nervous system • needed for normal growth • carbohydrate metabolism • female reproductive process (including foetal health) • healthy tissue • digestive system
BIOTIN	
• yeast • liver • eggs • whole grains • nuts • fish • brewer's yeast • wheat germ	metabolism of proteins, carbohydrates, unsaturated fatty acids. needed for normal growth • maintenance of skin, hair, nerves, sex glands, sebaceous glands, bone marrow
PANTOTHENIC ACID (B5)	
• Liver • kidney • brewer's yeast • sunflower seeds • buckwheat flour	• adrenal gland function • immune system • gastro intestinal tract function • carbohydrate and fat metabolism • energy production • health of skin and hair • healthy nervous system

PRINCIPAL FOOD SOURCE	MAJOR BODY FUNCTIONS
VITAMIN C	
• citrus fruits • rose hips • green peppers • broccoli • spinach • tomatoes • berries	• antioxidant and free radical scavenger • repair and healing of wounds and bones • tooth, bone, cartilage, skin and gums health • enhances iron absorption • mental health • immune system • helps maintain normal cholesterol levels
VITAMIN D	
• cod liver oil • halibut liver oil • milk • tuna	• calcium and phosphorus metabolism • bone health and growth • assists assimilation of vitamin A • aids thyroid gland • combines with calcium and magnesium
VITAMIN E	
• green leafy vegetables(cabbage, spinach, asparagus, broccoli, etc) • whole grains • safflower oil • wheat germ • vegetable oil **Vitamin E must not be taken within four hours of taking Iron or Calcium supplement. For easy absorption of Vitamin E within the system it is recommended that 100iu be taken for 30 days, then 200iu for 30 days, then 400iu or 500iu continuously.**	• antioxidant • nervous system and red blood cell health • protects Vitamins A and C from oxidative destruction • acts synergistically with selenium • normal blood clotting and health of small blood vessels • stimulates development and tone of muscles, including heart • maintains cell membrane stability
VITAMIN F	
• grains • nuts • seeds • lecithin granules • Udo's Choice Oil can be regarded as Vitamin F also Organic Choice 3+6+9	• composed of fatty acids • linoleic acid (LA) • alpha linolenic acid (LNA) • leads to hormone levels balance • immune and cell membrane health • body growth • anti ageing • brain and mind health
VITAMIN K	
• green leaf vegetables • soya beans • nuts • cheese • liver	• strong bones including joints and cartilages • teeth • normal blood clotting

NUTRIENTS

CO ENZYME Q10	
	• heart • circulation • gum disease • brain health • fatigue problems • anti ageing
CHOLINE	
• Brewer's yeast • fish • soya beans • liver	• nervous system function • liver, kidney and gall bladder function • immune system strength

V

PRINCIPAL FOOD SOURCE	MAJOR BODY FUNCTIONS
INOSITOL	
• bulgar wheat • brown rice • brewer's yeast • molasses	• prevents accumulation of fats in the liver • involved in control of blood cholesterol levels • helps maintain healthy hair
PABA	
• liver • eggs • molasses • brewer's yeast • wheat germ	• used by intestinal bacteria to produce their folic acid • skin and hair health • pain relief
BIOFLAVONIDS	
• citrus fruit • stoned fruit • rosehips • buckwheat • acerola	• antioxidant • proper absorption of vitamin C • maintenance of capillary strength • immune system strength

MINERALS

PRINCIPAL FOOD SOURCE	MAJOR BODY FUNCTIONS
CHROMIUM	
• shell fish • eggs • molasses • dairy products	• helps regulate blood sugar levels • helps insulin output • controls blood cholesterol
COPPER	
• liver • fish • green vegetables	• absorption and utilisation of iron and zinc • production of haemoglobin • formation of red blood cells • helps immune system
IRON	
• liver • red meat • egg yolk • raisins • molasses • whole grains • dried apricots	• transport of oxygen to tissues and release of energy from food • utilisation of oxygen • skin and hair pigmentation • normal nerve function • aids immune system • Must not be taken within four hours of taking Vitamin E
MAGNESIUM	
• milk • beans and peas • nuts • wheat germ • green vegetables	• activity of enzymes related to protein • production and nucleic acid • normal function of nerves and muscular system • arterial function • regulates blood pH • repair and maintenance of body cells • works in combination with Calcium and vitamin D.

PRINCIPAL FOOD SOURCE	MAJOR BODY FUNCTIONS
MANGANESE	
• whole grain cereals • egg yolks • green vegetables • tea • nuts • olives • oat flakes	• health of joints • female sex hormones • reproductive function • co-factor for vitamins B, C and E • healthy nervous system • connective tissue, ligaments and tendons
MOLYBDENUM	
• vegetables • wheat germ • liver	• balances body fluids • muscle tone and function • healthy nervous system
PHOSPHORUS	
• milk • cheese • eggs • cereals • meat • **Phosphorus is found in most foods.**	• normal bone and tooth structure • works with calcium and vitamin D • constituent of B complex co-enzymes • utilisation of carbohydrates, fats and proteins.
POTASSIUM	
• fresh fruit • vegetables • fish • meat	• balances body fluids • muscle tone and functions • healthy nervous system
SELENIUM	
• greens • beans and peas • whole grains and cereals • sea food • meat • nuts	• works synergistically with vitamin E as antioxidant and free radical scavenger • maintenance of heart function and circulatory system • protects against toxic minerals • healthy eyes, hair and skin • protects against body toxins • normal liver function • male reproduction capacity • anti inflammatory • immune system health
ZINC	
• sea food • kelp • mushrooms • pumpkin seeds • sunflower seeds • liver • wheat germ	• sense of taste and smell • male and female reproductive processes. • metabolism of pituitary, adrenal, ovaries and testes • normal prostate function • healing of wounds • skin and hair protein • health of bones and joints • Works in conjunction with copper which activates Zinc.
CALCIUM	
• dairy products • whole wheat flour • vegetables	• growth and maintenance of bones and teeth • normal blood clotting • muscle contraction • must be combined with magnesium

V

In this Encyclopedia many seek advice about better health, including **Peace Of Mind**. Any person who is not in close relationship with their God, their Creator, is missing out on much. The affinity, which many search for, often not knowing what they seek, is a tremendous asset in one's daily life. Imagine saying a prayer, talking with God first thing in the morning. Imagine saying: "O Dear God, I transfer my worries". Think of the Army General at the outset of battle as he said: "Lord God if I forget you this day do not thou forget me". The presence of God and indeed many things in life, are a mystery.

VITILIGO

White patches of depigmented skin are often normalised by change of Diet to pure natural foods. *Turn to DIET caption*. At the same time avoid foods, which you may be allergic to. These can include glutenous foods, dairy products, citrus fruit, coffee or chocolate. *See Allergy caption*. Take a Multivitamin, which contains Folic Acid, Vitamins B Complex, C, and E, with 30mgs supplement of Zinc to be taken each night for 10 weeks. Udo's Choice Oil is also recommended to help remove Vitiligo.

VOGEL Dr.

Dr Alfred Vogel (1902-1996) founded Bioforce who now produce an amount of natural health remedies which bring relief to so many in the present era. He was the modern Culpeper and Gerard who were such great herbalists. A Swiss naturopath, lecturer, author, herbalist and natural health giant, Dr. Vogel was responsible for a big awakening of the good of herbal medicine. Phytotherapy, as practised by Bioforce, one of the most important firms in herbal research, is proving to be of inestimable value as we search for better health. Should you wish to learn more about phytotherapy or this marvellous man *see Bibliography caption* for details of his natural health and healing book 'The Nature Doctor'.

VOMITING

See Nausea Caption.

VULVA – INFLAMED

Take Agnus Castus and Combination B New Era.
Change to balanced Diet to include natural additive-free food, fibre, fruit and vegetables combined with exercise. *Turn to DIET, Exercise and Sleep captions.*

WALKING

To attain better health, exercise is a must. One cannot ignore this advice if wishing to feel reasonably good. Before taking any kind of exercise consideration must be given to state of health, including physical mobility. Your medical advisor must be spoken to if with any health problem, which could be affected by exercise such as Walking - whether strenuous or otherwise.

By reading about Walking there is something to be learned. The retort might be: **"What is there to be known or learned about Walking?"** Read on and be surprised! Only a few years ago I would have ridiculed such an idea, on being told to read about Walking. Always being extremely active, believing that vigorous, intensive workout was necessary to maintain physical fitness, I have found this is not so. *Taking exercise now and again, not regularly, was a failing. Better little and often than trying to cram an amount in spasmodically.* Like that of all-too-many, the belief was, that in my daily duties, moving about, saying as housewives do: 'Don't I get sufficient exercise in what I do?' asking and answering the question at the same time, I was wrong.

In the UK the heart rehabilitation classes, where the nurses and physiotherapists endeavour to put heart patients who are convalescing on the road to recovery, are teaching the value of exercise, with much emphasis on Walking. Under their guidance, after use of the treadmill, those whom they have within their care gradually gain confidence in their ability to regain strength, leading to better health.

The advice given here on the simple exercise of Walking, when put into practice, can give much enjoyment.

A healthy walking session should last at least twenty minutes or longer, if able to do so. Break each session into three distinct parts - Warm up, Workout and Cool down. **Warm Up**. Walk slowly for five minutes. Gently loosen your joints as you walk, working from the feet up. Rotate or shake out you ankles, knees, hips, shoulders and elbows. Rotate your neck gently. Shrug your shoulders and shake out your hands. The warm up affects your heart, lungs, muscles and joints to prepare them for the next phase of your session.

W

Work Out. This phase should be at least 10 minutes to as long as you wish to enjoy yourself, depending on your level of fitness. Gradually increase your Walking pace until your heart is beating a bit faster (but not racing), you are breathing a little deeper and faster (but not out of breath), and are perspiring a little (but not sweating profusely). ***Stop Walking if you experience any unusual symptoms such as chest pain, dizziness or breathlessness.*** You gain most benefit by Walking at a pace where you are challenged but not overly uncomfortable, with some part of the route having an incline if possible.

Cool Down. Another five-minute phase. Gradually ease your Walking speed back down to a slow pace. Gently shake out and loosen all your joints again and do three full body stretches, reaching your arms up, holding each stretch for 10 seconds. As your level of fitness increases you can lengthen the period of time spent Walking for as long as you feel comfortable. Divide your Walk, whereby you warm and cool over two five minute periods, at the beginning and end of each session.

Some words of advice are offered regarding the need to wear clothing and footwear appropriate to the type of weather, time of year, and surroundings or terrain being traversed. It is important to keep warm, including the important area of the body - the head – the area of the body from where the most heat is usually lost. Keep the feet dry and wear comfortable footwear. Plastic trainers are not recommended.

Layers of light clothing are better than a combination of heavy items. Often Walkers, joggers, or those training for athletics and ball games can be seen in clothes and footwear most inappropriate for the weather conditions. This must take largely from the enjoyment. Purchasing a lightweight, breathable jacket and over-trousers means that the weather will not deter one from exercising. It is not realised that one of the main reasons for aerobic exercise such as Walking, to improve muscle condition, circulation and well being, is to reach the point of perspiring for full benefit. This need not be uncomfortable. *Keeping the heat in whether in the gym or in the open air is of primary importance, as the bodily warmth is used to help the circulation, joints and muscles, also in the release of toxic emotions, which affect our well being.*

A dog as a walking companion is like further therapy. *Read about this under Dog caption.* Another interesting thing to carry when walking is a Pedometer. Clip it to the belt and read off the kilos, miles or steps. If possible increase the number of steps daily, to reach better fitness and to help control weight. A Pedometer can be as a companion. Any sports shop will supply or order.

Enjoy yourself Walking to better health. It costs nothing, giving enjoyment to those willing and able to do so. Go at your own pace, do your own thing, set your own target. I used spend approximately 15 minutes walking when unwell but can now traverse many miles, spending many happy hours outdoors. Here it must be mentioned that I was cajoled into purchasing and carrying a mobile phone. This because of the experience of one man who, when walking in the forest, suffered a heart attack. His phone saved his life. *Part of this article on walking is reprinted with the kind permission of the Editor of that wonderful publication:* '**St Martin Magazine**', *42 Parnell Square, Dublin 1, to whom I am sure many will be grateful for the helpful advice.* Consumers Choice, **publishers of Walkways,** compiled this. *See Bibliography regarding both publications.*

WARTS

Apply one or two drops of Thuja Tincture or use Thuja ointment, gently rubbing in twice daily until cleared. I have found this to be the best remedy. In a few instances where the warts proved stubborn the Thuja was also taken internally, with success. Tea Tree Oil diluted has removed the unsightly warts but it takes some time. Verrcuae to be treated similarly, covering with bandage or sterilised plaster.

WASP STINGS

See Stings Caption.

WATER

Pure Water is to the body both drink and food, playing a vital role within all our systems.

Good Water, which was freely available, certainly cheap, has always been taken as a right for all. Sadly, like much which we took for granted in the past, it has been negligently interfered with by all too many, including those who have turned it into a money-making business at the expense of the user, to whom it was once free and pure. Our legislators have dictatorially forced on us the use of the toxic chemical Fluoride in drinking Water, with Ireland the biggest culprits, having made it mandatory as an additive. It is also being forced on the people of the UK, many of whom have stood up to the bureaucrats and said: 'No', so that only a little over 10% of the Water is Fluoridated. Over 90% of the rest of Europe have also said: 'No'. .

There is much more pollution of Water, including the use of Chlorine, but it is not my aim to highlight more here than has been written.

All need to be vigilant and to fight for pure Water, which is our right. We rely on Water for our bodies to function properly. *Research shows that only one in six people drink more than four glasses daily. We need eight glasses or more each day according to the World Health Organisation (WHO).* In warm weather we need more. It must be pure and free from the chemicals and toxins which tests show much of our Water contains.

Often one is actually thirsty when feeling hungry. This often occurs in hot working conditions or if overtired. *Those who wish to keep trim, not carrying extra weight, should bear this in mind. All should learn to drink Water, not just when thirsty, b throughout the day.* Dehydration is not recognised for what it is. One can be so without noticing the problem. This leads to ill health, as drinking copious amounts of pure Water acts as a detoxifier to kidneys, liver, the mucous membranes and other parts of the body. Avoid carbonated or caffeinated drinks, as they lead to osteoporosis, arthritis, urinary problems, indigestion and other illness. *Turn to Fizzy Drinks caption. THINK PURE, DRINK PURE.* A glass of tepid Water first thing in the morning acts like a cleanser on the stomach and body. Adding two teaspoons of each Cider Vinegar and Pure natural Honey makes an even better tonic or natural medicine.

Drinking Water is like an internal balm. It is as a stimulant. Without it our insides would be like a stagnant pool. Many think that alcohol is a thirst-quencher. It may be short-term, but if one is dehydrated the alcohol will do more harm than good. Drinking Water to quench thirst and avoid dehydration does much good and is as natural medicine. All children and teenagers, especially those at school and college, should be taught of the need to drink ample pure Water regularly, even when not required, also of the dangers of fizzy 'drinks' and alcohol. A bottle or container of pure Water should always be at hand for all. Because we cannot trust the Water suppliers, or be certain of its purity, bottled Water is bought in quantity. Some of this is of doubtful origin and may not even be as good as tap Water. Many of the Water filter jugs or other forms of filtration or processing, do little more that remove slight impurities. There is a twin filter system available, which provides purely pure Water, free from Fluoride and Chlorine. It is supplied by Simply Water Ltd. PO Box 164, FREE POST, Liverpool L15 4PU, UK or at Environment House, Brighton Green, Dublin 6. Or you can e-mail at info@simplywater.com or web, www.simplywater.com I hold no brief for Simply Water, only stating that what they supplied me with, also others to whom it was recommended, gives excellent Water, which has passed all tests successfully. Using the system can save much money, as well as providing pure Water, which as mentioned can be as medicine or food. *See Bibliography* for details of the excellent book: **'Your Body's Many Cries For Water'**. This is one of the most informative books ever. *Turn to Fluoride, also Chlorine captions.*

WATERCRESS

Another of nature's green gifts to all. The goodness of this herbal plant is little recognised. An excellent food, when grown under natural conditions. It is an extremely good source of Vitamins A and C, also Folic Acid. Contains Iodine, Calcium, Manganese and Iron. It is a good blood tonic. Take with salads or in sandwich form.

WATER RETENTION

This is a familiar complaint, which can be serious if caused by kidney or heart conditions. If combined with the latter it is often referred to as dropsy. Fluid Retention usually flares up, and is a fairly common ailment before and at time of menstruation, when ankles, feet and fingers become swollen, and the eyes may appear puffed. Fluid Retention can also affect men. It can be as a result of kidney, liver, heart or thyroid disorders, also if with diabetes or constipation. Medical advice should be sought to find and treat the problem if serious.

Hormonal imbalances at time of menstruation or being over-weight are the general reasons for Water Retention. As with much niggling ailment the root cause frequently is inferior Diet. Changing to natural additive-free nutrition, including supplements as suggested in DIET caption, has eliminated the problem and at the same time various other persistent complaints, helping to make menstruation carefree, and to lose weight. Drink four litres or more of water daily. Take exercise. The Diet will advise regarding avoidance of coffee and alcohol, also for the need to reduce salt intake and other things, which do not help. Aesculus (Horse Chestnut), Boldo, Waterfall, Agnus Castus, Potassium or a combination of some of these, also taking Vitamin B complex are all aids. They are listed in order of my preference. Drink Dandelion Root Tea, also using when in season fresh Dandelion leaves, mixed with salads. Dandelion, often regarded as a weed, is a safe, tried and trusted remedy, which has proved wonderful to remove excess Water from the system. A French remedy - and an excellent diuretic - which helps clear Fluid Retention, is to juice or liquidise a small bunch of watercress, then wash, chop and add three small carrots, three sticks of celery, some parsley and one apple to be taken as one or two servings when pureed. The health food store can supply Dandelion Leaf in Tincture form or as Tea, also any remedies mentioned here. *Turn to DIET and Exercise captions* which, when combined, can lead to better health including the problem of Water Retention.

WEEPING EASILY

If feeling weepy, sorry for oneself, or sensitive, take Pulsatilla or Bach Remedies Gorse or Rescue Remedy. They serve many purposes. *See Pulsatilla, also Bach Remedy captions.*

WELEDA

Weleda are well-known producers of homeopathic remedies, including Schüessler Tissue Salts, also an excellent range of natural body care creations, available at health food shops and some pharmacists. They have a very good reputation and their products are highly recommended.

WEIGHT PROBLEMS

See Slimming & Dieting Captions.

WETTING BED

See Bed Wetting Caption.

WHEAT FREE DIET

See Coeliac Caption.

WHITLOW

See Paronchyia Caption.

WHOLE FOODS

Whole foods are wholly natural, faultless, good, untainted, untreated, with none of the goodness removed. Little of what we are offered off the supermarket shelves is left unprocessed, therefore many have turned to the Whole Food or Health Food store for natural nutrition. Their personnel will provide answers to your questions regarding natural foods, which are wholesome. There will be no need to look at the ingredients labels when you examine their large range of all that is natural. The range of Meridian delicacies offered are an example of the kind of foods referred to.

WIND ON STOMACH

See Flatulence Caption.

WINE

Alcohol is an enemy of good health, best done without. Certain red Wines may be the exception. The type of grape, which has been used to make Wine, could be health giving. Antioxidants are in abundance in the skin of the grape, especially those used for making red Wines.

In recent years much research has been done, with high indication that red Wine may be good for certain health problems. We are reliably informed that there is indication that it can reduce the risk of heart attack, delay onset of Alzheimer's, slow the incidence of blood clots and may help to prevent cancer.

Many years ago I learned from an old herbalist of its goodness in the prevention or elimination of fungal attacks.

Chilean and Californian Merlot are high in antioxidants, also levels of tannins that boost circulation, and phenolic compounds that prevent clots. One glass daily is sufficient, certainly no more than two. Do not take alcohol, including Wine, with medicines or natural remedies.

WINTER BLUES

See SADS Caption.

WINTER ILLS

These are many and varied, being brought on by cold, damp and depressive-like weather. Safeguards against Winter Illness are proper intake of nutritive foods. *Turn to DIET caption.* Drink plenty of water, which we are not inclined to do in Wintertime. It is as medicine. Many do not realise the need for body warmth as they proceed from late Autumn into Winter, often clad scantily and wearing unsuitable clothes or footwear. *See caption on Body Warmth.* Echinaceaforce is one of the best natural Winter Ills safeguards ever formulated. It has proved to be a good health-giving remedy, also an excellent preventive of colds and 'flu. Because it is natural and with little advertising exposure, its use to replace the 'flu vaccination is little known. A further guard against Winter Illness is to take a tonic such as Floradix, Floravital, Biostrath or Salusan, alternated with a good Multivitamin supplement. Fortified with natural food and aided by one of the tonics suggested, makes for better all-round health and the strength to fight Winter Ills.

WOMEN'S HEALTH

While this Encyclopedia has been aimed at simple, natural remedies for all, it has to be said that if our Women folk did not care or worry about the health of all, we would be a much sicker nation. We know that all children must be guided towards what is best, but most men can seldom be led, driven or guided. They just want to do their own thing, all-too-often failing to accept advice about health or lifestyle. There is much advice for all in this Guide especially about Women's Health and I trust that all will benefit, including the caring women. Agnus Castus is probably a Woman's greatest friend, especially at menstruation or menopause time. Bio force, Quest, Optima, Solgar, Bio Health, Weleda, Gerard House, Lifeplan, Lanes, Vitabiotics, Natures Own, Hofels, New Era, Potters and Synergy are leading names in the world of natural medicines, all of which provide much which is good for Women's Health. Visit the health food store and you will be impressed by their knowledge and understanding. *'Think Natural, Eat Natural and Enjoy Better Health'.*

WORMS

Worms can be difficult to eliminate from the body, especially Round Worms. Garlic is the best remedy, which when taken with Caster Oil and Molasses seldom fails to remove the parasites. Take Garlic raw or in capsule form for seven days, then mix together and take two dessertspoonfuls of Caster Oil with one dessertspoonful of Molasses, each day for two days. This may have to be repeated for some weeks where round Worms are the problem.

WORRY

This is a form of stress almost always brought on by what often turns out later to be trivialities. No sooner is one worrying thing out of the way than another comes along. It is as if they are queuing up to enter the mind. Why allow them in? Because many love worries, they would not be without them. Worry is pointless. It destroys happiness, fuels ill health, and gets one nowhere. Most worriers seem to imagine the worst when thinking about family or friends. I was an inveterate worrier but learned many years ago to keep a diary, which included writing down of worries, problems, things to be done including those pressing. Next morning, immediately after breakfast, one of my first duties is to transfer what had appeared to be the important things of yesterday, the things left undone. The majority are usually trivialities, with the realisation that they were petty and unimportant, with no need to carry them forward. It took time to learn that it was a good idea not to worry. Just busying oneself with the things immediate, is the best way to forget this mindless existence. I aimed for better health, as suggested in this Encyclopedia. Better health of mind and body ensured that all brooding and fretting was shrugged off. Throughout this Guide I have repeatedly set out that if with reasonable health, then cares and worries can be cast aside or carried lightly. *Turn to DIET caption* to read of how to have better health of mind and body, with the ability to attain peace of mind.

WRITING

Writing is a powerful healer. The magic of conversation, just talking to each other, has disappeared for many since the advent of Television. Entering a home, seeing the goggle box turned on, with the resident trying to keep one eye on the visitor and the other on the television screen, is more than discouraging - it is downright bad manners. Far better either reach for the off button, or ask the visitor to leave. The art of letter Writing between friends and relatives has almost been abandoned. It is stimulating to receive a newsy letter, written as if it were the spoken word, as used in conversation, with no journalistic or other jargon – just written in simple form. It is as natural therapy to the writer, being even more so to the person who receives it. One can go further by keeping a diary, writing poetry, a novel, or one's life story, including anecdotes or snatches of stories of everyday happenings. You can become delightfully surprised at what you produce. There is the writing of a book in everyone - an ideal therapy factor.

THE FOODS WE EAT, THE DRINKS WE SWALLOW, IF NATURAL AND PURE, ARE AS
MEDICINE TO THE PARTAKER.

YEAST INFECTION

See Candidosis Caption.

YOGA

Here is one of the greatest aids to natural health and well being. It is a method practised for thousands of years, especially in India. Only in the past 50 years has it been accepted in the Western world for its physical benefits, with the ability to aid in the relief of many ailments. There are five different types of Yoga: Raja, Jnana, Karma, Bakti, and Hatha. It is the last system that is best known in the West.

Yoga has nothing to do with spirituality or religion, but somehow it brings about a much better mental attitude, when improvement in physical well being comes about through practicing the simple enjoyable Yoga exercises.

In India, school teachers and doctors teach Yoga, where it is the rule that all school children have lessons.

Gentle exercise, combined with breathing discipline, body posture and if so desired, spiritual features, including meditation, all make up this ancient system. It is an ideal, easy method of achieving fitness and resultant well being of mind and body. It can help to revitalise, as it brings all the muscles of the body into play, making one supple. It helps cleanse the system, having innumerable attributes, all leading to a feel good factor. Yoga is an excellent way to beat stress or depression, to help with emotional problems including calming of the mind. *Bill Feeney, director of the Yoga for Health Foundation, tells us: "Don't be put off by the idea that Yoga is strenuous. It is not. It can benefit people of all abilities and ages. We all have tools to help ourselves - breath, muscles, meditation, visualisation and relaxation. We just need to learn to use them".* There are many reports on how Yoga has helped renew relationships, to beat anorexia, those with multiple sclerosis (MS), arthritis, asthma and other illnesses, as well as its aid to the alleviation of minor, niggling ailments. Much could be written about this excellent, praise-worthy, easy, combined form of exercise and relaxation, which helps to bring about a huge difference in attitudes and health. ***Those with heart or serious health problems should check with their doctor before embarking on any exercise campaign, as should expectant mothers, those suffering from hypertension (blood pressure), or persons extremely overweight.***

Y

Find a class given by a qualified person. This is much more enjoyable than practising Yoga by yourself. The instructor will advise, help, teach, also offer full guidance, all of which leads to a relaxed body and mind. You will require light, snug-fitting clothing. Leotards are excellent or wear cotton tops and shorts. It is advisable to have a blanket or tracksuit when relaxing. **Those who consider taking up Yoga in order to overcome health problems, whether physical or mental, who feel they would not be able to do this, should carefully read the DIET caption in this ENCYCLOPEDIA.**

This all-natural, pure food and drink sustenance, combined with Yoga or other exercise, will bring about transformation of mind and body, giving added strength, zest and get-up- and-go feeling. I have yet to meet a Yoga devotee who was not in an exuberant outgoing frame of mind, always appearing energetic. They have explained how it is a good way to meet and make new friends, also how one feels so much better for participating. It all comes from the simple gentle exercise, which is YOGA. All age groups are catered for, from the very young to the very old.

YOGHURT

One need look no further than Yoghurt to realize what the 'food' manufacturers or producers can do to process and make good food bad.

<u>Pure natural unadulterated</u> Yoghurt is exceptionally good nutritionally. Acidophilus, which is found in concentrated form in natural Yoghurt, is extremely health giving. It assists in production of vitamins, being good for the immune system, skin and blood. It is prescribed for candida, fungal and many other health problems. Natural Yoghurt is a slimming aid.

We find that the food 'gurus' have turned Yoghurt into a money-spinning item. Yes, almost all are items, objects, and stacked in quantity on the shelves, which are colourfully produced, both in packaging and blurb printed on. The liquid they refer to as 'Yoghurt' is frequently coloured too, usually with factory-made pigment. Almost all are additive- filled, with much that is undesirable. Included can be: Sugar, Glucose Syrup, Starches, Flavourings, Colourings, Fruit concentrates, Stabilizers, Acidity regulators and much else.

'Yoghurt' which has been debased, adulterated, added to, one could fearlessly say spoiled, is not health-giving or nourishing. Using additives cheapens it. More additives means more profits. Those who purchase much of the processed stuff sold as Yoghurt often do so because the taste and colour is attractive. They would not dream of reading the ingredient labels.

The 'food' processors should be ashamed to have 'Yoghurt' printed on many of the containers. I repeat:" Natural Yoghurt is health giving. Read the ingredients labels and leave the additive-filled stuff on the shelf. Yoghurt should be pure, natural and unprocessed".

YOU ARE HOW YOU EAT, DRINK, SLEEP AND EXERCISE

Nutrition is knowing what constitutes proper and adequate Diet, taking age, weight, life and work style, also other factors such as smoking, alcohol consumption and medical history into consideration, then putting that know- how into practise. There is considerable flexibility in this matter, with the selection of whole natural foods and food supplements available today. Having said this it is only fair to say that all-too- many do not realise this. *The only way to better health and resultant peace of mind is by Exercise, proper Sleep pattern and the uses of Pure Unadulterated Additive - Free Foods and Drinks.*

MEN AND WOMEN DO NOT DIE - THEY KILL THEMSELVES.

ZINC

See Vitamins and Minerals caption. Those over the age of forty, male and female, should take this mineral. As one gets older the body does not make or provide Zinc, which is best when combined with Copper.

ZOSTER HERPES

See Shingles caption.

CONCLUSION

What is the answer to the health problems that are so prevalent?

It rests in our own hands. We are our own worst enemies. Learn to think NATURAL and eat natural foods, to use only natural products, READ THE INGREDIENTS LABELS. Leave anything that contains colour, additive, preservative, or chemical on the shelf. Let the 'food' processors know that we are not fools, that we will not accept their inferior products. Spread the message. Refuse to have anything to do with convenience and fast 'foods'. Decry the use of fizzy 'drinks' including 'energy drinks' and the overuse of much hyped alcohol.

YOU ARE HOW YOU EXERCISE, THINK, EAT, DRINK AND SLEEP

Some leave it too late.

All too many, particularly those with serious illness - turn to Homeopathy, as a last resort, often too late, when chemical medicines have failed. Had they visited a qualified homeopathist in the first instance the results might have been very much different. How often, even today, have I been told: "Oh, Homeopathy was tried. It was of no use". The full story was not told. It was too late. When the subject of Homeopathy was brought up on one occasion I was told: "I don't like it, I have never tried it". Sounds like the wording of the advert of old.

Homeopathy is now included as part of the National Health Service in Britain, even though many within the medical profession are highly critical of the therapy. With some the problem is that they are completely perplexed and baffled because it cannot be scientifically researched or studied. With many others anything by way of natural treatment is anathema to them. Homeopathy is recognised now more than ever for its healing and curative attributes. Using it as an afterthought is, as I have pointed out, 'often too late'. When using Homeopathic remedies always remember to stop the treatment when relief has been obtained. If the illness or ailment returns, recommence the natural medication. 'Like is been treated with like', hence the need for this advice.

BEWARE

Quite often in a supermarket, store or shop, which sells miscellaneous goods, in some magazines, and even on market stalls, one sees vitamins, minerals, herbal remedies or supplements, also pharmaceutical drugs and medicines, being advertised or offered for sale. The advertising is often gimmicky, with special offers and cut prices. Some of the manufacturers listed on the containers are unknown, whatever about their reputation. Here are instances bordering on quackery. Reputable manufacturers have their good name to uphold. It is in the interests of all to purchase from a health food shop or pharmacy. Remember it is the health of the partaker, which is of paramount importance. It is number one.

BIBLIOGRAPHY

The following books, magazines, periodicals and papers contain much which can help one to attain, regain or maintain reasonable health, through the use of homeopathic, herbal or natural remedies. Natural remedies can be complimentary or alternative to man-made drugs. I have derived pleasure also learning much from the writings hereunder:

These writings are not intended as a substitute for professional advice. Anyone who has a medical condition or is concerned about their health is advised to consult with a qualified practitioner, homeopathic doctor, herbalist, complimentary therapist or health food store personnel.

Alexander. Dan Dale ARTHRITIS AND COMMON SENSE, Worlds Work Ltd, Kingswood, Tadworth, Surrey, England. ISBN 457-00500-3.

Amziev. Alexis YOUR ARTERIES CAN CLEAN THEMSELVES! Pub. by Carnell Plc, 28 Eceleston Square, London, England. ISBN 1-85779-763-9.

Bartram. Thomas FWIMH, ENCYCLOPEDIA OF HERBAL MEDICINE, Grace Publishers, Mulberry Court, Stour Road, Christchurch, Dorset, England, BH23, 1PS. ISBN 0-9515984-1-4.

BATES METHOD FOR BETTER EYESIGHT, Obtainable from the Bates Association, P.O. Box 25, Shoreham-by-Sea, West Sussex, BN43 6ZF UK or Cygnus Books, as listed here.

BIOCHEMIC HANDBOOK ON TISSUE SALTS, Pub. by Thorsons, Harper Collins, ISBN 0-7225-0613-9.

BIOFORCE PHYTOTHERAPY COURSES, Bioforce UK Ltd, 2 Brewster Place, Irvine, Scotland. KA11 5DD UK.

Bricklin. Mark THE PRACTICAL ENCYCLOPEDIA OF NATURAL HEALING, Rodale Press, Griffin Lane, Aylesbury, Bucks, England HP1G 3AS. ISBN 087-857-136-1.

Bryan. Christopher FLUORIDE DECEPTION Pub. by Seven Stories Press, ISBN 1-58322-526-9.

Butmanghelid. J. Dr YOUR BODY'S MANY CRIES FOR WATER, Pub. by Tagman Press. ISBN 1-903571-49-9.

Cadogan. Mary and Shirley Bond. THE OAT COOKBOOK, Pub. by Martin Dunitz Ltd, 154, Camden High Street, London, England NW1 ONE UK. ISBN 0-948269-22-7.

Chance. Jeremy THE ALEXANDER TECHNIQUE, Pub. by Thorsons, Harpur Collins, 77-85 Fulham Palace Road, London, England W6 8JB UK. ISBN 0-00-711035-9.

Clark. Linda HANDBOOK OF NATURAL REMEDIES, Pub. by Thorsons, ISBN 0-7225-0612-0.

CONSUMER'S CHOICE 45 Upper Mount Street, Dublin 2, Ireland. Publishers of Walkways.

CYGNUS BOOKS
From UK; Cygnus, FREEPOST SS1193, Llangadog, SA19 9ZZ
From outside UK; Cygnus, P.O. Box 15, Llandeilo, SA19 6YX UK

DAILY TELEGRAPH, 1 Canada Square, London, England E14 5DT UK

Davies. Jill Rosemary SELF HEAL, Pub. by Newleaf, an imprint of Gill & McMillan Ltd, Hume Avenue, Park West, Dublin 12, Ireland. ISBN 1-85860-053-7.

ECOLOGIST The   Unit 18, Chelsea Wharf, 15 Lots Road, London, SW10 OQJ UK

Fleming. Dr Richard THE HEALTHY HEART PROGRAMME, Michael Joseph, an imprint of Penguin Books. ISBN 0-718-14593-3.

Fogarty. Ann O'Dowd EAT WITH JOY - ON A WHEAT FREE, GLUTEN FREE DIET, Pub .by A and A Farmer, Beech House, 78 Ranelagh Village, Dublin 6. ISBN 1-899047-73-5.

FOOD ADULTERATION AND HOW TO BEAT IT, The London Food Commission. ISBN 0-04-440209-0.

GRACE MAGAZINE. Quarterly by subscription from Grace Publishers, Mulberry Court, Stour Road, Christchurch, Dorset, England BH 23 IPS UK.

GREAT RECIPES FOR FOOD HEALTH, Readers Digest. ISBN 0-276-42104-3.

Griggs. Barbara GREEN PHARMACY. A History Of Herbal Medicine, Pub. by Jill Normon and Hobhouse Ltd, 90 Great Russell Street, London, England WCIB 3PY . ISBN 0-906908-841.

Griggs. Barbara THE HOME HERBAL, Pub. by Pan Books, Cavaye Place, London, England SW10 9PG UK. ISBN 0330-28147-X.

Groves. Barry FLOURIDE - DRINKING OURSELVES TO DEATH, Pub. by Newleaf, an imprint of Gill & McMillan Ltd, Hume Avenue, Parkwest, Dublin 12, Ireland

GUARDIAN. THE 119 Farringdon Road, London, EC1R 3ER.

GUIDE TO VITAMINS, MINERALS AND SUPPLEMENTS, Readers Digest. ISBN 0-276-42448-4.

Habgood. Jackie THE HAY DIET MADE EASY, Pub. by Souvenier Press. Also GET WELL WITH THE HAY DIET. ISBN 0-285-63535-2

Hanssen. Maurice CIDER VINEGAR, Pub. by Thorsons, Harpur Collins, 77-85 Fulham Palace Road, London, England W6 8JB UK. ISBN 0-7225-0576-0.

Hanssen. Maurice with Jill Marsden. E FOR ADDITIVES, Pub. by Thorsons, ISBN 0-7225-1562-6.

Healy. Martin F CURE YOUR ALLERGIES, ISBN 0-9536336-0-8.

Hoffman. David THE COMPLETE HERBAL, Pub. by Mustard, an imprint of Parragon, Queen Street House, 4 Queen Street, Bath, England BA1 HE

Holford. Patrick THE OPTIMUM NUTRITION BIBLE, Pub. by Judy Piatkus Ltd, 5 Windmill Street, London, England WIT 2JA UK. ISBN 0-7499-1855-1.

IRISH EXAMINER, Academy Street, Cork.

IRISH FARMERS JOURNAL, The Farm Centre, Inchicore, Dublin 12.

IRISH INDEPENDENT, Middle Abbey Street, Dublin 2, Ireland

IRISH TIMES, 10-16 Dolier Street, Dublin 2, Ireland

Kawalski. Robt. E. The Eight Week CHOLESTEROL Cure, ISBN 0-7225-2217-7.

Kordel. Lelord NATURAL FOOD REMEDIES, Pub. by WH Allen, London, England. ISBN 0-491-01742-1.

Lawrence. Felicity NOT ON THE LABEL, Pub. by Penguin Books. ISBN 0-141-01566-7.

Lockie. Dr Andrew THE FAMILY GUIDE TO HOMEOPATHY, Pub. by Penguin Books. ISBN 0-241-13572-9.

London Food Commission. FOOD ADULTERATION AND HOW TO BEAT IT. ISBN 0-04-440209-0.

Marsden. Kathryn   FOOD COMBINING (THE ORIGINAL HAY DIET), Pub. by Thorson, Harpur Collins, 77-85 Fulham Palace Road, London, England W6 8JB.

McKeith. Dr Gillian LIVING FOOD FOR HEALTH, Pub. by Piatkus, Ltd, 5 Windmill Street, London, England WIT 2JA UK. ISBN 0-74-99254-0.

McKeith. Dr Gillian YOU ARE WHAT YOU EAT, Pub. by Penguin Books Ltd, ISBN 0-718-14765-0.

McKeown. Patrick Close Your Mouth, BUTEYKO Clinic Handbook. ISBN 0-9545996-1-6.

McNeil. Ann A LITTLE BOOK ABOUT YOUR BACK, Pub. by Thorsons, Harpur Collins, ISBN 0-00-710661-0.

MEDICAL BREAKTHROUGH 2003, Readers Digest. ISBN 0-276-42728-9.

Mervyn. Leonard THE DICTIONARY OF VITAMINS, Pub. by Thorsons, Harpur Collins, ISBN 0-7225-0906-5.

Mindell. Earl SECRET REMEDIES, Pub. by Vermilion, Ebury Press, Random House, 20 Vauxhall Bridge Road, London, England SWIV 25A UK. ISBN 0-09-181644-0.

Moncreiff. Scott THE VITAMIN ALPHABET, Pub. by Collins & Brown Ltd, London House, Great Eastern Wharf, Parkgate Road, London, England SW11 4NQ UK. ISBN 1-85585-681-6.

Mortimore. Denise NUTRITIONAL HEALING - A STEP BY STEP GUIDE, Pub. by

Element Books Ltd, Shaftsbury, Dorset, England SP7 8BP UK. ISBN 1-86204-245-4.

PHYTOTHERAPY, THE POWER OF PLANTS, Herbal Health Publishers.
ISBN 1-870-40550-1.

Pickles. Hildesgard DEVIL'S CLAW, Reforma AG, Postfach, Switzerland 6300 ZUG.

Plant. Prof. Jane YOUR LIFE IN YOUR HANDS, Pub. by Virgin Books.
ISBN 0-7535-0850-8.

Sach. Penelope THE LITTLE BOOK OF WELLBEING, Pub. by Penguin Books.

Schlosser. Eric FAST FOOD NATION, Pub by Penguin Books.
ISBN 0-141-00687-0.

Smith. Dr Tom LIVING WITH ANGINA. ISBN 0-85969-749-5.

ST. MARTIN MAGAZINE, 42 Parnell Square, Dublin 1, Ireland.

THE TIMES, 1 Virginia Street, London, E98 1XY.

Thorsons. THE COMPLETE CIDER VINEGAR, ISBN 0-7225-1876-5.

Tyler. V. and S. Foster HERBS AND PHYTOMEDICINAL PRODUCTS, 'Handbook of
non prescription drugs, 11th Edition, American Pharmaceutical Association 1996:
695-713

Udo. Dr. Erasmus CHOOSING THE RIGHT FATS, Pub. by Alive Books,
ISBN 1-55312-035-3.
Also by the same author; FATS THAT HEAL, FATS THAT KILL.
ISBN 0-920470-38-6.

Vogel. Dr Alfred THE NATURE DOCTOR. ISBN 1-85158-274-6.

WELEDA REVIEW, Weleda Ltd, Heanor Road, Ilkeston, Derbyshire, England DE7 8DR
UK.

WORD FOR TODAY - YOUR QUIET TIME COMPANION, PO Box 255, Stoke on Trent,
Staffordshire, England ST4 8YY UK. or P.O. Box 784 Dun Laoghaire, Co Dublin,
Ireland.